FOOD
Energetics

"Nobody understands the power, magic, and impact of food better than Steve Gagné. Prepare to read, eat, and be transformed!"

JOHN DAVID MANN, COAUTHOR OF *THE GO-GIVER: A LITTLE STORY ABOUT A POWERFUL BUSINESS IDEA*

"This book is exceptional in the field of diet today. Steve Gagné's deep, informed perspective helps elucidate the thoughts of Michael Pollan and gives us access to a simple, user-friendly way of understanding food."

JOSHUA ROSENTHAL, AUTHOR OF *INTEGRATIVE NUTRITION*

"One of the most important insights for anyone who has personally experienced the diet/disease, diet/symptom connection is the awareness of inevitable food diet dogma—meaning, the initial tendency for any student of natural health to create fairly hard-edged principles around what is Right Food and Wrong Food and believe them as incontrovertibly true for the rest of their life and for all of humanity. Generally at that moment, a student of natural health will join one of the groups that best fit those beliefs, be it the All Raw group, or Vegetarianism, or Macrobiotic/Vegan/Natural Hygiene/Paleolithic or any other of the well-known food philosophies. Gagné gently helps dislodge this dogma and gets us to see a wider view of what food is, what it isn't, and how it has been used by healthy cultures throughout the world to heal and stay healthy. Whether you are just waking up to the realization that most of your symptoms are diet related or are an old salt in the study of the food and health connection, *Food Energetics* is simply a must-have book."

SCOTT OHLGREN, AUTHOR OF
THE 28-DAY CLEANSING PROGRAM

FOOD
Energetics

The Spiritual, Emotional, and Nutritional Power of What We Eat

Steve Gagné

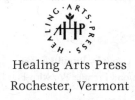

Healing Arts Press
Rochester, Vermont

Healing Arts Press
One Park Street
Rochester, Vermont 05767
www.HealingArtsPress.com

Healing Arts Press is a division of Inner Traditions International

*Note to the reader: This book is intended as an informational guide. The remedies,
approaches, and techniques described herein are meant to supplement, and not to be a substitute for, professional medical care or treatment. They should not be used to treat a serious
ailment without prior consultation with a qualified health care professional.*

Library of Congress Cataloging-in-Publication Data
Gagné, Steve.
  Food energetics : the spiritual, emotional, and nutritional power of what we eat / Steve
Gagné.— 3rd. ed.
      p. cm.
  Includes bibliographical references and index.
  ISBN 978-1-59477-242-9
  1. Nutrition. 2. Energy psychology. I. Title.
  RA784.G34 2008
  613.2—dc22

2008028563

Printed and bound in Canada by Transcontinental Printing

10 9 8 7 6 5 4 3 2 1

Text design by Diana April and layout by Priscilla Baker
This book was typeset in Garamond Premier Pro with Franklin Gothic used as a display
typeface

I dedicate this book to my children:
Taran, Shayla, Annette, Annika,
Madeleine, Brendan, Sofia, and Soren.

Contents

Part V. A Forbidden History of Food and Agriculture

Part VI. A Call to Common Sense

Introduction

Traditional foods and ancient cultural mysteries have long been a passion of mine, especially when viewed through the interconnected web of archaeology, anthropology, and the written and oral traditions of myths and legends.

Having had the opportunity to interact with numerous traditional cultures as I traveled and researched the globe both confirmed my ideas about food energetics and increased my knowledge of the continuity that exists with food traditions the world over. In fact, it could be argued that food may very well be the strongest cultural thread linking traditional peoples to their ancient past.

Moreover, the tremendous respect, reverence, and understanding traditional peoples have of the inherent energies and power of their food are examples of wisdom we can all use to help ourselves and each other in our awareness of health and happiness.

And it is this distinctive sense of being so intimately connected with their food, combined with their deep humility, that never fails to touch me deeply—nor to add to the growing store of lasting memories and images that have changed my life in ways I could never have imagined before my travels began.

The purpose of this book is to open the closed doors of the past and awaken our inner knowledge to the potential effects of our daily nourishment. Our food speaks a language through the science of nature that is very easy to understand and the benefits gained from this understanding can greatly assist us in healing both our planet and ourselves if we are willing to listen.

I hope you enjoy *Food Energetics* and that you find the material in these pages useful in your pursuit of health through natural and wholesome foods.

PART I

Energetics

1
Quality and Quantity
Beyond the Realm of the Senses

It is late September; the evening air is cooling rapidly. The elderly farmer sits quietly surrounded by the warmth of his wood-burning stove, his battered rocking chair creaking softly as he reflects on another long, full day's work. His field of organically grown rice is ready for the harvest; Mother Nature was generous this year. He knows there will be little rain for a few days, but this is fine: there is much to be done before winter sets in. The work is not a problem; he and his two sons will do whatever needs doing, for he also knows that all he gives to nature will be given back equally by her.

The hardwood fire in the stove pops and snaps. Lulled by its unpredictable rhythms, his mind wanders back over the acres outside. . . .

The quality of life has changed so much since his great-grandfather farmed this same land. There is plenty of demand today for the foods he grows, but he still prays for the day when more people will understand, as his grandparents did, the importance of simple, carefully wrought foods like his organic crops. "A stubborn old man!" That's what he's called by the neighboring farmers, because he prefers the old ways of farming to the new technology of big, loud machines, chemical sprays, and high-tech fertilizers. Their reasons for using these things never did make much sense to him; still don't. He silently prays that his sons will feel the same way he does when they get to be his age. But you never can tell, the way things are going these days. . . .

The old man's thoughts are interrupted by the sweet smell of freshly cooked rice—cooked to perfection, as usual. He returns to his rocking chair with a steaming bowl of rice, simple fare for this late evening—and to him, all that is needed to celebrate another good harvest. He closes his eyes and silently thanks the Creator for all that has been given to him and his family. He ponders the many satisfied consumers of his rice. He wonders if they know how much he really cares about quality, or if they, too, think he is just a "stubborn old man"—or if they even think of him and his farm at all. The warm bowl in his hands and the rising steam remind him it is time to eat. A smile appears on his wrinkled face, and he says to himself, "Of course they know—they eat the rice!"

And he is right: they do *know* it—whether or not they realize it consciously. This entire scene *is in* the food they're eating. In fact, it is as much a part of that food as the carbohydrates, fiber, and phosphorous that nutritionists analyze. In terms of human experience, it even may be considered the *more important* part of the food.

When they partake of that farmer's crops, the food's own experience is recorded electrically, through their digestive systems onto the awareness of their nervous systems. Their educated minds, distracted by a modern world of data and information, may not register the rhythms, melodies, and harmonies of the food. But every one of their cells catches that music—and dances to it.

This book is about that *knowledge*—not the information and data of lab analysis or nutrition textbooks, but the core experience of food, no fads and no nonsense. Chemical analysis might be considered "shadow knowledge," the echo of experience when it is dissected by the tools of man. *Food Energetics* is about true *knowledge,* the *knowledge* that foods impart to you when you eat and experience them.

This *knowledge* is as ancient as the lives of the plant and animal kingdoms. It is the same knowledge that informed the dietary wisdom of the great philosophical dietary systems of antiquity. Yet for many, it is utterly new and radical. The goal of this book is to make this *knowledge* yours.

Knowing Quality

Compare a head of organically grown broccoli, freshly picked by your local farmer, to the agribusiness-grown, chemically sprayed broccoli picked a week ago (or more) and shipped across the country in a refrigerated truck. You may not be able to see the difference between the two. You might not even taste the difference (though chances are, you will). But you can *know* that difference. That difference is *quality,* and the quality of something represents what is behind the scenes of any given *quantity.*

Quality means more than how "good" or "healthy" a food is. It also refers to a particular food's character and personality.

What we are doing is getting to *know* the living personality and character of the food—in much the same way you would get to *know* a new friend.

True *knowledge* of food, *knowing* the *energetics* of food, has to do with becoming familiar with the *quality* of food and how it relates to *quantity.*

Quality is not something you can see—yet it can be *known.* A food's qualities are an expression of the various stages of the process that winds up to the *quantity* of it.

Quantity, on the other hand, you *can* see—that is, you can measure it with your senses or with the physical instruments of science.

The study of energetics does not exclude technical, nutritional, or chemical information about a food, it simply acknowledges that these exist after the fact—the "fact" being the food itself. The *quality* of a food is its character or personality (or even its soul), and is affected by all of its experience. The *quantity* of a food includes only the various ways a food can be measured physically, such as in its nutritional composition, size, weight, water content, and even price!

"Well, then, how am I supposed to *know* quality, if not by using my senses to measure it?"

Aha—that's "information"—not *knowledge.* True *knowledge* is a human faculty that lies somewhere between the instinct that tells a newly hatched bird how to fly, and the inspired insight that tells Bach where to put the next note. How to gain a conscious, personal *knowledge* of the quality of foods is the reason for this book.

But to answer the question briefly: How you *know* quality is how you *know* when music makes you feel a certain way . . . how you *know* when you're in love . . . how you *know* what you want to do with your life.

By the way, focusing on the quality of foods doesn't mean being obsessively concerned with food to the point where everything you eat must be organically or biodynamically grown. That said, it certainly makes sense that consciously grown, naturally processed, chemical-free food is qualitatively superior to its mass-produced counterpart—and you *know* it! Dining at nature's table as directly as possible—without agribiz and its high-tech, genetically altering intermediaries—is a sensible way of reconnecting yourself with the earth. And no matter what Madison Avenue, Hollywood, or the American Medical Association tells you, the earth is your most direct link to the good life. The earth is our ultimate reference point for quality.

How many times have you heard the expression "I watch what I eat"? Anyone who works out, stays in shape, is lean, and has an outwardly good-looking or attractive appearance often has the opportunity to use this phrase. These people hear the question, "What do you do to look the way you do?" And they very often answer with, "I watch what I eat."

But do they really?

What does it mean to genuinely *watch* what you eat? Many of us think we watch what we eat but we are not watching closely enough.

A package of synthetic ingredients posing as food, torn from its packet, added to water and tossed back, does not constitute *watching what you eat*. Eating a piece of fruit on an empty stomach when your blood sugar is low is not *watching what you eat*. Eating low-fat foods is not *watching what you eat*. Eating salad because it will keep the calories low is not *watching what you eat*. All of these are examples of what people do when they have been told what to believe is good for them to lose weight and stay lean.

But genuinely *watching what you eat* is an art, a process that is simple yet takes conscious, careful observation. That is what this book is about: the opportunity to really watch, observe, comprehend, and digest what you eat.

2
The Decline and Fall of Energetics

The young man kneels by a makeshift fireside and acknowledges his appreciation as he cuts into the side of the deer he tracked and felled earlier today. As he arranges his meal, his thoughts go forward to the journey ahead across the plains. He will be traveling through unfamiliar territory, and he knows he will need to depend on a well-honed keenness of senses, a swiftness of foot, and lightning reflexes. He sits down to eat, grateful to be able to borrow those qualities from his brother the deer.

After he eats, he is aware of a sense of lightness and physical freedom, a soft wildness. The spirit of the deer becomes his. He also has prepared a small dish of gnarled roots and wild greens. He knows that these will give him access to the silent, earthy wisdom of the plant kingdom, an "inside knowledge" that the deer meat alone could not provide. From the wild roots, he absorbs a quality of tenacious rootedness, and from the sharp-tasting leaves, a pliant flexibility. To the plants, he murmurs his thanks as well.

Now he is ready for his trek.

Before the Fall

In times long past, among both tribal and high civilizations of a golden age, food was an integral part of the living philosophies that formed and developed human character. Long before the Industrial and Information Ages, we humans had a unified perspective of life borne of our regular interactions with nature. We learned from all these interactions with utmost care, since we knew nature both as our source, our partner in living, and the perpetual force that would answer our own needs and ensure the future of our offspring.

We did not perceive ourselves as something *other than* nature—we *were* nature. We knew that nature was simply humanity turned inside out—and humanity was nature turned outside in. When we referred to our individual characters as "my own nature," we *knew* this to be the literal truth.

Living closely with nature gave us the opportunity to observe, experience, and recognize many qualities in ourselves, qualities that corresponded with the growth processes and actions of plants and animals. Stirred in the pots of trial and error and heated by the fire of intuition and ancestral wisdom, our observations also revealed to us the many possibilities recorded in the plant and animal kingdoms, and how these possibilities corresponded to our own lives.

We learned to apply these living metaphors to every aspect of life, culminating in the extraordinary dietary philosophies that were handed down from the prehistoric golden age civilizations to the ancient Egyptians, Maya, Sumerian, Indian, and many other sophisticated ancient cultures. After the global cataclysm that nearly decimated the human species some 11,500 years ago, some of the survivors were able to salvage seeds and remnants of this ancient knowledge. Many of these ideas were later codified into formal systems of thought, such as the ancient Ayurvedic system of India, traditional Chinese medical systems, the Greek "four humors," the medicinal systems of Hippocrates, Paracelsus, Maimonides, and others. Perhaps the most well-known of these systems is the Medieval "Doctrine of Signatures."

The Doctrine of Signatures is a systematic viewpoint of nature wherein the structure or function of a particular plant or animal was taken as a signal from nature to man. These signals revealed the purposes the plant or animal could serve.

For example: watercress, a plant that easily thrives in its watery environment, was recognized as beneficial for patients with a water imbalance in their own internal environments. Walnuts, with their convoluted, hemispherical surface, physically resemble the human brain; today we have discovered that walnuts contain brain-supporting omega-3 fatty acids.

The Doctrine of Signatures observed such similarities and would (to take this last example) ascribe to walnuts a special effect on the human nervous system.

At their height, such systems became phenomenally complex and involved encyclopedic compilations of observations concerning health-promoting foods and remedies for specific illnesses. Yet the guiding principle was never complex at all, for all such systems are based on the *knowledge* derived from experience and ancestral wisdom.

The Decline of Energetics

Some time after the cataclysm of 11,500 years ago, a few survivors salvaged what remained of their great cultures and journeyed to new lands to reestablish civilization. Through years of hardship, these ancestors endured famine, sunless skies, and frigid temperatures. Finally, though deeply scarred (both psychologically and spiritually), they managed to begin again. Only this time, it wouldn't be a golden age, but one filled with warfare, strife, extreme environmental adjustments, and other related challenges.

Many who had reverted to a more primitive lifestyle remained fixed in that historical niche. Others rebuilt civilization, ever on guard from the dangers they faced from predators and fellow humans ready to conquer and destroy those nascent remnants of what once was.

For more than 10,000 years this cycle of on-again, off-again warfare and enlightenment prevailed, while most of humanity remained cloaked in a veil of amnesia concerning their true history. Even today, we desperately hold on to the beliefs and dogma that have finally culminated in the modern scientific and religious misunderstandings of who we are and where we have come from.

Yet even through these thousands of years, humankind at various stages of culture has maintained at least some connection with natural, wholesome foods and the *knowledge* of nature. It is only a comparatively recent occurrence that humanity has more fully disengaged from this intimacy with nourishing food and the wisdom gained from our ancestors. In the last hundred years or so, as food has become more refined and processed, people have become more segregated from the sources of their food, causing this food *knowledge* to fade, its currency debased to that of fragmentary traditions and empty imitation.

Some of the simple, early folk remedies, along with the herbs and foods upon which they were based, would later serve as the foundation for what would become modern pharmaceutical medicine; but while the ingredients and their physical effects were often handed down, the *knowledge* that inspired them was not. Later, even the ingredients were abandoned in favor of synthesized versions with dangerous side effects.

With the Renaissance and the Age of Reason came a mechanical view of nature and the world around us. Instead of being guided by a vision of a universe inspired by consciousness, spirit, and energetics, the new order saw the universe as a great cosmic machine, engineered by impeccable mechanics and oiled by infallible logic.

The very act of *knowing* was increasingly edged out and dominated by the supernatural god of religion along with the god of scientific materialism. Our new methods of "knowing" ourselves and our food are now, for the most part, either faith-based or the result of dissection, analysis, and linear logic.

The study of anatomy is based on the observation of dissected corpses—not of live people. Interestingly, the study of nutrition has also been based largely on the "dissection" of food "corpses"—the analysis of the ash left after burning a food in a laboratory. Such an abstract approach, divorced as it is from living reality, has little in common with energetic *knowledge*.

The Legacy of the Machine Age

The shift from a world guided by energetics to one steered by mechanics brought about one earthshaking change in our approach to life. Before the Machine Age we knew the importance of adapting to nature and living within nature. Once we'd bought into the simplified metaphors of the Machine Age, we came to believe that we could hop into the engineer's room and run this train ourselves. We even started to think we could *improve* on nature.

Advanced technology came married to a peculiar mentality—one guided by the audacity to think that the environment would or could adapt *to us*. This is the basic difference between some of the great civilizations and peoples of yesterday and the "advanced" civilizations of today. It is a difference that has uprooted the foundation of life as we *knew* it.

This confusion of the *many* for the *one,* of our human theories of life for life itself, has resulted in the dismemberment of a unified grasp of life into isolated branches of nutrition, medicine, science, religion, biology, psychology, *etcetera ad infinitum*—each with its human specialists trained to explore and analyze their particular branch alone.

With the atmospheric disasters created by the oil and coal industries in full view, with headlines blaring daily warnings about global warming, and with a litany of sobering events from the Dust Bowl to Chernobyl behind us, you would think we would have awakened from that Emperor's New Clothes fantasy, wouldn't you? But no! For the most part, we're still locked in that deep sleep.

Look at what is being funded today in the way of biotechnology. The Machine Age dream of Man the Divine Engineer is today's living nightmare.

The Informed Battleground

We speak of the modern epoch as the "Age of Information"—and it's true, amidst the dizzying babble of data, a Renaissance of true *knowledge* is struggling to emerge. But to a great extent, we still live within the conceptual prison of the Machine Age. The rise of mechanistic, analytical views on life meant redefining food, history, health, and human life in terms of concrete, empirical information and data.

In short, the value of quality was supplanted by a value of quantity.

In the Machine Age, the new model of health was based on warfare and aggression. Illness was seen not as our deviation *from* nature, but as an aggressive act *by* nature. The energetic approach to addressing illness by restoring natural immunity was replaced with a model that through its medicaments served to *weaken* natural immunity. Nature's aggression countered by man's aggression.

This aggressive bias is even evident in the language of modern medicine, which is essentially a *military* terminology. When our bodies are "invaded" by a pathogen, we are "under attack," and build up our immune "defenses" or take *anti*biotics, *anti*histamines, and *anti*congestants. Medical people speak of their "armamentarium" of medical weaponry, and of how well we are doing in the "war on . . ." (Fill in the blank.)

Healing in the Machine Age actually has little to do with wholeness or health. Rather than dealing with a sense of what health is, it has become a detailed cataloging of illnesses and their appropriate pharmaceutical countermeasures. Today, most "health care" is really "illness care" and "health science" is actually "illness science."

Genuine health care is relegated to the "secondary" health services—nursing, counseling, physical therapy, and rehabilitation—to actually deal with *health*—with recovering wholeness and not just vanquishing symptoms of sickness.

Our Confused Substance

Our modern war with food has resulted in much confusion, as evident through the many dietary programs available to choose from these days. Several decades ago, a popular book on natural health was published with the title *Are You Confused?** Unfortunately, the book's contents didn't clear up the confusion, and the answer today is generally the same as it was decades ago.

Ancient peoples, whether nomadic or agricultural, certainly were not confused on this point. They *had* to *know* nature—they *had* to adapt to their environment constantly in order to survive. In the process of doing so (and in a way humans seldom do today), they showed a great respect and gratitude for nature and her gifts. Along with that respect went keen observation and understanding.

Are you Confused? by Paavo Airola Published by Health US, 1971.

In those pre–Machine Age circumstances, we *knew* our food as the foundation of our blood, bones, and nervous system. It was the catalyst of our thinking and way of living. Food was the basic *substance*—a word that literally means "what exists behind, or the quality of, a stand or position." We *knew* that food was more than mere fuel—it was living experience incarnate.

Today, we have traded much of the intuitive wisdom and common sense of our ancestors for the technological ingenuity of sophisticated tools, chemicals, and other indulgences. Many of these new toys designed to improve our lifestyles are helpful and serve a useful purpose. Yet we continue to direct most of the progress gained through our newly acquired god, *science,* toward waging war with our environment, our food, our diseases, and most of all with each other.

This is especially true of modern cosmopolitan medicine, a medical model that has lost the slightest connection to its planetary roots. Happily though, the food folklore of our "unscientific" past finally is reemerging as the foundation of healing, and what was condemned yesterday as blind superstition is reappearing as today's validated scientific fact.

Like our ancestors, we have begun to realize that we too must learn to adapt to our ever-changing environment—and we may soon even grasp that our daily food, our *substance,* is a critical link in doing so.

If science can prove beyond a reasonable doubt that food is indeed our best medicine, then pharmacology just might be reunited with its past to become the healing tool it so desperately needs to be. For this to happen, though, there will have to occur a major shift in the way people perceive the conventional paradigm of food and health.

3
Enter the Age of Sanity

There is a growing awareness that proper nutrition and daily dietary habits have a profound impact on health. This is obviously good news: it looks like we are recovering our ancient understanding of the central importance of foods . . . right?

Wrong.

That's *not* what we're talking about. That's *quantitative,* the old paradigm.

It's not an issue of how many grams of fat you ingest, or of whether you will or will not acquire a particular symptom, such as high blood pressure, arthritis, or cancer. Choosing "the right stuff" to put in your mouth is not a simple true/false, avoid-the-bad-guys question. It's not even a standardized multiple choice. Neither high SAT scores nor an MBA will do you any good here. Making energetic food choices is an open-ended opportunity to exercise your human capacity for creativity.

The diet-health connection has created an important doorway through which many people are being reintroduced to an appreciation of *quality.*

True, most people who come to reexamine their diets because of health concerns are motivated primarily by fear, at least at first—and the grip of fear has a way of firmly keeping the blinders on. When motivated by fear of obesity, disease, or death, you are more likely to ask not "What is the true character of this food?" but "Is it okay or not okay to eat? Will it kill me or not?"

These are not the kinds of questions that open one's mind up to creativity and adventure.

Nevertheless, the new awareness of food-as-killer and food-as-healer has played a central role in exposing the limitations of the old paradigm and opening up questions of *quality*.

A Step in the Right Direction

"An ounce of prevention is worth a pound of cure," goes the adage. And many health-related organizations now say that diet may be instrumental in the prevention of major health problems.

Just how much of a role does diet play in the prevention of illness? Is it enough of a factor to warrant social and economic change in agriculture, medicine, and other political priorities? Are meditation, exercise, visualization, and positive thinking more important? Do some people need to eat in a healthy way and others not? How about money and social status? What are your priorities concerning the *quality* of your life?

Whatever your priorities, one thing is certain: to live on this planet, we all need a biological organism capable of adapting to the present and coming changes created by both man and nature. The biological nature of disease is one whereby one's internal environment alters itself to adapt to the problem at hand, while at the same time attempting to maintain its original biological integrity. Food is a powerful tool capable of altering the human biological organism toward or away from health.

How many people do you know of whose life work was cut short by diet-related problems, such as heart disease or cancer? But life goes on— and it does so driven by the patterns of nourishment that we choose for ourselves. Today, evidently, we have reached a point where we are learning some lessons regarding food quality and its relevance to health.

But there is a hidden limitation in this new awareness. Much of what is now considered "good food" is "good" only in reaction to what came before. What now constitutes the "healing diet," "natural foods diet," or "quality food" often is a highly *relative* evaluation—and that is not the same evaluation of *quality* we're talking about here.

"Eating Well"

To a generation of people who grew up during the Great Depression, "eating well" basically means eating *a lot*. That meaning is at the heart of such expressions as, "A steak on every table, a chicken in every pot," "putting some meat on the bone," or "Why don't you eat something that sticks to your ribs?"—a vivid image that brings shudders to indoctrinated fat-conscious diet-watchers. To people living in the early part of the twentieth century, the experience of eating simple, lean fare, void of nutrient-dense food, is the embodiment of deprivation. To them there's nothing healthy (let alone "virtuous") about it.

Not that long ago, people died of "consumption." And we're still doing it.

Back then, the word meant *you were consumed,* and it referred to the wasting away caused by tuberculosis infection. Literally, bacteria consumed you. Today, it is *our consumption of food* that kills us.

The model and the meaning of the word have changed—but it's not really that different.

The very idea of consumption is the problem. It is a mechanistic, quantitative concept that leaves little room for considerations of quality.

In *The Unsettling of America,* the farmer/philosopher Wendell Berry writes eloquently and persuasively that for the majority of the population, our divorce from nature at the turn of the twentieth century ended our role as producers and cocreators and created a new role as "consumers."

But "consume" is what a machine does—not what *you* do. A car "consumes" gasoline. You do not "consume" your food. You are not a machine, you are a life form—and your foods are life forms, too. The analogy of fuel combustion to eating foods is *not* a sound one.

When you choose, eat, digest, assimilate and absorb, utilize, and animate the cells of your foods, a process far more vital than "burning fuel" takes place. Indeed, in every sense you *merge* with those foods. They become you—and you become them, too. In the merging, what emerges? Not simply a well-fueled machine, but a slightly new you. It is not "consumption" but a *living union*—"consummation" might be a more apt term!

An alternative term to "consume" might be "nourish." In choosing your foods, you not only choose to be nourished, you choose specific qualities in your foods that nourish those qualities in yourself.

The energetic paradigm is one of nourishment, including nourishment on all levels of our being. What the world needs now certainly is not more consumption—but more conscious nurturing of life in all its forms.

Energetics: The Conservative Approach!

The conventional paradigm of food called modern nutrition is based squarely on the assumption that food is *matter*—strictly physical nourishment for the human body. This more left-brained, analytical viewpoint also holds that food is composed of many ingredients or parts called nutrients, including different groups of vitamins, fats, minerals, phytonutrients, antioxidants, and other molecular constituents that make up each and every food.

In and of themselves, these assumptions and conclusions don't pose a problem, and nutritional analysis can be useful. What *is* problematic is when this quantitative view of food is believed to be the total reality of food. People tend to take nutrition as the given rules and are led to believe they should think from these rules of isolated nutrients, i.e. calcium, vitamin C, phytonutrients . . .

While the twentieth century saw a tremendous amount of research in the field of nutrition, the conceptual paradigm of food still lacks nutritional *wisdom*. Analytical nutrition is sometimes viewed as the "conservative" approach to food and diet. But it's not conservative at all!

The word "conservative" derives from *conservare:* "to keep together, to save." Relative to food, the "conservative" is one who wishes to *keep together* a time-honored approach to food. True "conservatism" has little—if anything—to do with the modern nutritional paradigm of food.

Modern nutrition does not *keep together* or *preserve the traditional quality* of food. Rather, it fragments food into parts and disregards tradition as being of little relevance to the present. While this perception of food is neither conservative nor traditional, today it has become the *conventional* view. *Webster's* defines *conventional* as: "depending on or conforming to accepted models rather than nature; not natural, original, or spontaneous."

The Soul of Food

Neither nutrition nor modern medicine have any tools for understanding the following statement—yet it is a statement of truth: food is incapable of affecting only your body and not your soul.

Like religion, psychology, and medicine, nutrition has tried to peel away the spiritual from the physical. Therefore, talking about the soul and food in the same breath (unless you're talking about grits and chitlins) is nonsense, from a scientific standpoint.

And that's just it: *nonsense.* Nutritional science belongs to the senses, while matters of the soul are beyond physical quantification.

Today, with the budding science of neurobiology, science is beginning to scratch the surface of how foods affect mood and behavior. While studying "behavior" is still a far cry from exploring *the soul,* that line of inquiry may at some point bring biological science face-to-face with energetics.

A "conservative" (call it *traditional* if you wish) understanding of food employs a more balanced, right/left–brained perspective. This commonsense approach to food does not focus on the *parts* of foods. And it doesn't focus on the parts of *people,* either. Rather, it offers a comprehensive understanding of complete foods in their entirety and their effects on people in their entirety, from a *qualitative* point of view, embracing nutritional, physiological, psychological, and spiritual dimensions.

What energetics offers is a new paradigm that embraces the best of our past and present and opens the door to the possibilities for a brighter, saner future.

4
Your Most Intimate Relationship

Many people dutifully repeat "You are what you eat," and the next thing *out* of their mouths is data about bran, carbohydrate grams, antioxidants, calories, fat content, and other mindless drivel. *You* are not bran and carbohydrate grams . . . really, now!

"You are what you eat" does not mean that you are your concepts, or some narrowly defined, constantly changing scientific or pseudoscientific theories of what foods are. You *think* those things. They are what come out of your mouth—not what goes into it.

"You are what you eat" really means just what it says.

A dear friend of mine who is well versed in the ways of nature once said to me, "If you want to know anything about the nature of an individual, all you have to do is open his pantry doors and refrigerator and take a peek inside."

Sounds a little simplistic, doesn't it? It's not. In fact, this book is simply a detailed look inside that pantry and refrigerator—and inside you.

Why Are You What You Eat?

Bob is an angry, irritable person. His liver is congested and aching— though it is an ache he doesn't really notice—and his heart strains to pump blood through his gradually narrowing arteries. Every morning, he eats the same breakfast: eggs, sausage, and buttered toast. His mono diet includes a breakfast perfectly tailored to nourish his anger and irritability.

Billy is hyperactive. His nervous system is starving for trace minerals, and his blood sugar metabolism has gone half bananas—perhaps literally. When he gets hyper, his mom tries to calm him down by giving him more treats: sugar.

Jim is a door-to-door encyclopedia salesman. He is a nice guy—according to his friends, a little wimpy. Needless to say, he is not terribly aggressive in his job, and certainly not very successful. His intestines are waterlogged; so are his kidneys and adrenals glands. For that matter, so is his hand-shake. He loves diet sodas, date nut bread with cream cheese, Sloppy Joes, and ice-cream sandwiches. There's not much definition there, but that's what Jim likes to eat. . . .

All three of these people are classically what they eat. And yes, they are caricatures—but most people today are in fact *caricatures of their own limiting characteristics*—and they continue to nourish those limitations with the foods that match them.

For many, this self-perpetuating "vicious circle" of nourishment plods on until serious health problems develop—or until you wake up looking in the mirror one day and make a decision to change yourself, your diet, or both.

The problem is, it's awfully hard to alter only one side of the equation.

Just *try* to soften Bob's temper, calm Billy's moods, or stiffen Jim's backbone without changing their food. Billions are spent each year in the attempt, all the way from psychiatrists' offices to checkout-counter self-help books. The latest and most popular method is mass consumption of antidepressant drugs.

The effort doesn't last—or if it does, it does so only under the duress of trying *not to be* what you eat.

Try taking away Bob's sausages, Billy's candy, or Jim's wimp burgers—without their earnest commitment to change their behavior and personalities (or in Billy's case, his mom's).

Surprisingly, you may be more successful in this second effort. But it still won't work. Bob will find a way to charbroil his mung bean sprouts dripping in salt and peanut oil, and his temper will be back in full regalia. Billy's mom will slip him so much organic dried fruit and honey-sweetened carob bars he'll flip out. Jim will cook his brown rice in gallons of water, spread tahini on his oatmeal cookies, and become an *organic* wimp.

Just what is this mysterious sway food holds over our personalities? Why *are* we what we eat?

The answer to that question reveals the cardinal principal of food energetics.

Birds of a Feather

You are what you eat because: All things seek their own level, place, or plane of existence.

A rock thrown up in the air does not remain up in the air. Its natural plane or level is on the ground, and that is where it returns. Gravity? Well . . . not necessarily. The law of gravity is a mechanical explanation of the process—but it doesn't explain *why* the process occurs. The truth is, a rock is *out of place* in the air.

Here is a more dramatic example:

Plutonium and uranium originate deep under the earth's surface. For millions of years they sat there without any serious harm coming to the biosphere. They are utterly out of place aboveground at the earth's surface—so much so that they wreak havoc when brought here by forced excavation.

Where should we put them? Discarding them in space would be insanity—they are even more out of place there than on the ground. Seeking their own natural level, they are working their way toward being dumped in deep salt beds in Carlsbad, New Mexico. They're going there not by gravity, but by congressional mandate—but the means doesn't matter. The point is that they seek their own level.

Have you noticed the geographic dispersal of different ethnic groups in the United States? It's fascinating: When waves of immigrants flocked here and settled the country, they sought out regions that duplicated their native climates and terrain, creating colonies of Irish in Boston, Norwegians in the Dakotas, Spanish in Florida and Texas, and Germans and Dutch in Pennsylvania.

Have you ever noticed how people sit when they are in a meeting? Take a dozen people, say a board of directors, who meet once every few months. Put them in a different meeting room, even in different cities. Watch which places they each assume at the meeting table. Eight or nine out of ten of them will take the same position relative to the person chairing the meeting, even if there is no formal seating arrangement. They find their own natural plane of existence within the group.

I Eat the Body Electric!

Just as a rock is out of place in the air and plutonium is out of its element on the earth's surface, you would—I hope—be out of place smoking crack cocaine with a room full of addicts. Were you a weak and incoherent person, crack might entrain you so that you became a drug addict. Crack cocaine often does this sort of entraining; so do fast-food restaurants (in which I hope you also would feel out of place).

Here is a different sort of example: Internet chat rooms, where people can become sucked in to the point where they completely lose track of time, shirk responsibilities, and get lost, entrained by the subject under discussion.

Bill Cosby has a hilarious bit about cocaine. Wondering aloud what's so great about it, he's told that it "intensifies your personality." "But," he wonders, "what if you're an asshole?!"

There's a good point under the humor. It is not actually as simple as that you *become* what you eat (or in this case, snort or smoke); it's more that the character of what you eat or ingest can exercise dominance over you. In other words, your food can "entrain" you.

Entrain is an electrical term that means to "draw after or draw into." This is what greater systems do to lesser systems. The term *entrainment* is a perfectly descriptive one for food energetics, because electrical events are exactly what we're discussing! All your interactions, whether with foods or with other people, are at their essence *electric.*

A charismatic and vital speaker can easily entrain less charismatic and less vital individuals into his or her plane. In the process of doing so, the speaker gains power—and followers.

Can you recall a situation where you were either biologically or physiologically out of place? The first time you got on a bicycle or the first time you put on a pair of skis? How about dinner at a friend's house where you suddenly found yourself in the middle of an intense argument between your friend and her husband?

We've all had the experience of being out of place at some point in our lives. What did you do in these sometimes awkward situations? The process and situation either entrained you or *you entrained it* to fit your personal process.

It's no different when you are drawn into a relationship with another person. In the interaction, the two of you electrically merge to some degree—*and one entrains the other.* There is no such thing as a "neutral" human interaction. If it were neutral, there would be no basis for interaction or attraction—no more than a neutral electrical circuit would pass a current.

In a relatively balanced relationship, each person has the opportunity to be a greater system and each one alternates between *entraining* and *being entrained by* the other. Many relationships, however, are unbalanced in this way. One person is for the most part being entrained by the other person (compliance) or for the most part entraining the other (dominance).

Because an interaction is unbalanced does not necessarily mean it is an unhealthy relationship. For example, the positive, creative interactions of child and parent, student and teacher, or leader and follower all work precisely because of the one-sidedness of the entrainment taking place.

The Eater and the Eaten

Now, what does this have to do with food? Simply this: When you eat, either:

1. you entrain your food to become you, or
2. your food entrains you.

Normally, when you eat food, you step it up to fit your psychophysical process.

For example, let's say you like to eat carrots. A carrot, as everyone knows, grows downward into the soil. That simple observation speaks volumes about the essence of the carrot. It has an intense desire to penetrate the depths of the soil that supplies it with its vital nutrition. A carrot, once removed from the soil (its natural plane of existence), is out of place.

Eating the carrot doesn't void its desire to continue seeking its own level. The new medium into which you have placed the carrot—that is, you—has no soil, but low it goes anyhow, penetrating the intestines of your lower body, "planting" itself in your "soil." Burdock, parsnips, and other long root vegetables will do the same. Naturally, all foods are digested in the stomach, but it is the essence of the food we are talking about here.

Any food, when entrained by the human body, will seek its own *qualitative* level, the level where it can best express its native qualities, and resonate there. It will then be stepped up by your digestive system into a process that eventually becomes *quantified* as your body. This is not a difficult thing to do, if you are reasonably active and have a healthy digestive system.

Vegetables and plant foods of any kind all are inherently immobile. When removed from their plane and entrained into another, they must be *motivated* by what does the entraining—that is, by you, the eater. The motivating factors most commonly employed to do this are cooking and other food preparation methods, along with physical activity. The nutritional elements of the plant foods you choose to eat are not the only thing entrained by you when you eat. The *qualities* of the plants are entrained as well, be they frozen, raw, cooked, organic, irradiated, or chemical-laden plants.

Animal products, on the other hand, are not immobile, and they have their own nervous systems that have already served to record and step up the plant world into the animal's specific level. Animals are motivated in their own way, and they also seek their own level. The cow seeks the pasture, the duck water, and so forth.

Eating and entraining animal products is relatively easier for us, because animals require less transformation and motivation in the entraining process than plants. Yet, attempting to nourish and recreate your body on excessive quantities of animal foods can have its drawbacks, too.

The lesser is to the greater what the greater is to the whole.

The thinking and sometimes rational human system is greater than both the plant and animal systems—but the animal system is greater than the plant system. Animals eat plants. Plants do not eat animals (or only rarely!). Humans eat both, and the animal system more closely resembles that of humans.

Consider what happens when you regularly consume and entrain the *qualities* of hormone- and drug-saturated chickens and cows confined to man-made prisons, as opposed to living within their natural inclination for grazing and foraging in open environments. You, too, may easily be entrained to seek the same level as these poor creatures, which could manifest as paranoia and intense stress, depression, and other qualities of these confined animals.

The contrast of animal versus plant foods makes this point easy to grasp, but the question of whether you entrain or are entrained by your foods is not a simple question of animal versus plant. Any time *you become a lesser system in comparison to your food,* you become susceptible to entrainment. Humans can—and often do—eat just about anything, even if it isn't food.

In fact, we have always used this fact of entrainment to our advantage: when you are feeling a little off-kilter or "under the weather," you *want* your system to be entrained by that hearty bowl of stew, chicken soup, or any number of other traditionally nourishing preparations. But if you fall into a rut of *chronically* being a weaker system than your food . . . well, remember Bob, Billy, and Jim?

Bob, Billy, and Jim have all become locked in a cycle where *they are being entrained by their foods.* Their foods, you might say, *choose them.*

The study of the energetics of food is in reality an exercise in intuition and natural instinct. It is not a "system" of classifying foods so much as a way of training yourself to recognize the reality of what is in front of you—what is on your plate, so to speak. It also is the study of self-knowledge, for the qualities *of yourself* are what you will naturally tend to seek in the foods you choose. You must be able to recognize what you are—or what you would like to be—in order to consciously recognize the foods that will nourish that.

Eat, Think, and Be Merry . . .

The least important thing in your life is what you believe.

WALTER RUSSELL

One might argue that the mind or thinking is more important than food—but really, this misses the point. Thinking and food work together. They are two sides of a coin, and the coin is what and who you are.

Food affects the *quality* of your blood, which in turn affects your nervous system, which affects the brain—the organ that manifests thinking and records your reality. On the other hand, your thinking leads you to choose the food you eat, which in turn will affect your blood and nervous system.

Does it matter what comes first, thinking or food? Not really. Your thinking will decide what you eat and what you eat will nourish and support your thinking. Both thinking and eating are means of expressing, manifesting, and nourishing what you *are*. In a sense, it is not important for you to decide what to eat, or what to think. But it *is* important to decide and *know* what you are and what you want to be. Your eating and thinking both determine each other, and both are determined by what you are . . . *if* your own self-motivated identity is a stronger system than your thoughts and your food.

And that choice is always open.

The Quality of Nourishment

In part 2 of this book, you'll learn about the different criteria that guide our food choices. Part 3 provides a complete road map for discovering the different aspects of various foods' inherent characters and personalities. Part 4 explores specific personalities and qualities of each of the major food groups in detail.

But before considering a detailed understanding or refining your knowledge of food energetics, here are several simple and straightforward guidelines:

1. No matter what you eat, use the best quality you can. I can't emphasize this enough. You are *qualitatively* what you eat—so no matter what specific kinds of foods you choose, as much as possible choose natural unprocessed, organic, and biodynamic foods. You deserve it!

2. If you can, eat foods you grow yourself. This is a helpful principle, whether the amount involved is 80 percent of your total diet or 2 percent. If you do grow your own food (as free of toxic pollutants as possible), in a short while you will began to *know quality* because you will play a crucial role in determining it. Your *knowledge* will be realized through what you decide to grow, through what and how much you eat, and through your activity level. Growing your own food allows you to develop a more intimate relationship with your food, because you are in a position to experience its life process from beginning to end.

The first step in the process of changing yourself is *the desire to do so*. Once the decision is made, you will gather all the *quantitative* ingredients necessary to create a momentum toward changing yourself into the *qualitative* image you desire. Whoever or whatever you decide to be, food will, for better or for worse, influence your psychophysical being.

Food is a mirror: look into the mirror of what you eat, and you will learn to see yourself. This works the other way as well. Look into the mirror of yourself, and you will find a reflection of what you are eating.

PART II

Choosing Your Food

5
The Essence of Choosing

"Have you decided what you'd like to order, ma'am?" The waitress is waiting. You're scanning the menu a third time, pondering ingredients, trying to inspect your appetite for clues, mentally swatting away buzzing memories of how veal parmigiana used to taste when you were a kid, wondering whether you should order what you want to eat, what you ought to eat, or simply play eeny-meeny-miney-moe. Your friend ordered when you first sat down. It was easy for her—she just gets the same thing every time. Like clockwork, never even thinks about it . . . While the waitress waits, you're distracted by an uncomfortably nagging thought—who's doing the wiser choosing, you or your friend?

How do you make your food choices? How often do you choose foods that are supportive to your health? Once in a while? Often? When it is suggested to you by an authority on the subject? If your friends or peers consider a particular food healthy, do you follow suit?

Have you ever really considered how deeply your choice of foods can influence your physical, mental, and spiritual state of well-being? Have your methods of rationalizing food choices been effective in assisting you in creating the health you desire? Have your food choices really worked for you? Do they work for you now?

The way you choose your foods is a fundamental and personal issue that you face constantly, and will continue to face throughout your life. Obviously, food is a basic biological need; but more than that, it also plays a pivotal role in the formation of your relationships, your accomplishments, and your very character. And the choices you make as to how you'll nourish yourself not only profoundly effect *your* life—they also effect the state of the environment and all other life forms on the planet.

No one else can choose your food for you. You must do it—and do it wisely.

Essence and Appetite

No matter what reasons you have (or think you have, or think you *don't* have) for making your food choices, there are two essential reasons for choosing food: *hunger* and *desire*.

The word *essential* is chosen carefully here. It means that these two reasons form *the essence* of your choosing. There may be hundreds, even thousands of ways of interpreting hunger and desire. No matter how they're translated or what form they take, *hunger* and *desire* are the *essence* of what drives you to choose one food or the other.

Furthermore, *hunger* and *desire* are two ends of the same spectrum. The physiological sensation or drive of *hunger* is the most visceral, instinctive, automatic expression of your life force. The *highest* function of this expression is *desire*. *True* desire—not simply the desire of your senses, but the desire that fuels your entire existence—is your *appetite for life*.

This is the force—no matter how its variations are described by science or philosophy—that drives egg and sperm to join . . . that brings you up screaming from the womb . . . that drives all your cells and body organs to function . . . that brings you together with your partner . . . that drives your thirst for information and knowledge as you grow up.

It is the same appetite that pumps the pistons of aspiration as you seek success in your career and fulfillment in your relationships. If you have fallen into the grip of a terminal illness, it is the "will to live" for which doctors and healers eagerly watch—since they know that *it* is the only force with the ability to make you truly whole again.

At times, people have tried to tell us that desire is an evil and that a cardinal rule for living in society is to curb your desires. I've watched many people attempt to follow this "path." You know what? It doesn't work. In fact, I believe that this "desire-is-the-problem" attitude is an unfortunate detour in the story of human development. It stems from a misunderstanding of the true scope and majesty of human desire—and from the fact that desire, while it is a simple thing, does not always express itself in simple ways.

Human beings often appear as complex things, no doubt about it. However, we have only one *true desire*—to love and to be loved. And while this one desire expresses itself in a kaleidoscope of forms, dimensions, and languages, it is still easy to get hung up in feeding it on only two or three levels.

For example, if you eat up your time satisfying your desires for tasty food, good sex, and fine grooming, then guess what you're doing?— You're losing out on the fulfillment of so many other levels of your desire. It's like finding a cursed magic potion: the more you drink, the thirstier you get. There are so many different examples of this trap. Like Charles Dickens's Ebenezer Scrooge, you might spend your whole life glutting your appetite for financial and corporate power, and never take the opportunity to quench your thirst for companionship and personal involvement—a classic case of "cutting off your nose to spite your face."

Or (and this example will be closer to home for some) you might spend years in dutiful pursuit of physical health and spiritual refinement, only to find that you've been squelching your "more base" appetites for sensual love and material success. But they're not "more base" at all. No level of desire is any more true or more noble than any other.

The purpose of food energetics is to help you align yourself with your desire and to remove the obstacles and limitations that stand in the way of that alignment, whether they are barriers of concept, attitude, lack of information, or sheer inertia.

Choosing the Real Thing

Most of our food choices appear to have little to do with the food itself, more often being based on something *we think* about the food; something someone else thinks about it; some circumstance surrounding the food; or (most commonly) something as blind as mere habit.

In other words, these choices are dictated by something *extraneous* to the food itself.

In the sections that follow, you'll notice some common criteria for food choices that seem almost completely extraneous. Numbly pulling a certain food out of the freezer at the end of a long day because a TV commercial told you to—that certainly seems an open-and-shut case of extraneous choosing. By contrast, selecting a food in order to gain its specific sensibilities (like the example of the young Native American man described in part 1) is about as clear an example of *essential* choosing as you might find.

But by and large, your real food choices tend to be motivated by a mix of impulses, usually of both the "essential" and "extraneous" variety. Knowing food energetics can help free you from extraneous choices and further assist you in choosing essence as much as possible.

Cultivating the art of choosing—at least as far as it applies to foods—involves three simple stages.

Calling Your Own Bluff

The first stage is to recognize what is extraneous—in other words, *irrelevant*—in your food choosing.

Choice by habit is a good example. With habitual choices, often you'll find there were *originally* underlying essential reasons for making what has since become blind habit. But those reasons are of the past, and choice is of the present. For example, "I like this particular food, have always eaten it, so therefore I will continue to eat it!" Okay . . . but have you ever stopped to ask yourself if that particular food likes you? Have you really thought about how it makes you feel? Do you really enjoy all it has to offer, both negative and positive qualities?

Another example is a food choice dictated by the influence of *media advertising* (discussed in chapter 12): You choose a food because someone else told you to (because it would make you sexy and smart and build your body twelve ways—and their bank accounts twelve more).

This stage is fun, because when you recognize each extraneous choice for what it is, chances are it will simply disappear. It is the very fact that you're *not conscious* of why you're making that kind of choice that allows it to keep its grip on you in the first place.

Listen to the Questions You're Asking

The second stage is recognizing *what it is* that you truly *are* choosing—to take an informed look at your essential choices, at what qualities you are actually choosing when you select one food over another.

Are you attracted to a certain taste or texture? What character does that confer on you? Or are you seeking a more general personality in a food that is harder to pinpoint, but just as strongly attractive? What does that attraction mean—what *quality* is it you're after? What qualities in *you* are you responding to, or seeking to nourish?

This book will help you take that "informed look." (We'll supply the "informed," and then it's up to you to take the look.)

The third stage is simply a further development of the second: teach your choosing to be guided by energetics in all its dimensions.

Experience unfamiliar foods, further explore previously unseen qualities in *familiar* foods, and be aware of foods that sound a resonant note to your own character—or to the character you seek. Practice new choices, refine old ones; get to know foods and choose them as carefully as you would a business associate or a lover—for in reality, they are both!

As you master the art of choosing foods to support and fully nourish your life, you will also learn to recognize many new and exciting qualities in yourself, perhaps some you never knew existed.

6
Habit
Appetite's Nemesis

If desire is the fundamental driving force of your choosing, and certainly the foundation of all aspects of *essential choosing,* then its opposite is *habit.* Habit is the archenemy of desire. It is the epitome of unconscious choice and *extraneous choosing.*

The thing that is so insidious about habitual food choices is that over time, they can make quite a dent in your state of health, not to mention your relationships with foods and eating in general.

Imagine you are driving straight down a road. You've got a good reason to do so: the road happens to be going in a straight direction. After five minutes, your mind drifts and you continue on out of habit. Now the road curves into an intersection. Still driving out of habit? If so, you've got a problem.

A ridiculous example? Maybe—but it happens all the time with food. The hospitals of America are full of Bobs, Jims, and Billys who kept on driving straight through their habitual meals, failed to notice some curves in the road of their own physiology, and hit intersections labeled "Cataracts," "Carcinoma," and "Coronary." Not all of those intersections in the road are health related, either. Some are labeled "I Hate My Job" and "Bored with My Life." So much for habit's straight and narrow path.

A Doughnut Odyssey

I vividly recall being in the seventh grade, an age where one decides pretty much for oneself what to eat for breakfast. Being an active teenager, I wasn't deeply concerned with what I ate for breakfast. In fact, here was my criterion: if it didn't require any time to prepare, I'd eat it.

It so happened that for two years, I had the honor of living next door to a doughnut shop. How convenient. Every morning, before setting out on my long trek to school, I would indulge in a cup of coffee and a couple of doughnuts.

Now, there are a number of reasons I may have had for starting out on this doughnut odyssey. One reason was that they were simply there, in my immediate environment. (We'll revisit this reason in a few chapters when we explore the idea of "circumstantial choosing.") My blood sugar may have thought the daily sugar fix would put my pendulums into the right swing. Maybe a psychologist would say that doughnuts evoked my teenage idea of female companionship because they were soft and sweet.

Whatever my reasons, my morning visits to the doughnut shop soon became *habitual*. The habit continued for the rest of the two years I lived near the doughnut shop.

During that time, I had not the slightest idea as to how this food was influencing my mental and physical health, nor did I care. It wasn't until I changed residence that I realized I could no longer tolerate eating doughnuts! The very *thought* of eating another doughnut repulsed me. Obviously, I had eaten too many for too long: the association of doughnuts and breakfast became a negative one.

For the next few years, doughnuts were mercifully gone from my diet. I did not delete them consciously so much as by automatic reaction to the O.D. of those doughnut-fed morning treks.

As I got a little older, I became more aware of healthy foods and the importance of health in general. And then a peculiar thing happened. I started to want to eat doughnuts again. But this time, they would have to be "healthy doughnuts" made from quality ingredients. The world of health foods offered three or four versions of what were supposedly healthy alternatives to the junk-food doughnut. I tried them all.

Another negative experience, worse than the first. Whole wheat doughnuts were heavy and simply awful. I thought, "If these are healthy, then who needs them!" It wasn't until after extensive experimentation that I realized a natural doughnut could be made in my own kitchen. After a few experiments with homemade doughnuts I finally reached the conclusion that my quest for the perfect doughnut was rooted in my past and was the result of a negative experience. What's more, doughnuts were in fact something about which *I could care less*. Yet today, if someone were to offer me a homemade doughnut made with natural ingredients, I wouldn't turn it down.

Light at the End of the Doughnut Hole

My choice to eat doughnuts for breakfast in my early teens came about as a result of convenience and availability. This gradually became a habit that could have led to a variety of outcomes. When I changed my diet to natural foods, I could have maintained a secret habit of eating junk-food doughnuts (I mean, no one would have to know). Or I could have sworn off doughnuts completely, and lived with a secret fear of what might happen should I again indulge in them. I could have continued eating a healthier version of doughnuts (which I eventually realized didn't really exist); or I could have substituted something else for doughnuts (which doesn't really exist, either: a doughnut is a doughnut).

All would be rationalizations to continue doing something that really didn't work for me. Instead, I chose to simply let my doughnut experience be.

By just letting it be, I eventually reached a point, some years later, where I could manage an average of two nights a week of peaceful sleep without haunting nightmares of doughnuts dancing around my head. I still wake up in the morning with the shakes because of intense cravings, and it is only when I realize that I am no longer in the seventh grade and don't have to go to school anymore that I can pull myself together and attempt to be a responsible human being. Other than that, I'm handling the whole experience quite well. . . .

Okay, I just made up that last paragraph. None of it's true. But it could be.

I've seen this sort of thing happen to people just like you and me, more times than I can count. The shrapnel of blind habits can leave some pretty impressive damage—and past and present food associations can have powerful energetic influences on our lives.

The point of the doughnut story is that an original method of choice—in this case, simple convenience—can gain considerable strength and momentum through sheer habit. This applies to all methods of choosing, whether it's your parents' choosing for you, sensory preference, advice of others, cultural and traditional preferences, or nutritional "knowledge." Choices that are not consciously reexamined easily become a habitual part of your paunch's palette. And "too much of a good" thing for the wrong reason—be it whole grain, wild game, salad, or organic fruit—can and will produce adverse effects, regardless of what one might like to believe.

When considering what and how you eat, you'll find that your choices of food are influenced in some way by one or more of the factors we'll explore in the following chapters. Consider how much these factors influence your choice of food, and then decide for yourself *if and how they work to support your life.*

It is important to remember that the same food can and often does have different intensities of effect on different people. This can be determined by when and how often a particular food is eaten along with one's overall dietary patterns.

It is more *your relationships with certain foods* that determine your experiences than the foods themselves. Your relationships with food are some of the most intimate relationships in your life. How you interact with food can determine a great deal about who and what you are!

Let's explore a few of the common choices people use to determine how and why they eat the way they do.

7
Choosing with Your Senses

In a moment, I'm going to ask you to close your eyes and picture the foods of your fondest memories. (Don't close them yet—you need to read the next paragraph first!) As you see them in your mind's eye, let yourself recall the flavors, aromas, and the way you feel as you savor them.

> . . . The smell of fresh baked bread on a cold winter's day . . . the taste of crisp sautéed vegetables, lightly flavored with soy sauce and a dash of hot pepper . . . the captivating sight of a holiday feast with a steaming turkey centerpiece surrounded by oyster stuffing, candied yams, fresh green salad, fluffy mashed potatoes and gravy, deep red cranberry sauce, grilled marinated wild mushrooms . . . that first glass of perfectly smooth semidry wine . . .

Now go ahead, close your eyes, taste, and smell . . .

Your Sensory Signature

There's no doubt about it, no matter who you are or how educated you are, Rhodes scholar and road worker alike have powerful sensory associations with foods. They have nothing to do with your reasoned thought—they are visceral and compelling. And the truth is, those sensory associations comprise one of the most common ways people choose their foods. How a food looks, tastes, smells, and feels as you eat it, whether it is cold or hot, crunchy or soft—all these physical characteristics of a food have tremendous sway over both your feeling for it and how it affects you.

We usually think of this association in terms of "taste"—yet the sense of taste per se is only a small part of the hypnotic sensory associations foods can hold for us. Physiologically, the sense of smell actually has more to do with how a food "tastes" than the sense of taste itself. And that sense of taste/smell rarely stands alone in our palette of preferences; most often it combines with other physical features of food, such as its texture, in determining our likes and dislikes.

Your sensorial preferences in food are quite specific and unique, much like your fingerprints.

Each of us has distinct preferences for foods with certain flavors, textures, temperatures, and colors. Here are some of the many shades of variety that color our choices:

- Flavors: sweet, sour, bitter, spicy, or salty
- Textures: soft and moist, watery and viscous, hard and dry, crunchy, soft and chewy, heavy and dense, light and crispy, greasy, slimy, pasty, etc.
- Temperatures: cold, cool, warm, hot, or room temperature
- Colors: bright, dark, pastels, and often specific colors: red, white, yellow, etc.

These factors all represent physical qualities of food—but they can have both physical *and emotional* effects on us by energetically influencing our vitality, moods, and feelings.

- Soft and creamy foods: puddings, some fruits, and soft cereals (porridge), are often associated with small children and the elderly. You may have a preference for these foods because they nourish a soft, childlike innocent quality or a passive, easygoing nature.
- Hard and crunchy foods: crackers, toasted or crusty bread, and

some types of cookies are often associated with anger, anxiety, irritability, or frustration. These are often eaten aggressively, so you can hear the crunch and feel it as you eat them.

- Heavy and dense foods: thick deli sandwiches, hearty stews, or peanut butter sandwiches on heavy whole wheat bread are often associated with procrastination, resting, inertia, or maintaining the status quo and a general lack of physical motivation.
- Light and crispy foods: raw vegetables, salads, some raw fruits, chips, or popcorn, are often associated with lack of self-control or spontaneous emotional expression, or can also relate to freshness, fun, and carefree energy.

These are just a few of the food choices people make based on texture. Yet even these textures rarely stand alone as a choice; they are usually combined with a particular flavor, color, or temperature.

For example, a person who chooses to eat milk chocolate desires the sweet flavor but also a soft and chewy or soft and moist texture. Another person with a taste for potato chips, corn chips, or rice cakes desires the salty flavor in addition to a light and crunchy texture. Bread with peanut butter will tend to have a sweet flavor with a heavy and dense texture, and pickles can have a sour flavor with a light and crispy texture. The person who wants plain corn chips is making a very different statement than the one who prefers corn chips with guacamole and salsa. A person who eats most of his food cold, directly from the refrigerator, is either consciously or unconsciously supporting an emotionally cold personality and is likely to suffer from digestive distress, compared to the person who takes the time to warm his food for easier digestion.

Do you see the volumes you can learn about yourself already, just from these past few paragraphs? Here are some more examples—more food for thought:

- When you regularly choose to eat bitter foods, you can develop a bitter edge to your character.
- Hard and dry foods can contribute to a hard and dry character.
- You may find an especially heavy, sticky food irresistible (or

habitual) because it supports a procrastinating inertia you aren't ready—or don't realize you're ready—to let go of.

Some people *think* they dislike a particular food, even though they've never actually tried it. This is common in children, and adults often insist it's "not reasonable"—yet we adults do it more than we realize, too! And in fact, usually there is indeed a very good "reason," even if we're not aware of it. How so? This sort of "blind dislike" may be based on a single quality, whether appearance, texture, temperature, color, or some other physical association. People may have no "rational" reason not to eat that food—*they may simply not want to become that way themselves.*

The dislike of a particular food often can be altered by preparing the food in such a way as to change one or more of its qualities. Oatmeal is a good example. Alone, oatmeal is a boring, passive, pasty, and neutral food. Add some roasted almonds, raisins, a little fresh cream, and some natural sweetener and you have something quite enjoyable to eat, with a variety of flavors, textures, and energies that not only raises the nutritional profile dramatically, it also makes oatmeal worth eating.

How about those dark green vegetables, the ones so many of us have a hard time with: kale, collard greens, dandelion greens? Steam them? Boil them in plain water? No, thanks! No one ever ate these foods like this and intelligent people with any taste for food are not about to start now. It is no wonder how few people want to eat these highly nutritious foods. But ask someone raised in the Deep South how to cook collards—or ask anyone else who has had these foods in his or her diet for generations. They'll show you how to enjoy and benefit from these "bland" leafy greens.

Choosing Colors

A food's color has a subtle yet deep influence on us. Light creates colors and contributes greatly to the mood and quality of our temperaments. In fact, light *is* food to the photosynthetic plant kingdom. A food's color is its most direct way of telling you about its own preferences and character.

Here are the six basic colors from which all others are derived:

- Warm to hot colors: yellow, orange, and red
- Cool to cold colors: green, blue, and purple

Each of the warmer colors has a complementary cooler color, and vice versa. For example, red and green are complementary, as are the pairs purple/yellow and orange/blue. When these paired colors are placed side by side, each causes its complement to appear brighter. In other words, they enhance each other's energetics.

One may like or dislike a particular food simply because of an association that a color denotes. For example:

- Red foods—tomatoes, red peppers, rare beef, lamb, and red apples—have associations of strength, sensuousness, defensiveness, intensity, and heat (though they do have varying other energetic qualities, too).
- Green foods—leafy green vegetables, green beans, green peppers— often have associations of coolness, openness, independence, and spontaneity.
- Brown foods—mushrooms, wheat bread, chocolate—tend to denote earthiness, security, comfort, boredom, and blandness.
- Black foods—including some beans; some sea vegetables; burnt, grilled, or charred foods—have associations of distress and melancholia, and at the same time, dignity, strength, and power.

Creative chefs implement a balanced color scheme in their preparations to create appealing and satisfying meals. The most energizing meal is one that includes a mix of both warm-colored and cool-colored foods. A more warming meal will tend to highlight darker, more warming colors, and cooling meals will tend to emphasize lighter, more cooling colors.

A variety of colors in a meal give it a wide spectrum of energies. The result can be a deep sense of physical and emotional satisfaction.

Another physical example of food is its shape. The two basic shapes, from which all others are derived, are the *cube* and the *sphere*.

- Foods that are round and smooth (spherical) express qualities of sensuality, attraction, comfort, serenity, and satisfaction.
- Squared, jagged, or odd-shaped foods express a character of inquisitiveness, restlessness, challenge, excitement, or repulsion.

I attended a wonderful dinner party several years ago where our host, an extraordinary natural foods chef and baker, was asked by a guest why she baked only round cakes, and never square or rectangular ones. She replied without hesitation:

"In my experience, I find round cakes evoke a sense of harmony."

These are only several examples of the many possible variations of foods' sensory attributes. It would be easy to fill an entire volume detailing them all. However, the best way to learn them is to experience the foods themselves with an open mind.

Let's go on to explore some other dimensions of choosing food.

8
Circumstantial Choosing

You've been in flight for an hour and two drinks and are just starting to get mildly hungry. The flight attendant has worked her way down the aisle and reached your seat. She asks, "What would you like for lunch, ma'am?"—and both your mind and your stomach draw a blank.

"What are my choices?" you mumble.

"Chicken à la Nebbish or the Macaroni and Cheez-Food plate," she responds.

You hear yourself say, "I'll have the Nebbish . . . thanks."

As powerful as sensory preferences are, there is another and even more immediate criterion for choosing: choices dictated by your circumstance. Aside from simply taking what's offered or what is on the menu, here are some other examples of such circumstantial choosing:

- The foods that were in your surroundings while growing up
- The foods your parents taught you to eat
- The foods that are available in your neighborhood
- The foods that are in your pantry or refrigerator when you get hungry
- The foods that are readily available at this time of year
- The foods you decide you can afford

When Sir Edward Mallory was asked why he had climbed Mt. Everest and explained the motivation for his quest with the immortal words "Because it was there," history added an entry to its page of timeless quotations.

Somehow when you give the same reason for consuming Chicken à la Nebbish, it seems less impressive.

However, choosing according to circumstance—unlike choosing by pure habit—is not necessarily a *blind* choice. There are both essential and extraneous shades of circumstantial choosing.

Availability

The choice to secure food crops indigenous to your own locality or region in order to establish an ecological and energetic relationship with the region is an example of choosing according to your circumstance— yet it is far from blind. It is also a choice that goes directly to the *essence* of your food and your environment. Learning and applying food preparation styles that are traditional in your locale can also help you catch the flavor of where you live in a very profound way.

On the other hand, allowing your food choices to be *limited* by your circumstances or locale is often a nonchoice, with all the creative potential of the blind habit.

For most of us, the "availability" of foods is a highly relative term— that is, relative to *how much and what kind of effort you want to expend to get it.* Most of us these days actually have access more or less to whatever we want and need. It is fairly easy, if you take the time and effort to research sources, to find foods of the best quality. A friend once showed me how to create a gourmet meal entirely out of foraged, wild foods from abandoned lots—in a Boston suburb.

Price and Priority

The issues surrounding circumstantial choosing are best clarified (as so many issues are) by considering the matter of cost.

"I live on a fixed and severely limited income, so my range of choice is pretty drastically limited—right?"

Wrong. Just about anyone with a job can "afford" to eat an interesting, varied, and exceptionally high-quality diet. For most of us, who have some disposable income to spend on food, it is more a question of what we *think* we can "afford"—or more accurately, what we *choose to afford*.

The price you pay for your food will depend on how important *quality* is to you. Many people think foods that contribute to health are expensive, and therefore may seek cheaper versions of these foods. While this can be true, the adage "You get what you pay for" is quite fitting when considering quality foods.

Yet high quality does not *necessarily* mean high cost. If you enjoy eating meat, you can purchase a smaller *quantity* of an exceptionally high *quality* of pasture-raised, unadulterated, chemical-free beef, cared for with devoted attention, and while it will cost more than what you'll pay at the supermarket, you will be far more satisfied eating half or one-third the amount. Net cost: pennies to dollars *less*!

The "health food" business is just that. It is a business, and like any business, it has its share of concerned individuals as well as opportunists. It is your business to determine the price you must pay for quality.

And you do pay, one way or another. Your health is your greatest wealth, and skimping on quality just might cost you more dearly than you intend. Why? Because poor-quality foods do not support your health and many are known to contribute to health problems. The evidence for the nutritional superiority of naturally raised foods continues to increase. Meanwhile, there's no reason to wait for science to catch up to what common sense tells us: quality matters.

Common sense tells us that it only takes a few ingredients to make a loaf of bread. Flour, water, salt, and leavening. Why on earth would I want to purchase from the local supermarket and consume a loaf of bread with twenty-five ingredients when twenty of them are not even edible and some have been proven to be deleterious to health? While this loaf of commercial bread may cost one-third the cost of a real loaf of bread and I may have to go the extra mile for the real bread, it is simply a matter of quality.

The bottom line of circumstantial choosing is this: harmonizing with your circumstances is one thing. Being controlled by them is quite another.

9
Choosing with Your Personality

Beyond choosing a food for a specific feature, many people make food choices based on the overall character of a food, a side dish, or even an entire meal. You may choose a *character* or *personality* of a particular food that, in some way, echoes your own or one that you seek to acquire.

In part 3, Working Models, we'll systematically go through the various ways of assessing a food's personality. In part 4, The Cast of Characters, we'll look at some of the personalities of dozens of specific foods in detail.

For now, to give you a general picture of the idea of food personalities, let's look at two types of contrasting, complementary food personality types.

Dominant or Compliant?

While a food's personality is determined to a great extent by its physical qualities, a food also may have an overall more *dominant or compliant character* that is made up of a range of individual qualities.

- A dominant personality in a food may include: a stronger flavor, especially strong energetic effects, a more pronounced color, and more limitations as to how it can be prepared and with what other foods it can be prepared.
- Compliant foods are usually milder in flavor and color, softer,

49

more yielding to a wider range of preparation styles, and are able to combine more easily with a wider variety of other foods.

Obviously, dominant foods tend to entrain compliant foods. Chefs often use dominant foods to more clearly distinguish a compliant food's personality. Compliant foods, on the other hand, are useful ingredients to absorb and soften a dominant food's extroverted qualities.

You can evaluate a food's dominant or compliant character relative to the food group to which it belongs. For example: relative to cereals, buckwheat, corn, and amaranth have more dominant personalities, while rice, barley, and oats have more compliant personalities. Among leafy vegetables, dandelion, chard, and watercress have dominant personalities compared to the compliant personalities of lettuces, Chinese cabbage, and bok choy.

Other dominant-personality vegetables include parsnip, tomato, celery, burdock, and rutabaga. Among dairy products, those with dominant personalities include hard and sharp cheeses, butter, yogurt, and goat products—compared to the compliant personalities of cow's milk and soft, mild-tasting cheeses. Beef is a dominant food relative to poultry, yet among poultry, pheasant is a dominant food compared to chicken.

Here are some other dominant and compliant foods relative to their particular groups:

- More dominant: game meats, red-fleshed fish, garlic, spices, chocolate, berries, and citrus fruits
- More compliant: tofu, cabbage, oatmeal, rice, white-fleshed fish, eggs

The two personalities complement one another, just as do complementary pairs of colors. Compliant foods *need* the leadership of dominant partners to help define them and give them dynamics. At the same time, dominant foods *depend on* the more genial temperament of compliant supporters to absorb and buffer their strong personalities.

For example, a plate of pasta (more compliant) comes to life with the addition of garlic, tomato, and olive oil, all more dominant foods. Adding a bit of onion or watercress to a plain lettuce salad gives it just enough punctuation to give the salad some character.

While both affect one's personality, dominant versus compliant is not a question of "better" versus "worse." Both characters are cardinal requirements for achieving a good balance of foods and a harmonious personality in the eater. Neither is preferable over the other; a one-sided emphasis on either can lead to an imbalanced personality. Both characters are essential ingredients for maintaining physical health as well as a flexible personality.

The Spice of Life

Diet experts tout the benefits of a "well-rounded" or "varied" diet— but many people, perhaps even most people, actually eat within a fairly restricted sphere.

Sometimes this is obvious, such as with the person who literally eats the same meat and potatoes or the same deli salads every night. But sometimes it is not so obvious.

Many people have a tendency to eat meals that may involve a fairly wide selection of different foods yet still repeatedly emphasize the same *food personalities*. This often goes unnoticed because we have not been taught to recognize food personalities. Yet what may appear to be a "well-rounded, varied" menu plan may in fact be about as heterogeneous and pluralistic as a Daughters of the American Revolution fund-raising steering committee luncheon.

For example, people often eat from one side of the dominant/compliant spectrum without realizing it.

- A diet that relies on rice, oatmeal, cream cheese, white meat, fish, eggs, tofu, and various steamed vegetables may *look* varied—but it is nearly 100 percent *compliant*.
- By the same token, a diet of meats, onion and tomato salads, topped off with chocolate and citrus fruit, is *dominant* in the extreme.

If you choose to eat a diet primarily composed of compliant foods—essentially a diet with minimal seasonings, bland foods, and limited preparation methods—then your personality will become similar to your chosen diet. Just as compliant foods are dependent on more dominant foods, a diet based on large proportions of compliant foods can create a state of physical weakness, pale complexion, and emotional dependency in the eater.

On the other hand, a diet consisting solely of dominant foods—foods with strong personalities—can support the human personality traits of self-righteousness and even arrogance and isolation.

A healthy, fulfilling, and satisfying diet not only includes a wide variety of foods, it also includes a variety of satisfying preparation methods. Most importantly, you need to know that you choose and eat foods with your entire personality—and not just with your mind or your taste buds.

Now take a look inside *your* pantry and refrigerator!

Who do you see?

Choosing by Association

Most of us have learned to choose our food by associating it with feelings, events, people, places, or other images—especially those of the past.

When you were a child, your dietary choices were made for you, for the most part, by your parents—based on whatever were *their* particular criteria for choosing. Gradually, your learning how to choose for yourself began to overlap with, and often to conflict with, the influence of your parents' food choices. In fact, this form of choosing is one of the earliest and most common expressions of a child's independence.

The memories of particular foods also form some of the most recognizable landmarks in the scenery of our past. Thanksgiving or other holiday dinners with family or that special birthday dinner just for you at Mom's or Dad's favorite restaurant are a few examples of these memories.

We thus develop an entire vocabulary of food-as-symbol—a vocabulary that usually has little to do with the essence of foods, but more to do with our own views of, and feelings about, our own experiences.

You may recall as a child having a dislike for a particular food because of how or with what you associated it. Maybe it became boring to you because it was served too often. Maybe you disliked it because you were forced to eat it, and that set up an automatic resistance to it. Or maybe that particular food led you to recall a particular emotional experience every time you ate it—perhaps you once ate too much seafood and got sick, and the association of seafood with that experience of sickness created a mental block against seafood. And seafood is an arbitrary example: for you, it might have been that party where you ate too much cake or pizza. For me, it was doughnuts on the way to school.

Food has an uncanny way of touching our psyche, affecting how we perceive our world and ourselves. We perceive some foods as having a positive influence in our lives, and see others in a negative light. Some have both positive and negative influences; at times a certain food feels right to eat, while at other times the mere thought of that very same food makes you feel nauseous.

Learned Choosing

Psychologists often use the term *learned behavior* when referring to behaviors that are not motivated from the inside but taught from the outside. In choosing your food, there are choices that come from what you've been taught. These are "learned choices."

It's not always easy to recognize the symptoms of learned choosing. There may indeed be some essential qualities about the food that make it "right" or "not right" for you at the time. However, it also may be "all in your head." Uprooting those food associations that stem solely from your past can be a liberating experience.

Learned choosing can begin as early as when you were being nourished in utero and continue on through childhood into maturity.

If your mother was addicted to chocolate, it would not be surprising if you grew up with a strong preference for chocolate. Since the chocolate contributed to the quality of your formative, embryonic nourishment, it would have contributed to the actual development of your cellular body and nervous system—a sort of "biologically learned" choosing. In that case, the choosing has already been done for you by your mother and will have been recorded in your nervous system as a learned choice of chocolate.

Learned choosing also develops later in life and can easily degrade to a pattern of habitual eating. You may consume a pint of ice cream every night at precisely 8:00, or a bag of chips whenever you watch TV. A well-established learned choosing may become deep-rooted enough to become a food addiction.

A pattern of being controlled by learned choosing can be the result of factors that shape your character into a chronically compliant mold: a suppressed childhood, lack of attention from parents, too much attention from parents, peer pressure in school, dissatisfaction with your job, poor body image, etc.

Learned choosing can also develop as an outgrowth of circumstantial choosing. An elderly fellow may choose and prefer strawberry ice cream to any other ice cream because he has learned to choose it through many years of exposure to it. It is familiar to him. If chocolate raisin mint ice cream is not familiar to him, it's doubtful that given the choice, he'd choose to eat it.

On the other hand, give a young child the opportunity to choose between an exotic fluorescent-colored ice cream and vanilla or chocolate ice cream, and he will often choose the more exotic—because he is familiar with these colors through Saturday morning cartoons and weirdly colored breakfast cereals.

"Familiar foods" tends to mean "safe foods," and they are often associated with comfort and assurance: "Mom and Dad ate them, they've been around for a long time—what could be wrong with that?"

Well, Mom and Dad were taught about their food, too, and likely by teachers who didn't know much more about food energetics than they did! (On the other hand, your great-grandmother probably *knew* her food: nature and *her* parents' common sense were still her teachers.)

While the past has in many ways influenced how you choose your food, you needn't depend on it to make quality choices today.

More often than not, learned choosing is based on *reason*—and reasoning does little more than allow you to continue making excuses for doing what you are doing. It is important to learn how to choose your food through *knowing* as opposed to reason. Knowing your food intimately requires trust in yourself.

I *trust* that you *know*—do you?

10
Choosing from Reaction

Choosing a particular food out of reaction is a more driven action than choosing by simple association. In reactive choosing, you are looking to the food for help in solving a problem or to compensate for an uncomfortable or upsetting situation.

There are two aspects to choosing from reaction. The first is choosing out of *physiological* reaction. This is where your body actually is striving to achieve homeostasis or a state of productive equilibrium. The second is when you choose a particular food out of a more *emotional* or *psychological* reaction.

Choosing from Physiological Reaction

Physiological reactions occur regularly within your body on hundreds and thousands of different levels. Your body is a vital organism in constant motion, with a wide range of dynamic capabilities of *expansion* and *constriction*. Every cell, muscle, nerve, organ, and tissue in your body expands and constricts with varying degrees and frequencies.

Some of these rhythms and functions are more obvious than others. Your heart beats with a steady, pulsating rhythm that differs from the slower flow of respiration in your lungs. More subtle cycles of expansion and constriction include the various integrated rhythms of hormone secretion, the alternating electric currents of your autonomic nervous system, and the cycles of venous and arterial blood circulation.

The rates and rhythms of these bodily functions strongly affect your food choices. An imbalance or lack of dynamic interchange between expansion and constriction in any of these cycles can contribute to desires and cravings for foods.

A classic example is hypoglycemia: when your blood glucose level is chronically low you will feel a reactive desire for food or drink to force that level up. Sugar, anything sweet, alcohol, and overeating are common targets of that reactive choosing.

But here is the ironic part: in most cases, the imbalance itself is caused, or at least, heavily contributed to, by an imbalance in your prior eating! Recalling how easily people construct a one-sided diet out of personality preference, association with past circumstance, or sheer habit, it's not hard to see how that can happen.

The most common type of choosing from physiological reaction occurs when one is consuming a diet lacking in important nutritional components. Diets lacking in a variety of quality protein sources, fat sources, carbohydrates sources, or vitamins often lead to reactive eating, which manifests as compulsive eating or overeating in order to compensate for nutritional deficiency. The person then feels temporarily satiated, but because the nutritional deficiency was not and cannot be met through quantity or substitution, the cycle is doomed to repeat indefinitely until the problem is recognized and reconciled.

Cycles of Reaction

Overly tight and constricted physiological functions often result from a reliance on foods that produce *constriction*.

- Foods that cause constriction include salt, meats, poultry, eggs, salty and hard cheeses, and dry, baked foods (such as crackers and dry, crunchy cookies). These foods can set up a physiological reaction where the body in turn desires—*demands,* actually—a compensating *expansion*.
- Food that cause expansion include sugar, sweets, milk, alcohol, spices, fruit, coffee and soft drinks, and a preponderance of raw foods.

This process works in the opposite way as well. When physiological functions become expanded, you'll react by craving foods of a constrictive nature to recover a sense of balance. The extent or degree of expansion or constriction in your physiology determines the extent of the reactionary desire for its opposite.

The problem with reactive choosing is that one-sided conditions tend to lead to one-sided reactions, which lead to one-sided conditions. . . . It's quite easy to work into a cycle that grows to destructive and compulsive proportions. Such reactive cycles not only cause physiological wear and tear, they can also play havoc with your psychology and personality. Your mind, thinking, and moods are affected by the swings of constriction and expansion as surely as are your blood cells and digestive system.

Alcoholism is a perfect example. There are a host of psychological, emotional, and spiritual dimensions to the character patterns that develop with alcoholism—but underneath it all, there is also a physiological pattern that stems from a reactive food cycle. Behind a compulsive craving for alcohol (and you can substitute sugar, chocolate, or drugs here if you like), there is lurking an overemphasis on heavily constricting and drying foods, especially meats, eggs, hard, salty cheeses, and salty snacks.

Opposites React

What is the opposite of reactive choosing? It is *proactive choosing*. You can't stop constriction and expansion from occurring in your body, if you want to keep on living and breathing. But you can break some of those devastating cycles of reaction. The key lies in taking an active part in choosing your foods with creativity, adventure, and openness to change. The moment you get stuck in a rut, you set the stage for reactive choosing.

Balanced dynamic interchange of expansion and constriction from *proactive* choosing will produce a balanced and stable condition in your metabolism.

"What on earth does *balanced dynamic interchange* mean?"

Let me explain. Opposites react together, and when they do, the interplay between them can produce a temporary state of balance—*more or less*. What dictates just *how* "more or less" this is? The answer lies in this question: Just *why is it* that opposites react together, anyway?

Despite the commonly held view, opposites do *not* attract.

For example, in human interactions, two people do not really attract each other: *one* actively attracts the other, and that other *is attracted*. Only one of the two does the attracting; that one also *entrains* the other.

An example from food is the natural combination of a dominant personality food and a compliant personality food. They may combine well together—but they don't attract each other. Only dominant forces have any power to attract. A compliant or passive entity has the power only to respond to being attracted; it cannot itself actively attract.

The same goes for the so-called positive and negative poles of a magnet—there's no mutual attraction there, either. A negative electrical charge has no capacity to attract—no more than a quiet, depressed, and timid person attracts other people. Makes sense, doesn't it?

This heretical viewpoint was pioneered by Walter Russell, who provided an answer to the question "Why do opposites react together?"

Opposites do not attract; rather, they unite for the sole purpose of voiding their differences.

Two people who are romantically involved are not attracted by their oppositeness. In fact, it is precisely what the two have in common— *their sameness*—that provides the possibility for coming together with any degree of harmony and enjoyment.

Their differences are not attractive—in fact, as time progresses, the two will do everything they can to void those differences and become *more* similar. Just look at a happy, content couple in their eighties: they've had so many decades of opportunity to void their differences that they have become remarkably alike, even though they may at times complain about each other. (As you have already guessed, the commonly held corollary idea that "likes repel one another" is also untrue.)

Proactive Choosing

How different two opposites are before they interact will determine what kind of reaction takes place. Interplay between two foods, personalities, or forces that are more equivalent (less radically different) will result in a milder, smoother reaction: there's less difference to void.

For example: whole cereal grains and fresh vegetables are two groups of foods that are relatively equivalent—they exhibit only mild differences and are generally classified as carbohydrates. When eaten together, there is little basis for strong reaction, and thus they produce little reaction in one's metabolism.

A less equivalent and more unbalanced interplay between two opposite foods results in a stronger reaction. A diet including wild game (on the one hand) and spices and alcohol (on the other) produces more dynamic opposition. The wild game produces powerful constriction, tension, and heat, while the spices and alcohol tend to create balance by enabling the game to unwind and release that constriction—that is, the spices and alcohol create expansion, relaxation, and cold.

If one half of the equation is eaten without the other, a reactionary desire or compulsion is created for its opposite. And when the opposite *is* consumed a powerful reaction takes place. The extremes between the two are voided and a degree of balance is established.

Neither one of these patterns is "better," in and of itself. It takes two to tango.

A broader range of oppositions gives a greater edge and more dynamic spark to your character, as well as a more active metabolism. And for those lacking in dietary dynamics it could lead to important changes both in temperament and physiology.

A more mild, narrower range of dynamic opposition with diet might seem easier to handle; however, it can lead to monotony and a yearning or craving for excitement.

Obviously, both have their benefits and their drawbacks. And just as obviously, how you design your patterns of dynamic opposition is up to you. One way or another differences between the two must be voided. With foods, the differences or extremes of stronger personality foods are voided or balanced with weaker personality foods. And vice versa.

Second That Emotion

This same process of expansion and constriction (opposition) occurs on an emotional level. Psychology and physiology are two sides of one coin.

For example, when experiencing stress, it is not unusual to choose foods of a relaxing, expanding, and unwinding nature to help balance the pressure—that is, the *constriction*. Sugar, alcohol, chocolate, fruit, and other foods with expanding natures all have the capacity to unwind tension and release accumulated heat from the body.

Another common reaction is to choose more constrictive foods, in an effort to "pull yourself together," when you feel the situation is "coming apart."

Unfortunately, choosing and eating foods out of emotional reaction rarely works to your benefit. During emotional upset, you likely are experiencing confusion, frustration, fear, depression, or other negative feelings that can interfere with your common sense, intuition, and other well-balanced sensations of joy, happiness, and love.

Ever notice how emotions are usually discussed in a negative context? "I'm getting emotional about this." "She is too emotional." "Control your emotions." There's a reason for that.

"Emotion," from the Latin *emovere,* means *to move out, stir up, agitate,* any of the various complex reactions with both psychical and physical manifestations. The *e* in emotion means *out*: emotion is an *out motion* or motion *outward,* an unwinding centrifugal motion, a motion away from the point or center.

This form of motion negates things, takes them apart. The opposite force in nature is the positive force of coming together or winding into a point. All emotions have an out motion behind them, a motion that negates. Emotions negate life and take it apart. That is why so much time, money, and effort is spent on trying to resolve or cure emotional problems and put things back together.

This is not to say that one shouldn't experience emotions! (That would be unrealistic, wouldn't it?) While emotion is a negating force, this doesn't mean emotions are negative in the sense of being bad to have. It's simply that emotions express the "getting away from the point" half of a natural cycle.

We do need to be clear on the fact that emotions negate the inspiration of life, which is expressed, for example, as *love*. Love is not an emotional experience. Love is inspirational, beyond emotions. It is a *lack or loss of love* that is an emotional experience. Joy, happiness, enthusiasm, love, and compassion are *not* emotions—they are naturally occurring nonemotional states that are experienced when one is *inspired* with life.

Unlike anger, fear, and other emotions, the natural states of love, joy, and happiness do not need an excuse or reason to be. The charge or inspiration in our lives is discharged and negated through emotions.

Emotions, however, are dependent on excuses. I am angry *because* . . . I am depressed *because* . . . I am scared *because* . . .

Naturally, then, when people choose foods through emotional reactions, they usually choose foods that *negate life,* junk foods, or foods that are particularly negating for them—that is, foods that do not support their own individual health, balance, and peace of mind. A person suffering from depression might choose to eat a quart of ice cream, while the person suffering from resentment and hatred might choose processed foods high in trans fats: pizza, burgers, fried chicken, and other items from fast-food chains.

Can you think of a time when you were feeling emotionally unstable but also hungry, so you prepared yourself a healthy, balanced meal? I don't think so. It doesn't happen that way, even though that would be the beneficial thing to do. Unfortunately, that is not how we feed our emotions.

When you grab a food out of your emotional state, you are *seconding that emotion*—you're using foods to re-create and perpetuate that emotional imbalance and record it physically into your body. When it repeats over and over, like a broken record, it can lead to the pattern known as *addiction*.

Choosing Addiction

The word "addiction" derives from the Latin *adducere,* meaning *to lead toward.* When you are addicted, whether it is to a food or a type of situation (or for that matter, to another person or type of relationship), it means you are led toward that food, situation, person, or relationship. Compulsively led. *Reactively* led.

So, if you are being led—who or what does the leading?

You do.

There are no addictive foods—only addictive behavior patterns.

Yes, you may be entrained by a situation or a food. But don't forget the dynamics of entrainment:

The lesser is to the greater as the greater is to the whole.

In an addictive pattern, you may have allowed yourself to play the role of lesser. But you wrote the script—and you are still writing it. And the role of "greater system" is still available for recasting.

Much of this reactive choice comes from the simple fact that emotional experiences are draining and exhausting (negating). Usually, the reaction is intended—whether consciously or unconsciously—to replenish, recharge, and emotionally satisfy oneself with a favorite food. But reactive food choices not only support the present emotion, they also prepare the psyche for more reactions that will continue to negate your life. The next time you experience an upsetting emotional problem, try eating small quantities of wholesome healthy foods, breathe deeply, get physically active, and watch what happens to your emotional state.

If you find yourself regularly choosing extreme foods through reaction, you are out of control with food. When you are out of control with food, you will not be satisfied, nor will you be nourishing yourself. Eating a quart of ice cream when you are depressed will not nourish you, inspire you, or improve your depression. It *will* feed and increase your depression.

The essence of proactive choosing is simply to really choose your food. Don't let it choose you—or control you—and do not underestimate the power of food, because if you let it, it *will* entrain and control you.

11
Choosing from the Bigger Picture

All the criteria for choosing we've looked at so far are very personal: they have to do with you and specific areas of your life. Yet there is another dimension of choosing that has to do with the bigger picture of life on earth.

The earth is our ultimate nourishing organism and we all are plugged into this common source. For some of us this is a more direct and conscious connection, while for others it is less apparent, depending on our individual lifestyle and perspective.

Your universal environment is the same as mine and everyone else's. Your bloodstream has its counterpart in the earth's oceans. Your lymph stream corresponds to the fresh waters of the earth. These, along with many other correspondences and resonance, are part of the basic constitution of the human species and all other organisms.

In fact, everything we've been talking about so far having to do with recovering our direct experience of foods and our sense of *quality* of life has its logical culmination in our living a life of proactive choosing as integrated parts of the total earth environment.

In these turbulent times, many people have unplugged themselves from this planetary circuit, whether consciously or not. For that matter, we have become unplugged from each other as well. There are many reasons for this growing alienation and distancing, including our modern lifestyle. But the root of that disconnection lies in our severance from real unprocessed food, through all our habitual, reactive, and other nonessential methods of choosing.

The larger goal of food energetics is to reunite with our true source by consciously and proactively choosing our foods and living their effects.

Environmental Impact

The idea of your personal diet having a significant environmental impact has gained a more widespread airing, and this is on the whole a wonderfully positive trend. It certainly will affect our chances of surviving intact well into the future, and it has numerous fringe benefits as well.

But most importantly, the budding food-ecology idea is helping us become more receptive to discovering *quality* in our own lives, in our food, and in our planetary surroundings.

However, many people have missed some critical points in the whole issue of choosing food from the bigger picture.

The idea of "environmentally sound food choices" really has two aspects: your impact on the environment, and your environment's impact on you. The first is what's talked about these days. The second is what we've been looking at all along here.

The ecology movement, while it is championing some important issues, tends to suffer from the same susceptibility to dogma and one-sidedness as does the natural foods community. For example, many of us have become aware that the production of fast-food burgers destroys acres of tropical rain forest; that you could float a destroyer in the amount of water it takes to raise one steer; that it takes twenty times the acreage of land to feed someone on factory-farmed beef as it does on grain; and so forth. Consequently, the idea of eating ecologically is often equated with vegetarianism, and eating meat is often dismissed categorically as "bad for the environment."

These points of view are dangerous oversimplifications, because they do not take into account the all-important distinction of *quality*.

It's quite true: support your local fast-food burger joint, and you support the genocide of tropical critters, plants, trees, Amazonian natives, and a fair-sized chunk of the planet's atmospheric balance.

However, you can eat meat *and* be a paragon of planetary stewardship at the same time. Not *despite* the fact that you eat meat—but *because* of it. If you take the trouble to find a source of meat that raises its animals in a conscious, highly ecological manner, pasture-raised or grass-fed on land not suitable for raising crops—as has been the norm in traditional farming communities for thousands of years—then your food choice will actually contribute to conscious partnership with Gaia rather than the blind plundering of fast-food burger chainsaws. Besides, the farming of soybeans (considered natural health foods by many) is one of the biggest contributors to rainforest destruction in the twenty-first century.

It's not so much what specific *species* of foods you choose that helps or harms the ecology; it is the *quality* of those foods.

Now even if you eat the very highest, most consciously produced quality of beef, it still is true that it would be ecologically ruinous for everyone on the planet to eat the amount of beef that average Americans eat. And that's just the point. If you choose to include the highest quality naturally raised beef in your diet—and you learn to *know* the qualities of your foods overall—you're not going to consume huge amounts of meat for breakfast, lunch, and dinner.

Just as there are quality foods, there are quality eating patterns; one leads naturally to the other.

Backyard Investment

We all eat higher or lower from the same planetary food chain; but we each choose a different spectrum from within that total environment. Choosing from the bigger picture also brings up the issue of regional quality.

In addition to each individual food having its own quality, each bioregion also imparts its unique character profile to the foods that originate there. This is determined by such factors as climate, terrain and soil type, weather, agricultural history, and so forth. Every society is colored to a surprising extent by the personality of its local environment, which is recorded into its collective experience through its local cuisine.

One of the critical elements that modern technology has introduced into diet has been the capacity to eat foods gathered from great distances—not as imported luxuries, but as daily fare. The effort to restore a sense of regional integrity to the food supply is often termed *bioregionalism*.

The issue of bioregionalism has powerful political and economic dimensions as well. The infrastructure of society today is shot through with powerfully vested interests in the status quo of food. This includes a frightening dependence not only on chemicals but also on channels of distribution, on food production's economy of scale (e.g., mass farming, even including some "organic" operations), the fossil fuels industry, and so forth. Restructuring of our entire food system—which will be the ultimate, inevitable effect of a widespread appreciation of quality—has profound implications.

Today many major food corporations are investing seriously in organic. At the same time, they are investing *far more heavily* in biotechnology. I won't even begin to discuss the energetic quality of a food artificially synthesized in a laboratory, or of foods cloned from one stud gene. I'll let you use your imagination. (Don't think about it too carefully; it could well give you nightmares.)

As a society, we need to give more critical consideration to the value of regional supply as a necessary step for planetary awakening and even survival. However, it makes no sense to turn this challenge into another set of rigid rules.

In America much of what is currently eaten in the way of organic vegetables comes from California, involving phenomenal expenditures (in both money and petroleum) to transport them east several thousand miles. In one sense, this is highly unecological; yet in another, it does support the fledgling organic industry, which in turn lends support to the value of bioregionalism. Eating locally or regionally, like every other aspect of choosing, is only one factor of many to consider.

You Are as Big as Your Environment

On the personal level, bioregionalism also need not become a straight-jacket. You are free to embrace a geographically wider or narrower bioregion in your choosing and eating. Again, no one pattern or parameter is preferable, in an absolute sense. You are free to choose a more cautiously limited environmental larder, or a more adventurously large one. How big an environment can you or do you want to manage within your body and character?

The possibilities of eating according to your environment are limitless. Any limitations you set are based on your individual ability to interact and create balance with your environment.

All the foods you need are available to you to create a working definition of your environment.

You are as big as the environment you define for yourself.

12
Big Picture or Big Brother?

Between our external environment and our internal physical environment lies our social environment—and this is where you'll find some of the most persuasive "extraneous" influences on people's food choices. There are both essential and extraneous sides to this coin, but on the whole, these external influences tend to serve as distractions from developing your own, personal ability to *know* and choose your own foods.

"Relax . . . We'll Tell You What to Eat!"

The advertising of foods through television, radio, magazines, and newspapers has a powerful, even *hypnotic* impact on how you choose your foods. Catchy slogans and persuasive images that promote food products in the media utilize the skills of highly trained people who understand how to appeal to our sentiments through music, color, sex, and virtually any other means to get the message across.

"Milk is a Natural," "Milk—New York's health kick," "Real food for real people," "Coke is it," and "It's the real thing" are just a few of the buy-our-food mottos that have wormed their way into the American consciousness. The addition of celebrities to advertising campaigns has influenced an entire generation of young people who now choose one sugared, caffeinated soft drink over another.

It *does work*—and this is not a criticism of the advertising industry.

Quite the contrary, much of their work is entertaining and impressive. But wouldn't it be great to see a celebrity promote something healthy for a change? To date, unfortunately, the best we've seen is wholesome-looking singers promoting "health foods" such as refined, nutritionally flaccid breakfast cereals.

When more people begin to perceive their daily food as something more than a convenience, when food is more clearly understood as a vital link in the entire human experience, then media will no doubt reflect that change of heart and mind.

Until then, advertising and the public promotion of food is simply a business helping to make choices for those who are not making their own. They are just doing their job. Your job is to determine how much you make this business your business.

What is truly fascinating about food advertising is that the most effective advertising works simply by creating the illusion of your having a personal conversation with someone you know. The only way advertising works is if the illusion is stronger than the reality. The tremendous sway food advertising has on people today is so powerful only because most people have no fundamental conversations about food on their own.

Suppose your husband comes home from work, takes one short, understanding look at how tired you are, and says (or your TV says): "Hey, honey, you deserve a break today. . . . Let's go out to McNulty's for burgers." What happens if this is your response: "Yes, but do I deserve hypertension and an acid stomach?" Suddenly, the television isn't quite so powerful.

Ghosts of the Past

Many of us choose our food according to an inherited, cultural, or religious background, which may include dietary laws based on religious beliefs. This way of choosing may be based on mere learned habit or on a conscious sense of pride or respect for one's cultural background, perhaps viewed as "getting back to my roots." However, in the practical reality of the current global community, unless you are living in a traditional environment close to nature, choosing food according to a dietary or religious tradition is an influence with virtually the same value as TV advertising.

For one thing, choice by tradition rarely offers the opportunity to exercise *your own judgment* in discovering what is best for your personal situation. For another, the circumstances under which these laws and codes originally existed are seldom found today. The guiding principles of the great food traditions are gradually being resurrected in a modern, transcultural renaissance of general dietary wisdom. But the geographic and genetic particulars of specific traditions are—*history*!

For example, the principle of bioregionalism, which implies that both our agricultural economy and our human physiology work best when following the dictates of our own region, is a modern restatement of a dietary rule of thumb that was second nature to historical traditions. The dietary laws of past generations originally were based on the availability of food, the character of a people's particular environment and trade with other cultures. It makes no sense to transplant an ecologically sound dietary tradition from the ancient Mideast to modern Manhattan without modifications.

What's more, one has to wonder: did these dietary laws *really* work? Were these people happy, healthy, and free—or were they suppressed by dictators and religious fanatics? And if the dietary laws *did* work, do they *still* work, and can they meet an individual's personal needs in the society he chooses to live today? People who choose their food through traditional methods of the last thousand years or so need to take a hard look at these questions.

That Was Then—This Is Now

"Tradition" derives from the Latin *traditio*: "a surrender; a statement, opinion, or belief handed down orally from one generation to another." What works is what works in your present situation, and if you are not in a traditional situation—which few people in the twenty-first century truly are—then it is important to physically, mentally, and spiritually move beyond tradition.

There is an exception to this statement: the most important aspect of traditions, and the one to retain with your own diet, is where you find universal consistency in principle. We'll discuss this idea later on in some detail.

What is *your* opinion, *your* statement, and *your* belief? How important is another person's opinion from the past? Will you not allow yourself the liberty and freedom to choose your food by exercising *your own judgment,* free of dogma?

Selecting foods according to food traditions is often simply an example of learned choosing, one by association with familiarity.

A man of Italian heritage prefers to eat Italian food, a learned choice from birth. He meets and weds a lady of Irish descent who, let's say, has had Italian food only on occasion. However, she does enjoy potatoes. (Another learned choice, by the way, since potatoes are not originally a traditional Irish food, but a fairly recent addition to Irish cuisine.)

Together, their food is comprised of both Italian and Irish traditions with a few additional foods that their traditions have accepted as a result of familiarity. The newlyweds not only exchange vows, they also exchange in-laws and family recipes. The two cultures of food are joined. A child is born, and she is nourished by food from both of her parents' traditions.

As she grows up, she begins to learn about the food from the school cafeteria (if you want to call it food), which is different from what she eats at home. Hamburgers, hot dogs, and other new and exciting pseudofoods are introduced into her choosing and are learned, consumed, and recorded into her nervous system.

She finally reaches the age where she decides to get married. (How she was able to reach this age never ceases to amaze me, what with the food from the school cafeteria and the educational system and all) and marries a man of Jewish descent. A whole new world of food is introduced to her. Kosher food (another learned choice—and man, has this one been through some changes since the days of the ancient Hebrews) . . . cream cheese, bagels, lox made from farmed salmon and preservatives, none of which have anything to do with any true tradition. The pattern continues in their offspring, and theirs, and theirs, and theirs, until the original principles of tradition are all but lost. Not only are they lost, people begin to believe that all their new "foods" are actually part of their tradition and heritage.

Putting Tradition in Perspective

With each generation remnants of dietary traditions are salvaged along the way, but for the most part, all the traditions have been replaced by total dietary confusion. Over the past few generations, many new foods, some natural but most artificial, have been introduced and accepted, yielding a new dietary "tradition" and along with it, a new species of human life.

It is often said that if food is blessed by a rabbi, priest, guru, or some other self-proclaimed or otherwise chosen master then that food can do no harm. Another way of saying this is, "If you pray and are grateful for your food, then anything you eat is okay."

The truth is, anything that is wholesome and healthy to eat is *already* blessed by God through nature. Do you really need an intermediary or middleman to confirm that? And blessing or prayer are *qualitative* factors that affect the *quantity* (the food itself)—but they do not necessarily delete all of the *other* qualities, no matter how much anyone would like to think or believe they can.

There are many religious people who pray before eating or eat blessed food who also suffer from serious health problems and rationalize their problems as being of the body, and therefore not important in the greater spiritual view. How sad. What a dualistic view of life! The body is not separate from the spirit; it is an *expression* and *celebration* of spirit!

Prayer and blessing of food, while often helpful, are neither the only factors nor the ultimate pathway to ensure health, whether you term it "physical" or "spiritual" health. In reality, there is no such thing as "physical" or "spiritual" health: both are simply quantitative ways of viewing the ever-changing *quality* of health.

When it is *you* that chooses your life, then you will also choose your food. When you're not, you are *choosing under the influence.*

13
More "Choosing under the Influence"
Concepts, Advice, and Dietary Trends

Today, more than ever before in history, people eat with their brains—especially that part of the brain that remembers and follows what one has been told to do or not do.

Food pyramids . . . macrobiotics . . . acid/alkaline . . . raw foods . . . low carb . . . vegan . . . vegetarian . . . paleo . . . instincto . . . fruitarian . . . Bible diet . . .

All of these are more or less elaborate concept structures that we ultimately end up reducing to the granddaddy of choice concepts: *good and bad.*

While there is always at least a germ of truth to a concept system, and often a large amount of value, the bottom line is that despite the best intentions, choosing foods according to conceptual systems often does not consider your individual needs as a whole person. Leaving little room to exercise common sense and intuition with foods not suggested in their guidelines can make such programs extremely difficult to maintain with any consistency, and in many cases downright dangerous.

Standard dietary guidelines, such as the government's RDA and mainstream nutrition's pyramid of "basic food groups," are created by people who appear to have little concern for the quality of food but plenty of concern for quantity. All their suggestions are based on their supporters: the dairy industry, meat industry, agribusiness, and chemical companies. Having these people around your food is hazardous to your health. The proof of the pudding is in the eating: with all the advances made in nutritional and medical research, the mainstream approach to food and health has left a legacy of increased incidence of cancer, increased medical care, obesity, and rampant malnourishment.

For the past 150 years, this approach to food has culminated in the foundation of the biggest fad diet of them all, the standard American diet. And you *know* this one doesn't work! Not only does it not work— it is getting progressively worse, with newly improved (and *approved*) artificial foods, such as synthetic fats, synthetic sweeteners, synthetic fibers, soy products made from the residue and waste of manufacturing, etc. These blatant examples of food madness have created so much confusion, it is no wonder we have so many reaction diets.

Much of the reasoning behind the natural foods and progressive nutrition approaches, while embracing an awareness of the complexity of nature and of the importance of better quality foods, is also severely limited by its fascination and indoctrination with quantitative nutritional analysis.

A Brief History of Dissection

The history of modern nutritional analysis is a relatively brief one—and it is the story of a field of study with two distinct threads or influences. On the one hand, it has been characterized by a genuine scientific investigation into nutritional components, their behavior and function, and relative value in human health. On the other, it has also been driven by the agendas of large corporations who through the power of funding have bought their own scientists to back their claims for their latest artificialized food fads. This schizophrenic nature has made modern nutrition almost a scientific Jekyll and Hyde, "pure" science contrasting and conflicting with "commercial" science. In the battle between the two natures, truth has too often been a casualty.

Food has been viewed from a strictly left-brain point of view only since the 1800s. From the 1800s through the 1950s modern science began to explore and exploit the basic components of food, including such breakthrough discoveries as these:

- Discovery of the elemental composition of foods (carbon, hydrogen, nitrogen, and oxygen) and how to measure them
- Discovery of the basic chemical makeup of carbohydrates (sugars), proteins (amino acids), and fats (fatty acids)
- Discovery of vitamins, including fat-soluble vitamins A and D
- Mass production of vitamin-enhanced foods and the beginning of the large refined-food and processed-food corporations

From the 1950s to the present, progress continued in the following areas of food science:

- Continued detailed analysis of micronutrients and macronutrients and their effects
- Increased processing and refining of whole foods, with the addition of preservatives and synthetic vitamins
- The rapid increase of artificial foods designed to increase corporate profits, while at the same time decreasing the quantities of traditional natural foods

During this period of nutritional "progress," malnutrition and obesity have increased, along with the incidence of degenerative diseases, in part due to this new way of understanding and presenting food.

Nutritional science continues to progress today, with new discoveries that go beyond the world of vitamins and macronutrition in the exploration of the great diversity of micronutrients, such as the study of phytonutrients and antioxidants.

Phytonutrients, also known as *phytochemicals,* are components that give plants their particular smell, taste, color, and immune properties. Many are used by the body to assist in making hormones and neurotransmitters. Some common phytonutrients include phenols, polyphenols, tocopherols, tocotrienols, and flavonoids.

Antioxidants are free-radical scavengers that help protect the body from cellular damage and contribute to the prevention of disease. Some antioxidants include vitamins E and C and the carotenoids betacarotene, leutin, and lycopene. There are more than six hundred antioxidants naturally produced by plants, but most in current usage are synthetically produced for inclusion in the formulation of multivitamin and antioxidant supplements.

There is no doubt that these and other nutritional discoveries have been extremely important in educating ourselves about the composition of food. But the one-sided perspective of nutritional research has culminated in a direction that *is* cause for concern: the foolish attempt to improve on nature.

Genetically modified organisms (GMOs) have been shown to destroy biodiversity and create sterile land by eliminating vital microorganisms and soil nutrients. This leads to the destruction of natural genetic information vital to a food's integrity. And this doesn't stop with the contamination of maize and indigenous cereal crops. We now have herbicide-resistant soybeans, corn, and a host of other highly questionable pseudofoods, such as fruits and vegetables laced with animal DNA. . . . The list goes on.

This is an absolutely insane direction. It is essential that we rediscover the energetic approach to food so that we grasp what it is we are doing to our food supply.

The Misleading Power of Analysis

Modern nutrition determines the healthiness of a food by isolating its vitamins, proteins, minerals, fats, and other constituents. Choosing your foods based on the results of nutritional analysis, while it may help you become more aware of your health needs, does not help you to know food intimately. It is not the betacarotene found in squash or carrots that makes these vegetables important food choices. Vitamin C is not a valid reason to eat citrus fruits, nor should lycopene be the reason for eating tomatoes.

Can you imagine eating a food solely because it contains some single element that's "good for you"? Well, many people do. People eat skinless chicken breast because it is lower in fat than beef, oranges because they contain vitamin C, salad because it has vitamins or enzymes, and—most absurd of all—bran because it is a source of fiber!

Eat bran? What about the rest of the grain? First we are encouraged by experts to eat grain that has had the fiber removed and discarded, then the same nutritional science suggests we eat the discarded bran separately, and after years of consuming refined and processed grain we end up back where we started, with the current suggestion to consume grains in their whole form. And then, to top it all off, a new nutritional fad sweeps the nation that discourages using carbohydrates, especially grains, altogether. All because of a few generations that consumed refined grain products—products that became what they are through advances in nutritional science.

For thousands of years, grains were consumed in their whole form or ground into meal. Why take a food that has a nutritional track record of sustaining traditional peoples for thousands of years, and through scientific "advancement" make inferior products that end up wreaking havoc on people's health and the environment?

A good question—and one we all need be attentive to, since this has for the most part been the legacy of nutritional analysis. Add this ingredient, take away that ingredient, lace it with preservatives . . . basically, screw with it until it has completely lost its original identity.

How about milk, because it has calcium? Is that really a good enough reason to drink milk? The positive of calcium hardly outweighs the negatives of pasteurization, homogenization, or lactose intolerance.

Nutritional concepts focus on the ingredients of a food to the point where the food itself is less important than the one or two essential ingredients it has in it. Drinking milk for the calcium and orange juice for the vitamin C is missing the whole point of what a food is really about. This way of looking at foods does little to help us understand how to nourish ourselves. The concept is backward and limited to a kind of linear thinking that completely disregards essential *qualitative* factors.

To *know* food, you must perceive the food as a whole, before even considering its parts.

Choosing Professional Advice

More and more people today are opting to choose their food through the advice or recommendations of a dietary or health counselor. Western culture teaches us to depend on professional advice when coping with problems of any kind—physical, psychological, or spiritual. We have asked for and been given guidelines for living based on tradition, morals, economy, spirituality, and numerous other value concepts that are supposed to improve our lives and make the world a better place.

Some of our cultural maps for living are practical; others are outlandish, especially those that have to do with how we should eat and maintain our health. Our past dietary guidelines have been so ridiculous and unworkable that we have produced a desperate need for professionals and experts in the field of nutritional and health counseling—"qualified" people with enough experience to guide and reeducate the confused masses on how to eat.

Some health counselors have degrees and are medically or nutritionally qualified to do what they do. Other counselors have no degrees, but are qualified through years of experience and their knowledge of food. Some counselors are very strict with their advice while others can be very loose; some offer simple and practical advice, others complex and thought-provoking advice, and others outrageous and completely off-the-wall advice.

A counselor who has studied conventional nutrition at a university may have received a document certifying one's diligent work in memorizing the many intricate details of vitamins, amino acids, and other food constituents. However, this information and experience, while it may warrant degrees or signify a status of Certified Nutritionist, has little to do with the qualities of food—only the quantities. Furthermore, this person's advice may not contribute to creative experimentation and responsibility on the part of the client.

On the other hand, the counselor who holds no degrees and is not recognized by an institution or medical doctor could have a wealth of experience in the energetic nature of foods from having lived with an indigenous tribe in the Amazon rain forest, yet little experience when it comes to technical nutrition.

Both forms of advice can be and often are helpful, but it is the client's responsibility not to become dependent on the counselor and his or her suggestions.

When you go to a counselor, all you are doing is choosing his or her *advice*. After you go home, *you* still need to choose your food!

Fear and Health

Perhaps the most common reason people seek the experience of dietary counselors is the hope that the advice will heal a health problem. Dietary counselors often work from the belief that health problems, from mildly irritating symptoms to severe degenerative diseases, are caused partially (or even largely) by certain foods or food groups, and that dietary change can help the body heal itself.

No doubt about it—a healthy diet can help adjust the human body into a healing mode by enhancing immune functions. And certain foods can resonate with or energetically affect a particular organ in the body. But it is a specious oversimplification to assume that it is solely the food that is actually doing the healing. And "resonating with or energetically affecting" does not necessarily mean *healing*.

At this extreme, the theory of healing an illness with certain foods is not unlike the "magic bullet" theory of modern medicine. If I had a quarter for every time a client has asked me what specific food "is good for" a particular symptom, I could buy Manhattan and move it to Maine for a vacation home.

Drugs themselves, as I hinted at in part 1, are hyperspecialized, synthetic descendants of herbal remedies, which are themselves extensions of the healing lore of ancient food energetics. And just as drugs have their desired effects (eradicating or changing symptoms) and their undesired side effects, the same can be true for some specific "healing foods" and their effects, when consumed in excess.

A dietary counselor might say, "Brown rice heals the intestines; you should eat brown rice every day to heal your constipation, diarrhea, or enteritis." Theoretically, according to traditional Chinese medicine, rice resonates with or affects the large intestine. And besides, it's got bran.

But what if your intestines refuse to be nourished by brown rice because of your past eating habits? If your system is accustomed to large amounts of trans fats and processed animal foods, and has gotten its carbohydrate mostly from Twinkies and Wonder Bread, the *resonating* that brown rice does may turn out to mean that your large intestine is precisely where it creates lots of gas. For that matter, what if you just cannot stomach brown rice? So much for theories and concepts.

The healing power of any food is enhanced when it is placed in a context where it can work synergistically with other supporting foods. All foods are dependent on other foods for nutritional support; therefore, healing begins with balanced overall nutrition, not with one food for a specific problem.

Another common misconception among health practitioners is the promotion of a particular food or herb based on the idea that it "stimulates the immune system." Stimulating the immune system is very different from *supporting* the immune system or *enhancing* immune function. Almost every toxic substance *stimulates* the immune system—but none *support* it. There are many scientific studies that have shown certain foods or supplements stimulate the immune system—but that doesn't mean that particular product is "good for you" or that it *supports* your immune system.

To be healed, you must first have the desire and will to heal yourself. To create a foundation for healing to take place, you also need to nourish yourself with foods that work for you through your own capacity of absorption and assimilation.

And what is "healing," anyway? It is not something separate or distinct from *normal living*. Everything in this world is in a constant state of change. In terms of health, this means that you are always moving forward or backward in some way—and often doing both at the same time on different levels. If you are living your life proactively, choosing and eating your foods with purpose, adventure, and constant new discovery, you are living.

Doing something that is truly "healing" simply means that you're *moving forward*. That's what choosing your food wisely is all about.

A physically, mentally, and spiritually nourished individual *is* healing!

Choosing Dietary Trends

Dietary trends have been around for years. Each new nutritional discovery becomes the catalyst for a new trend: iron, calcium, bran, phytonutrients, antioxidants, enzymes, vitamin C . . . each term represents a mini era in food fad lore.

The Standard American Diet (S.A.D.) and modern "health care" system are the principal reasons for these modern dietary trends. With their extreme imbalances and high-tech, low-touch qualities, modern conventional diets and medicine have served as the impetus for the many, sometimes rational, sometimes irrational, usually reactive, spin-off dietary trends of today.

And certainly, there is much cause for reaction.

Today's "health care" system, which isn't a system of caring for health so much as it is a system for dispensing pharmaceuticals, is cracking under the pressure arising from the rampant overuse of surgery and drugs, not to mention the creation of designer diseases formulated through the practice of chemical warfare, along with artificial foods, genetic manipulation, and irradiated foods. The rampant and deepening disorientation festering in many of society's leading scientists, politicians, and members of our health care system can only further intensify the natural reaction of a "call to arms"—or more accurately, a *call to farms*—by responsible individuals who wish to reclaim their freedom from this social madness.

If enough people had the desire to eat in a more natural, qualitative, and balanced way—and put the effort into doing so—it would have a powerful impact on society. In fact, it could literally redirect the course of destiny for the planet. Now *that* is revolutionary.

But are these nutrition-inspired dietary trends an avenue for effecting such a change? How effective *are* dietary trends at influencing positive change?

Unfortunately many of them, while they may represent an improvement over the S.A.D., suffer from much of the same quantitative shortsightedness as their mainstream nemesis. These "alternative" diets often rationalize their position with promises of guaranteed weight loss, cures or recovery from minor and major health problems, antiaging, or increased spiritual awareness.

How valid are these claims? Are their rationalizations for following a particular diet sensible or even realistic?

Let's observe some of the pros and cons of a few of the more popular and most commonly followed dietary trends.

The Vegetarian Idea

The vegetarian approach has been around for a long time; vegetarian organizations and publications produce impressive lists of famous vegetarian people through history. However, it is within the past several decades that vegetarianism has gained a widespread following. Historically, this newfound popularity of avoiding meat follows the post–WWII era, with growing awareness of the conditions under which animals were being factory-farmed and subsequent reactions to excessive consumption of these animals among various subcultures.

Interestingly, energetics reveal that this is as much a *physiological* response as it is a historical and social one.

To say that vegetarianism, as a lifelong way of eating, is superior to a diet including animal flesh dangerously misses a critical point: people vary widely in their basic psychophysical constitutions. Most people simply are not well suited to a diet completely devoid of animal protein (or even one including dairy or eggs, which some forms of vegetarianism allow).

This is not to say that vegetarianism is without significant value. But a strong *undercurrent of reaction* does contribute to the driving momentum for vegetarianism.

Vegetarianism has emerged as a key lifestyle response to the prevailing global environmental crisis. However, as I pointed out in chapter 11, this is an overly broad generalization. There is nothing inherently "bad" about including a variety of animal foods in one's diet—neither physiologically nor environmentally. The importance and "rightness" of vegetarianism is to some extent colored by our individual place on the pendulum of dietary change.

Vegetarian Diets

The lacto-vegetarian diet includes a variety of raw and cooked vegetables, grains, fruits, seeds, nuts, dairy products, soy products, and, in the case of lacto-ovo-vegetarianism, eggs. Though dairy products are of animal origin, they are often rationalized as being supportive supplemental nutrition (i.e., calcium and protein) in an otherwise plant-based diet—and besides, you don't have to kill animals to get them.

A vegetarian diet can theoretically be nutritionally satisfying if practiced with a wide variety of whole foods. In practice, though, many vegetarians follow a diet based on industrially produced fast foods that actually contains far fewer vegetables than the vegetarian diets of the sixties and seventies. Unfortunately, this modern version is inferior to the earlier forms of the diet, where advocates regularly consumed more carefully thought out, balanced meals of whole foods.

The lactovegetarian diet has a long history in India, where many believe the diet supports nonviolence and spiritual development and is the ultimate diet for those seeking the path to enlightenment. Part of this philosophical leaning is due to the traditional sanctity of the cow in India (its flesh is forbidden food by some widespread religious sects).

This may be partly a spiritual issue, but anthropologist Marvin Harris points out, it is also a practical lifestyle choice. In densely populated India, the cow is far too important for its role in agriculture to allow it to be used as a food. India's population relies on cattle for heavy labor in the fields. To consume them would put an impractical burden of labor onto its people, causing further stress on the already heavily stressed population.

Let's consider some pros and cons of the vegetarian diet.

Positive Qualities

The diet introduces people to a variety of whole foods and seasonings (herbs and spices) and appetizing and inventive ways to prepare them. Recipes incorporating a wide variety of plant foods from around the world help expose people to new preparation methods and tastes.

Negative Qualities

Health problems that arise among vegetarians tend to focus around allergies, *Candida* (a systemic yeast infection), and lymphatic problems. These problems can be due to an excessive consumption of dairy products and carbohydrates; or they can arise from the modern version of vegetarianism, where the original food sources of protein and fat (dairy and eggs) have to some extent been replaced by large quantities of less healthy soy products, plant oils (soy, canola, and safflower), and margarine. Strong cravings for sweets often lead to excessive consumption of sweetened flour products (cookies, cakes, pastries), dairy and soy-based ice creams and sugar, acceptable foods in many vegetarian diets that also contribute to health problems for vegetarians.

The Vegan Diet

The vegan diet is essentially the same as the vegetarian diet, only without any dairy products and eggs; some vegans also consume only raw foods. Followers of the vegan diet are generally strong supporters of animal rights. They believe animals are sentient creatures and thus not meant to be eaten by humans, and that humans also should not take the milk of another animal, as that milk is designed for that animal's offspring.

For many vegans, the ideology of veganism can take precedence over the quality of food they consume. This is evidenced in the large quantities of packaged foods and soy-based products, along with stimulants in the form of lattes, coffee, and chocolate, that often make up a large portion of vegan diets. Naturally there are exceptions, and some vegans do attempt to consume meals of more consciously prepared foods; but many lean toward the convenience of processed and packaged foods as their main sources of nutrition.

Positive Qualities
Introduces one to whole natural foods and how to prepare them.

Negative Qualities
Vegans, especially children, often suffer from nutritional deficiencies, including vitamin B_{12} deficiency, hormone problems (especially thyroid), tooth decay, hair loss, loss of bone density, chronic yeast infections, fatigue, loss of muscle tone, digestive distress, weight gain, emotional instability, and compulsive eating habits due to lack of nutritional satisfaction. A lack of traditional whole foods very often leads to dependency on stimulants (coffee, tea, etc.) and an excessive consumption of sugar and chocolate for energy support. Quality foods are often replaced by "natural" processed soy foods and other poor-quality protein substitutes.

Vegans can be extremely defensive, often to the point of being hostile toward those who question or expose the often faulty logic surrounding some of the sacred principles of the vegan diet and philosophy.

Raw Foods Diet (Plant-Based)

This particular vegetarian approach to food includes a diet composed solely of uncooked foods, particularly vegetables, fruits, seeds, nuts, and sprouts. Animal products of all types are avoided, as are cooked plant foods. Proponents of this diet use the following reasons, among others, to rationalize their belief in raw foods:

- Raw foods are superior to cooked because they are *alive*; cooking kills.

- Animals should not be used for food because taking the life of an animal is inhumane.
- Animal foods inhibit one's spiritual development; vegetables and fruits do not.
- Raw plant foods are the foods of our ancestors and thus the ideal foods for us.

A raw foods diet can be an efficacious approach for cleansing the body of accumulated wastes resulting from the overconsumption of processed animal products and excess dairy products. However, there is no historical evidence that human beings ever existed or thrived on a raw foods diet, especially a plant-based raw food diet.

As with any conceptual system, there are holes in the concepts. For example, cooking does not "kill" foods—at least, no more than eating them does. And that statement is not flip: cooking actually is an *extension* of the eating and digesting process. While cooking may destroy some enzymes, enzymes are not the only substance in a food that is important for health maintenance. In fact, traditional cultures derived ample amounts of enzymes from both raw and fermented food used in combination with cooked foods.

Toxic components often found in some raw foods are neutralized through cooking. Cooking is also known to enhance bioavailability of some nutrients, especially phytonutrients. Cooking food can make many foods easier to digest by breaking down cellulose fibers and altering or changing the cellular and nutritional components of many plant foods, making them more suitable to the internal human environment. The manipulation of food molecules and nutrients through cooking (real cooking, that is, and not factory processing) is more of a process of transformation than one of destruction.

Raw foods certainly have a place in the human diet—but all food gets "cooked" one way or another. If it is not cooked externally through conventional cooking methods, it must be done internally through vigorous digestion.

Ingested food is digested and metabolized at relatively high temperatures in the heated environment of your digestive tract until it is ready to be used as nutrition. The ability to digest (cook internally) largely depends on the vitality of your digestive system and your degree of physical activity. The majority of animals that exist on a raw food diet have these abilities. They chew their plant food for long durations, eat continuously, and are active. They also have radically different digestive systems from ours (even apes and monkeys, considered by many raw food enthusiasts to be our ancestral links, and both of which regularly consume small animals and insects).

Cooking some percentage of your food simply reduces much of the work and effort required by the digestive system, and thus results in improved digestion and metabolism overall.

A raw-food vegan diet has a cooling effect on the body and can temporarily be balancing for overheated conditions or for those with an extensive history of heavy animal food consumption. However, in such cases, after one has cleansed much of the accumulated excess from one's body, one may tend to become oversensitive to cold weather, often to the point of becoming very thin and less adaptable to environmental changes.

As far as the killing of animals and inhibition of spiritual development is concerned, it is instructive to remember that even within many spiritual traditions, animals have long been used for food. In cultures with an awareness of the *quality* of life—including both nomadic and settled, traditional peoples—taking the life of an animal was done with respect and gratitude for the animal and the environment.

On the other hand, the way potatoes and lettuce are mechanically slaughtered en masse for fast-food chains and the frozen-food section makes me shudder. Now *that's* murder in the kitchen. The same goes for the way chickens, beef cattle, lambs, and other animals are "raised" and killed for modern mass-food appetites.

There are as many definitions and qualifications for spiritual lifestyles as there are people, and it is not unusual for followers of a particular dietary trend, especially those who advocate natural foods, to have their own spiritual belief system. Some Buddhist monks who live in the mountains, estranged from the busy life of urban dwellers, eat a vegetarian diet, and it works for them in their spiritual quest. Additionally, some Tibetan monks thrive in their spiritual development on a diet that includes animal products, both flesh and milk. On the other hand, a businessman living in the city with a desire to supply the masses with a needed product may choose to eat a nonvegetarian diet, yet he may experience spiritual fulfillment from his business venture by simply being of service to people.

Diet alone does not determine a person's spirituality. Some people believe that living in isolation from others is more spiritual than living and working with others. While this may work for some, it does not work for others. Both need be ready spiritually to change their position on whatever they believe, for *change* is a spiritual and dietary certainty. It is not so much a matter of belief as it is a matter of choice, and one's choice is always susceptible to change.

Another form of raw foodism is a diet comprising both raw plant foods along with high quantities of raw animal foods. Compared to the plant-based diet, however, this animal-based raw foods diet has received little attention and has fewer followers. This is partly due to the taboo placed on animal products because of their saturated fat content, an issue that finally has come full circle and turned out to be more hype than hope for the big refined vegetable oil companies. But the raw-foods animal-food diet is as unrealistic as its opposite, and far too expensive for most people to follow using quality foods.

Positive Qualities

In addition to introducing one to a wide variety of edible plant foods high in enzymes and vitamins and highly creative ways of preparing them, the raw foods diet encourages the very important practice of consuming lacto-fermented vegetables and it extols the health benefits of coconuts, including the beneficial health aspects of coconut oil, a highly saturated fat. The raw food diet generally discourages the use of processed soy foods, poor-quality oils, and other unhealthy foods so commonly prevalent in other plant-based diets.

Negative Tendencies

Raw fooders tend to suffer from many of the same nutritional deficiencies and health problems as vegans, although the causes are different.

Like vegans, they are under the delusion that children can thrive on such a diet. Another common trait among raw food groups is a lack of hygiene, and this can affect their attitudes toward food. Some believe food should be eaten raw directly from the soil, tree, or whatever source it comes from without washing it. Parasites are common among raw food advocates and many have to resort frequently to strong toxic pharmaceuticals in order to remedy the problem, only to find it returning for another round of toxic treatment.

Constipation due to reduced peristalsis or overworked intestines is common. Binge eating and eating disorders in general are also common within these groups. Most raw fooders consume high quantities of sugar in the form of fruits; other sources of sugar are also common, especially chocolate. Coffee is another indulgent substance.

Some extremist followers of these diets believe the ultimate form of raw foodism is to consume only fruit. Every food cult has extremists, but the raw food groups may have the most extreme of all of them. Like vegans, raw fooders can become highly defensive when their sacred beliefs are exposed or questioned by others with valid points of view.

The Macrobiotic Enigma

A macrobiotic *way of eating* differs from what is conventionally known as "the macrobiotic diet" or dietary regime. *Choosing and eating foods* macrobiotically means consciously choosing and managing one's diet in a way so as to create balance within oneself and between oneself and one's environment. Since a basic premise of macrobiotic eating is to nourish oneself properly and to adapt flexibly with one's environment, the possibilities can be endless.

The "macrobiotic diet," on the other hand, represents a set of specific dietary guidelines emphasizing a circumscribed variety of whole foods, some of them chosen according to season, and plant based, with the exception of fish and seafood, which can be eaten on occasion if one's health permits.

Most people who decide to incorporate the "macrobiotic diet" into their lives do so because they perceive it to be a natural means of regaining their health. However, there are also people who perceive macrobiotics to be more than simply diet alone. These people see macrobiotics as a broad-based philosophy that they believe is a viable and commonsense way to live and further develop their spiritual awareness.

There is no doubt that a diet primarily consisting of whole cereal grains, vegetables, sea algae, beans, fruits, nuts and seeds, and fish and seafood, can be instrumental in establishing a sound foundation for health. However, like other dietary trends that promise spiritual enlightenment and freedom from disease, macrobiotics tends to attract its share of fanatics and blind believers who refuse to question pertinent issues. (This is ironic, as one of the basic tenets of macrobiotics as it is generally taught is having a spirit of "noncredo.")

Though it is based on a practical approach to eating, macrobiotics is often criticized for its limitations. The macrobiotic diet is an experiential diet that, depending upon personal interpretation and one's individual ability to assimilate the food, can provide a sound foundation from which the responsible person can *begin* to discover his or her individual dietary needs.

However, when taught or interpreted as a fixed set of guidelines, with its experts, authorities, its "rights and wrongs" and "good foods and bad foods," the "macrobiotic diet" becomes just like any other conceptual choosing: *choosing under the influence.*

Moreover, because of the diet's present association with health recovery and the fear-of-illness mindset that often accompanies its practice, followers are especially prone to abdicate their own proactive choosing and to follow the rules and dictates of others whom they perceive as knowing the truth.

Unraveling the Macrobiotic Dilemma

In the sixties, when macrobiotics was first gaining a following in the West, its adherents were associated with fanaticism and zeal. There still exists today a subcurrent of fanatic zeal, and a significant number of those seeking to recover health are encouraged to cling to eating guidelines that are impractical and overly strict. Perhaps this is due to the assumption common among many followers of macrobiotics that all illnesses tend to be caused by *excess* and that people who are ill therefore need to follow strict dietary guidelines in order to discharge excess accumulations or fat, protein, and other wastes in their bodies.

While many people who suffer from serious illness *do* indeed have conditions of excess, and a strict macrobiotic diet can temporarily be beneficial, there are equally as many people who suffer from conditions of *deficiency*, and unfortunately, if these people follow strict macrobiotic guidelines, this can result in their becoming more malnourished than hale and hearty.

This is not, strictly speaking, due to anything inherent in macrobiotic principles per se. True, a strict "macrobiotic diet" tends to create a dry and cold condition due to a lack of reasonable amounts of fat and protein. But the cause of people becoming unbalanced through the "macrobiotic diet" is the same as with any other dietary trend: people choosing their food from an extremely dictated, limited set of criteria.

Those who intuitively have a sense of the qualities of food might use macrobiotic principles and adapt them to their own needs and desires and can do very well, indeed.

While macrobiotics does claim to have its philosophical basis in global dietary traditions, it tends to lose this essence and sensibility when its proponents relegate many traditionally healthy foods to the "bad" food category.

The idea of "civilized" agricultural peoples who based their diets on a variety of whole foods (both plant and animal) in remote antiquity is a well-established fact. In fact, the practice of agriculture (and especially that of growing grain) is something that historians are consistently updating from the originally held theory of 10,000 years ago as an original timeline. What is important to understand, in the context of macrobiotics, is that animal products of varying types also played an equally important role in global food traditions as plant foods. Whether this is something macrobiotic adherents have missed out of simple ignorance or is something intentionally skipped over because it doesn't fit their set of preexisting guidelines, it is a point of historical fact that strains the macrobiotic "traditional diet" claim.

Macrobiotic food is often described as bland and tasteless and rationalized as such by its proponents as a "sensitivity" issue—meaning that spices, herbs and other seasonings (except for a chosen few, such as scallions, ginger, raw radish, and a few others) are either overstimulating or simply unnecessary for good health. In other words when one has eaten "well" for some time, one's taste will become more refined and purified to the point where one will no longer need or desire such interesting, flavorful, and satisfying food preparations.

In this regard, the vegetarian diet has more to offer in its embrace of genuinely global cuisine.

When macrobiotics goes global—that is, away from its typical Japan-centric focus—proponents tend to substitute tofu for dairy, carrots for tomatoes, and wheat gluten for meat. (In other words, when it goes global, it doesn't really.) This does little to improve its reputation for bland and flavorless foods.

In fact, substitutions of traditional natural foods with less nutritious ingredients mimics the extremism of the agenda-driven science of the natural foods industry, where junk foods disguised and labeled as "natural" are created from soy products to produce soy hot dogs or soy cold cuts.

If it is true that, as macrobiotic followers commonly claim, "Man can eat anything," then the only real problem with macrobiotics lies in the interpretation and often dogmatic beliefs of its adherents.

Positive Qualities

Macrobiotics has a strong focus on traditional methods of food preparation. One of the few natural diets that stresses chewing well, regular whole meals, and fermented foods.

Philosophically, macrobiotics has its own interpretation of the principles of traditional Chinese medicine, especially yin and yang and the five elements theory. These serve as helpful educational tools for followers and offer important ways of understanding food and its relationship to health. Macrobiotic proponents also discourage the use of pharmaceuticals and other drugs unless necessary.

Negative Tendencies

There is a tendency to have a limited understanding of the role of animal products in traditional diets that leads to classifications of foods in terms of good and bad. (For example, fish is good and most all other animal products are bad.)

Another area lacking in understanding among macrobiotic adherents is that of fats and oils. Healthy tropical oils are misunderstood as being bad and saturated fats are called "cancer-causing," whereas poor-quality and nutritionally inferior vegetable oils (canola, soy, safflower, corn, etc.) are considered okay to use in moderation. All animal fats are considered bad.

This kind of weirdly limited understanding also holds true for many herbs, spices, and garlic (considered extreme yin and stimulating). This misunderstanding of herbs and seasonings in traditional diets fails to acknowledge the antiviral, antibacterial, and other beneficial qualities of these essential ingredients.

Macrobiotic practitioners have a tendency to binge eat, especially with sweets and overeating in general. Coffee and other stimulants are also common indulgences beyond moderation.

14
Five Familiar Faces

Sharon Leibowitz is forty-three, married, doesn't work outside the home, and leads an active social life. She plays tennis regularly and when she doesn't she either jogs or takes a vigorous walk.

Sharon is hip to the latest trends in diet—has been for years—and she and her friends are all into eating "lite." Sharon and her two (sometimes three) friends have lunch together daily at one of their three favorite restaurants. The restaurants differ in what they have to offer, but Sharon's and her friends' food choices are always limited to salads (chicken, tuna, or plain) and sometimes broiled or steamed fish, with no oil or butter—and no salt. Dinner is not much different: broiled chicken (without the skin) or broiled fish and more salad. When the ladies are together and want a snack, fruit is the food of preference because it's high in fiber and low in fat.

These ladies want to keep the fat off and they believe this diet will do it, for so they have been told. They are all eating right 'cause they're eating lite.

Sharon has some problems, though, most of which she can share with her friends. But one problem she cannot share, lest she expose her carefully guarded secret lifestyle.

Yes, she freely shares the fact that she feels cold—chilled to the bone, in fact, most of the time. She also tells her friends how she feels tight and tense, especially in her stomach, and suffers from severe constipation. Also, she is nervous and rather high-strung, although she is emotionally cooler when and if it comes to sex with her husband—and these things, too, she freely shares, because her three friends can all relate: they have similar experiences. "From stress," they tell each other.

What Sharon doesn't share with her friends is *what she eats when she is alone* and away from their company. God forbid they should see or know what she does! Little does she know that her friends are doing the same.

A half-pound of cheese with crackers, lots of butter spread over bagels, a half-gallon of frozen yogurt or low-fat ice cream at one sitting (one *standing*, actually), and more of the stuff she is not supposed to be eating but is compelled to indulge in to secretive excess to compensate for her extremely limited and nutritionally deficient "looking good" diet.

Sharon's mom, a generation older and a helluva lot wiser, does not quite get her daughter's lite food trip. If this "lite diet" is so great, then why is her daughter's hair so dry and brittle? Why is her skin looking papery and not vibrant? And those hips, oy veh!—all that diet and exercise, but they really haven't changed a bit! But she holds her tongue: experience has taught her, Sharon wouldn't listen anyway.

Is there a little Sharon in you?

Hank Thomson, fifty-two, a determined winner of an attorney—more concerned with money and the law than he is with justice—is an aggressive, robust fellow with a red face, quite a bit overweight, and considered a "type-A asshole" by others in the business.

Hank is married. His wife dislikes him immensely but stays with him for the money. His two kids don't think much of him, either. He is loud, domineering, and demanding—characteristics he uses (he thinks) to his advantage when dealing with his adversaries: his family, other attorneys, or naive juries.

His wife cooks his bacon and eggs every morning (she feels she has to) and she never questions him about where he eats dinner because it's not worth being yelled at. The kids have to have breakfast with him, but at least they don't see him on weekends. He spends that time with his girlfriend, and Mom doesn't even know it, or maybe she does but chooses not to see it.

Bacon and eggs for breakfast every morning with lots of coffee, hamburger or steak for lunch with a couple of scotches-on-the-rocks, and for dinner, more meat, potatoes, and more alcohol. Lots more. Hank's diet consists of high protein, fat, and some carbohydrate in the form of white toast or potatoes. Vegetables are out of the question. (And dessert? Her name is Julie.)

Hank is killing himself, but if he has his way about it, he'll take down those around him first.

Bill Tanden is sixteen, on the high school basketball team—great player too, and much appreciated and liked by all his classmates. Bill is a good-looking guy who loves the girls but doesn't have any luck with them.

It's his face. The acne. And not a little: lots and lots of it. He has lots of gas, too, but he usually hides that more successfully than the zits.

Both Bill's parents work, so his food at home consists of whatever he can grab. Bill doesn't really think in terms of "meals"; his biological clock is a combination stopwatch and alarm clock. Bill's notion of dietary planning is "getting something into my stomach"—a meal to Bill is often milk and cold meat sandwiches or pizza, hot dogs, TV dinners, and sometimes just milk and cookies.

The dermatologist says it's a common skin problem Bill will grow out of and prescribes a topical that only produces large craters on Bill's pizza face.

Poor Bill. He's fermenting, and he doesn't know what to do about it.

Jill Cameron is an attractive lady, even though she is a little thin, a little pale, and looks somewhat older than her twenty-six years.

A vegetarian for ten years, she tried the raw foods and vegan diets but couldn't stick with them, so she settled on what she believes is a healthy compromise. Jill often may be found preaching the religion of "good foods and bad foods." She spends a large amount of time trying to convince people that her diet is the diet for them—going so far as to say it will make them more spiritual, more clear, and most of all, it will make them healthier and more energetic than they ever thought possible.

Jill talks a good game; her sweet mannerisms make her all the more convincing.

Jill started her health regimen years ago because she was told she could cure her severe *Candida* (systemic yeast infection) problem with the proper diet, especially if she avoided animal flesh and substituted soy protein for animal products. Her belief in vegetarianism is so strong she is unwilling to consider any connection with her diet and her condition of low thyroid, severe digestive distress, and low energy. For energy, she hits Starbucks a few times a day for her lattes, unaware of how great a role this stimulant plays in her overall diet.

While she calls herself a vegetarian, her diet actually contains few vegetables. It consists mostly of "natural junk food"—soy products, sugar, chocolate, muffins, scones, bread, and other flour products made with free-radical-producing vegetable oils, all of which conspires to throw her into deep depression, exacerbated by feelings of profound isolation. So par for the course have these feelings become that it never occurs to Jill that they could be connected in any way to her fanaticism about diet.

In ten years, her yeast problems are still not actually cured. In fact, they are worse than ever, but she now has a prescription from her doctor for the problem.

Jill has become a prisoner of the Unreal Zone, a place where people go who are food-obsessed and diet-dependent. She is a believer and—despite what she thinks and feels—she is not alone.

Mrs. Margaret Page is sixty-four, a widow who lives alone, though her three grown children visit her regularly. Mrs. Page is a sprightly lady with a few problems. Her blood pressure is slightly elevated, and her bones are fragile. She has been told by her doctor not to worry, just to continue taking her blood pressure medicine, drink lots of milk, eat bananas because they are high in potassium, and take extra calcium. She's always been a good patient and does everything her doctor says. Nothing has changed—at least, not for the better.

Margaret eats mostly vitamin supplements, prescription drugs, chicken, sugar, and lots of dairy products ("for calcium"). What this poor, sweet lady has not been told is that all those drugs and sugar are actually contributing to her lack of calcium, and taking all the calcium supplements in the world won't do any good. While her three to four bananas daily may be high in potassium, they are also high in sugar, which is depleting her body of the vital minerals it needs to correct her problems. They also are quietly helping to make her feel cold—and increasingly, strangely depressed and fearful—at night.

It's so difficult, isn't it?

I mean, who are you supposed to believe? Everything is so confusing!

PART III

Working Models

15
Character Study

Once you begin to recognize your patterns of *extraneous* food choices, you start to pave the way for deepening and broadening your adventures with the *essence* of food. Vanquishing your acquired concepts, you're freer to develop direct *knowledge* of a full palette of foods and their energetic characters. The essence of foods can be recognized on a range of levels, from the most visceral and sensorial to those of more lofty social and environmental concerns. Now it's time to explore some specific approaches to recognizing a food's energetic essence.

The following discussions are not intended to comprise a "method" or a complete, systematic "school of thought" on food energetics. They are not set down here as pigeonholes for categorizing foods. Rather, they are *tools for observation,* meant only as a starting point to help you sharpen your direct experience of the uniqueness of each food you encounter.

Any one of these aspects of food energetics could easily be developed further to fill an entire volume. That's not my purpose. These brief observations are offered as a ladder you can use to climb up to a better vantage point. Once you've scaled the wall, you can throw away the ladder!

The various aspects of foods' character described in what follows can serve as the basis for your determination of food energetics. Collectively, they form a single picture that will clarify your *knowledge* of food energetics. No single feature, in and of itself, can give you a complete picture of any particular food. Taken together, and mixed well with liberal doses of your personal experimentation and exploration, they'll tell you many a fascinating and enlivening story—stories you can use to recreate your own life.

To begin, then, let's take a look at foods' essential character, both as unique entities each with its own *overall signature* and as characters as expressed through their *direction of motion, rhythm,* and *temperament.*

16
Food's Essential Character

The "essential character" of a food is its *essence*, original nature or constitution, what the food is born or bred to be. Before looking at that character or at any particular aspect of it, know that every food has its own signature, and that signature is *synergistic*. A food's essential character will always be more than the sum of the parts you can observe and describe, whether you are using this book alone or in combination with other systems of food observation.

All types of food, whether animal, vegetable, or mineral, have essential characters that can be described yet which also surpass description. This essence describes what a food *is*.

A duck is a duck is a duck—because of the characteristics that make it a feathered, webbed-footed creature with a bill that spends half its time on land and the other half in water and goes quack quack. No matter how it's raised or how you cook it, a duck cannot be a chicken or a cow.

This quality exists in people as well. You and I each have a constitution with which we were born. Some people are tall, others short; some have large hands or feet while others have small hands or feet. The physical shapes of our body constituents, the physiological rhythms, patterns, combinations of strengths and weaknesses, the inborn tendencies of our nervous systems, and tapestries of ancestral experience and behavior . . . these many characteristics make us who we are—an essential character that not only defines us both as humans but also defines you as "you" and me as "me."

Cereal grains have similar qualities that group them together under the title of "cereal grains," yet each one has its own individual constitutional makeup. Some grains are very small, some larger, some take an hour to cook while others may take only fifteen minutes. Moreover, each grain has its own historical background. Corn has been extensively bred by humans, while quinoa is relatively untouched. Buckwheat has a background of rough, rocky, and marginal soils in which it has learned its hard lessons of survival, while rice has been graciously penned in irrigated, weed-free environments by humans for thousands of years.

Pick up a catalog of natural, heirloom seeds and read the descriptions of the different types of cabbages, carrots, or pinto beans, and you'll begin to grasp the tremendous diversity of the plant world.

Each food is truly unique!

Poetry in Motion

The first step in grasping a food's particular character is to understand and appreciate that every food got where it is today through its own unique process. Plants sprout from a seed and grow within a particular environment; some animals are hatched from eggs while others are gestated, born, and nurtured from infancy to adulthood. Each history is unique and rich with energetic implications.

The pattern of motion that creates a food tells you a great deal about that food's character, because that food is in fact *the result of how it got there.*

Motion can be described through its two different aspects: *direction* and *speed.*

The speed of a food's origination is a fairly simple thing to describe. Mushrooms grow very quickly—sometimes even sprouting up in a matter of hours—while ferns and asparagus take slightly longer. By comparison, carrots and parsnips spiral their way down into the soil at the speed of a snail. Chickens are small, compact, and quick little creatures. Cows are large, expanded, and slow-moving creatures. Lettuces tend to grow rather quickly, compared to many other leafy vegetables. Burdock roots take a longer time to grow and mature than carrots, and they are more tightly wound, more dry and longer—that is, more deeply penetrating—than carrots.

Smaller, more compact plants and animals tend to have a faster character than larger, more expanded plants and animals. The story of the tortoise and the hare is somewhat instructive here: slow, steady growth can produce an effect of steadiness and groundedness in the individual who eats those foods. However, the harelike speed of a fast-growing plant or animal, and the agility of temperament that implies, can have a stimulating and motivating effect on the person who eats it.

As in all contrasted characteristics, various speeds all have their beneficial points as well as their drawbacks. Foods that are more rapid tend to contribute to faster reactions and to a more unwinding and releasing effect, assisting in the discharging of stored energy. Slower foods tend to contribute to a building, accumulating, storing, and charging of energy reserves in the body.

The variable of speed in foods also has its energetic impact on your own behavior, including your thought processes and expression.

What do people say about you? Are you slow and methodical, too slow sometimes, or high-strung and hyper . . . ?

It is possible to choose foods overall with a similar speed as yourself, or you can choose foods with speeds that are vastly different from your usual pace. You can even choose foods that express a huge spectrum of different velocities. No particular style is "best"—it is all a matter of personal style and desired quality. This is your life!

Patterns of Growth

Direction of growth is another way to understand the energetics of a particular food. There are multitudes of different shapes and directions foods can grow. Briefly, we can narrow these growth directions down to four basic directions from which all others originate. Any animal or plant will grow:

- downward or upward
- inward or outward

Furthermore, each gravitates or levitates to *its own specific level*. Thus, radishes and pears both grow downward, but pears seek their level hanging up on a tree branch before beginning their downward growth, while radishes start at seed level and penetrate the soil to seek subterranean territory.

One broad, sweeping way to combine all possibilities of direction is with these two images:

- motion winding to a point and coming together
- motion unwinding from a point and coming apart or dispersing

Anything can be perceived as being dominated by a combination of these four directional tendencies.

Observing Identities

Understanding a food's identity through how it grows and develops is easy when using the following figure as a model. Here we have four basic variations of energy that describe both the general energy of a food and the potential effects it might have on us.

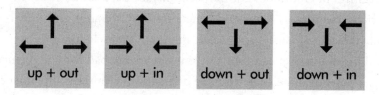

Four Directions of Growth

I will use vegetables as examples for ease of understanding and consistency as we learn how to observe a food's identity, but please understand that these principles apply to any food, whether plant or animal. I will also give examples of human temperaments that fit these four models to show how foods can influence our behavior and emotions.

Up and Out

Broad leafy greens like chards, collard greens, leafy lettuces, and bok choy are just a few of the many plants that fit this energy pattern.

These plants help to release stored energy in the upper part of the body, especially the heart and lungs. Green plants are high in chlorophyll and are known for their active practice of photosynthesis, taking in carbon dioxide and releasing oxygen. Closely observe a leafy green and you'll see a fine network of veins in the leaf, branching out gradually from a thicker base stem. This network is the plant's circulatory system, through which it distributes minerals, water, and other constituents throughout the leaf.

The leaf itself represents a plant's *circulatory and respiratory system* and has a direct correlation to our corresponding physiological systems. While leafy green plants take in carbon dioxide and give off oxygen, our lungs do the opposite, taking in oxygen and releasing carbon dioxide. Therefore, leafy green plants energetically resonate in our respiratory and circulatory systems, and tend to release stagnation in these systems in an upward and outward direction.

Other examples of foods with this *upward and outward* energy include tree fruits, cream, milk, and chocolate.

Excessive consumption of foods with this energy pattern can result in feelings of emotional and physical instability, mental disorientation with an inability to focus and concentrate, cold hands and feet, being easily influenced, timid and weak, and loss of muscle tone.

This does not mean foods of this nature are bad for you. It means that if you consume them in large quantities, without complementary foods from the other three energy patterns, it can lead to an imbalance that will tend to manifest in the ways mentioned above.

Up and In

Kale, mustard greens, dandelion greens, chives, and green onions are just a few of the many green plants that fit this energy pattern. Some of these green plants have serrated edges, while others are long, straight, and smooth. The long, smooth structure of green onions and chives, along with their spicy flavor, have a strong releasing, dispersing effect on the upper body systems, while the tightly serrated and bitter flavors of the kale and mustard greens have more of a drying and tightening effect on these systems.

Being green plants, these variations of greens with *up and in* energies still resonate in the same systems as the *up and out* green plants, but in different ways. Overall, green plants tend to lighten and enlighten the one who eats them.

For the purposes of natural healing, you can see how effective it would be to use the first group of leafy greens (*up and out*) for releasing heavy stagnation in the lungs. For example, a person with a nagging dry cough could benefit immensely by consuming the large, moist, oxygen-carrying leafy greens from the *up and out* category. On the other hand, a person with a damp cough, heavy with excess mucus, would be more likely to benefit from the dryer, more bitter-tasting and tightly serrated leaves from the category of *up and in*. Kale or mustard or dandelion greens would help to dry and purge the excess mucus.

Other examples of foods with *up and in* energies include coffee, chicken, toasted seeds (pumpkin, sesame and sunflower), and crackers. While all natural whole foods have positive qualities, excessive consumption of foods from this category can result in the following negative symptoms: increased erratic energy, hyperactivity and obsessive behavior, and uptight and inflexible attitude.

Down and Out

Turnip, rutabaga, radish, onion, ginger, potato, sweet potato, and yam are just a few of the many rounded or irregular-shaped root or underground plants that fit this energy pattern.

Not all of these foods are actual root plants; however, they all do have the same kind of energy pattern, although the intensity of the energy in each varies greatly. Potatoes, sweet potatoes (no relation), and yams are tubers. They are texturally different from root vegetables. Ginger is used more as a seasoning and has a spicy flavor, while sweet potatoes and yams have sweet flavors.

Root vegetables represent the digestive system of plants. Their purpose is to penetrate downward into the earth where they can absorb and assimilate water and the vital essences needed to grow and support the total plant. Unlike the uplifting and exposed qualities of leafy plants, roots are private plants that perform their work in secrecy, hidden beneath the earth. Roots evoke the feelings of stability, grounding, and security, all characteristics of a healthy digestive system. The energetics of root plants and those that grow underground also resonate with other organs and functions of the lower body, i.e. reproductive organs, bladder, prostate, ovaries, uterus, etc.

The *down and out* category of plants affects the lower part of the body with a relaxing and unwinding energy. For example, soft-cooked rutabaga and turnip have a slow and relaxing effect in the lower body, while raw ginger, onion, and garlic have a rapidly dispersing effect in the lower body resulting from their spicy flavor. Cooked garlic and onion have a sweet taste and therefore have a slow and relaxing effect in the lower body. Sweet potato and yam have a soothing and relaxing effect in the lower body, while potatoes, bland and lacking in flavor, need other foods to give them definition. You can easily see how each of these foods, while they all resonate in the same area of the body, has its own unique way of doing so.

Other foods with *down and out* energies include: soft ripened cheeses, soft baked products (cake, muffins), and any foods or combinations that tend to be soft and heavy.

While reasonable quantities of *down and out* energy foods are very supportive to health, excessive amounts of these foods can result in feelings of, well, down and out: sadness, depression, insecurity, and melancholia.

It is important to remember that foods love company. To better understand this simple but important point, seek out traditional combinations when eating specific foods. Don't just eat a big hunk of cheese. Add some raw vegetables or fruit, wine, capers, olives, bread, crackers, and other traditional accompaniments. You will enjoy it more and it will have added health benefits. And more importantly, these accompaniments all have their own unique energetic properties that balance and support the cheese. The same goes for most other foods.

Down and In

Carrots, parsnips, salsify, and burdock roots are just some of the many long and tapered root plants that fit this energy pattern. Unlike *down and out* root plants, *down and in* roots have a more penetrating quality. With a focused determination, these roots penetrate deep into the earth, performing the same functions as other roots but with more intensity and tenacity.

These roots tend to contain less water than round roots, so the way they affect the lower body will be different from rounded roots. Long roots tend to have a gathering and tightening effect in the lower body. Just as they ground and stabilize the plant, roots carry their energetics to our complementary systems, where they support lower body functions, each one in its own private and unique way. These types of roots are stabilizing foods that help to gather one's energy in the lower body, and give one a sense of presence and thoughtfulness.

Let's consider an example of how root vegetables can be supportive to the lower digestive tract.

A person who has been dealing with constipation for a month would like to do something right and natural to relieve this problem. A couple of options would be cooked round roots (turnips and onions) or cooked carrots and parsnips. Since the problem is constipation, does the individual need long downward and inward roots that tend to constrict and penetrate, or round soft roots that help to relax and soothe the intestines? Exactly—the question yields the answer. Cooked turnips and onions would be more beneficial for this problem. How about if we add a bit of fresh grated raw ginger (strongly dispersing down and out energy) to the turnips and onions? This would enhance the *down and out* effect by stimulating the energy.

Other *down and in* foods include eggs, hard dry cheeses, grilled meat, smoked meat, and fish. An excess of *down and in* foods can lead to the following symptoms: self-centeredness, stubbornness, repetitiveness in speech and action, physical and mental stagnation.

Again, I cannot stress enough the importance of accompaniments. For example, in order to avoid the strong *down and in* effect of eggs, it would behoove you to add some *up and out* energy, in the form of black pepper, to balance this energy. Most people try to balance eggs with salt, toast, and coffee. It simply doesn't work.

Other Plants

Then there are all the other vegetables that grow on the ground, other than roots and leaves. Each of these vegetables also has one of the four energetic patterns predominating. Cabbage, broccoli, cauliflower, celery, cucumber, squash, pumpkin, string bean . . . these represent what you could call the "social group" of vegetables.

While each has its own unique energetic qualities, this group of plants generally affect the middle of the body and all the organs that reside there. The liver, gallbladder, spleen, stomach, and pancreas are the organs that strongly influence our social lives and these plant foods are helpful in healing and maintaining those biological functions. For example, the liver has long been associated with anger and frustration, so it makes sense that foods biologically soothing and supportive to liver function could be psychologically helpful in dealing with anger issues.

There are also water plants to consider. Watercress, lotus seeds and roots, algae (both fresh and salt water), etc., tend to be supportive to blood, lymph, kidneys, and bladder.

You can easily see how each category of food could become a book of its own; the possibilities are truly endless. Imagine what you could learn by expanding your food horizons to global proportions. Thai food, Lebanese food, Japanese food, Guatemalan food, African food, Iranian food, Vietnamese food, Turkish food, Indian food, Native American food . . . Go on, observe, identify, and experience! You have nothing to lose, except perhaps some long-standing limitations that most likely could use some adjusting anyway.

Rhythm: It Don't Mean a Thing if It Don't Have That Swing!

Motion has direction and speed—and it also has rhythm. Like you and me, all foods have their own unique rhythms of life. Our metabolisms reflect our personal rhythms. Likewise, plants' and animals' growth and behavior patterns reflect their rhythms.

Rhythm includes speed but is a more complex characteristic. There are as many different rhythmic profiles as there are people, melodies, plants, and animals, but for the sake of including this feature in these guidelines, we'll focus on the two generalized categories of "more regulated" versus "more irregular" rhythms. And because rhythm also includes the characteristic of speed, we'll look at four possible combinations:

- a fast, regulated rhythm
- a fast, irregular rhythm
- a slow, regulated rhythm
- a slow, irregular rhythm

The rhythm and tempo, that is to say, the *behavior* of a food, can have a profound effect on your biological and psychological behavior. For example:

- Alcohol has a *slow, irregular* rhythm that produces an unwinding effect when ingested. The more you drink the more unwound you become.
- Coffee has a *fast, irregular* rhythm, an effect that is noticeable as soon as it is ingested.
- Cheese has a *slow, regular* rhythm with variations among each type.
- Whole cereal grains have *slow, regular* rhythms also with variations among them.
- Spices have *fast, irregular* rhythms, as witnessed in their rapid dispersing qualities.
- Eggs have a *slow, regular* rhythm, as evidenced in the way they affect the body with a gradual sinking and settled sensation.
- Chickens, on the other hand, have a *fast, irregular* rhythm, as evidenced in their behavior patterns.

These few examples of food rhythms are enough to show that monodiets or a lack of diversity in diet cannot support vital, dynamic health, and neither can a diet consisting of chaotic combinations of foods.

What type of rhythm do you want? Which do you *have*? Have other people expressed to you (either directly or indirectly) how they feel about your usual rhythm? Have you heard it, and have you done anything about it? They could be wrong about their perceptions of you—but then again, you could be wrong about your perceptions of yourself. After all, you are accustomed to your particular rhythms.

While food is not the sole source of your biological and psychological rhythmic patterns, you do eat what supports and maintains them. Intestinal irregularity, fatigue, the psychodramas in your life, irritability—you name it, it has something to do with how and what you eat.

Eat foods with *fast, regular* rhythms and you can easily get ahead of yourself, accomplish a great number of things—more than the average person, but just don't let anyone get in your way!

Eat plenty of foods with *fast, irregular* rhythms and you will be able to do many things, albeit haphazardly—even to stimulate your imagination beyond what you thought possible—but be careful not to get in your own way!

Eat plenty of foods with *slow, regular* rhythms and you can become more stable and less erratic, not necessarily the most exiting or dynamic person, but at least more reliable.

Eat plenty of foods with *slow, irregular* rhythms and relax, take it easy, get frustrated, and create a desire for more stimulating things to do.

Whatever you do, get rhythm—lots of it—and get to know and play the food symphony like the best conductor would render Beethoven's Ninth! What matters is to catch the rhythms of what you eat, know when the tune goes up or down, when it's rich or dry . . .

17
Food's Temperament

In addition to direction of growth, speed, and rhythm of motion, a food's essential character is also colored by an inborn *temperament*, expressed in terms of its *moisture* and *temperature*. These two factors can be expressed in terms of four grades of temperature—*hot, warm, cool, and cold*—and two basic moisture gradients—*damp and dry.*

Naturally, these are only broad categorizations: in living reality, there are many, many subtle grades and shades of these factors and an infinite number of possible combinations. But these six "shades" and the eight possible combinations will suffice to describe different foods' temperaments—enough to give you the idea and help you learn to recognize each food's unique temperament and the effect it can have on your own.

Each food's constitutional character (a food's original nature) is strongly colored by one of the following eight combinations of temperament:

- Hot and damp
- Cold and damp
- Warm and damp
- Cool and damp

- Hot and dry
- Cold and dry
- Warm and dry
- Cool and dry

Like *observed identities,* these inherent or constitutional temperaments of foods are tendencies and are not fixed. They are relative to a given situation and must be experienced and intuited.

The Temperaments of Animals and Plants

Specific foods may be compared to other foods according to their inherent temperaments. Chicken, for example, has a *warm and dry* temperament relative to duck, which lives partially in a water environment, is higher in fat and has a *hot and damp* temperament. The meat of a chicken is drier relative to duck meat, which is greasier. Both chicken and duck are animal foods, which gives them both a *warm to hot* temperament.

Beef has a *hot and damp* temperament and eggs have a *hot and damp* temperament as well. However, their essential characters are quite different. An egg is a whole, undeveloped, and inactive animal, while beef is a portion of an active, fully developed animal. An egg has a thick and creamy texture whereas beef has a solid and sinewy texture.

Venison (deer meat) is less fatty than beef, and deer are also more nimble and active than steer, so venison has a *hot and dry* temperament relative to beef's *hot and damp* temperament.

The realm of vegetable foods also offers a huge spectrum of examples of these varied constitutional temperaments of foods.

Tofu is high in protein, wet, and soft, and has a temperament that is *cold and damp*. Hard winter squashes (acorn, butternut, buttercup, etc.) have a *dry and warm* temperament compared to summer squashes (yellow squash and zucchini), which have a *cool and damp* temperament.

Among whole grains, millet is *warm and dry,* buckwheat is *hot and dry,* whole wheat is *warm and dry,* and so on.

By the way, some of these categorizations have been popularly disseminated through a revival of interest in traditional Chinese medicine. But they are mostly taught and practiced in a fragmentary, theoretical way. For those who are familiar with these concepts from traditional Chinese medicine (or from any reinterpreted system based on similar ancient systems), note that these aspects have no meaning or value when considered separately, in isolation.

Say a person has a hot temperament—does that make him or her particularly loud, or especially volatile sexually? You can't tell unless you also know *at least* about the dampness or dryness of that character. *Hot/*

damp and *hot/dry* are very different, indeed—and the same goes for all such semiparallel combinations.

The Temperaments of People

As in all energetic descriptions, applying these to people can make them more vivid.

People, too, have temperaments that can be *known* as hot or cold, warm or cool, and damp or dry. And of course, the foods you eat, along with their particular temperaments, will have a powerful influence on the temperamental aspects of your behavior.

The weight-loss fad so prevalent in America is a good example of how easily one can develop a *cold and dry* condition. The fear of fat and other healthy, traditionally nutritious foods has resulted in a broad range of physical deficiency and eating disorders, as well as the plethora of mental symptoms that accompany them. Insecurity, emotional instability, fear, and insensitivity are just a few of the common symptoms that often result from taking such an important dietary element (i.e., fat) out of one's diet.

When you feel *cold and dry,* it requires more stimulation to generate heat and warmth for sexual satisfaction; therefore, relationships can be seriously affected. Intense cravings inevitably lead to guilt and depression, just a few of the symptoms that arise simply because of a temperament that could so easily be adjusted through commonsense nutrition.

The British, noted for their exceptionally dry sense of humor, live in a damp climate—and consequently, have traditionally chosen a preponderance of dry or drying foods (such as toast, chips, and tea). The most obvious contrast would be the French, noted for their rich sensuousness of expression—and, naturally, of cuisine. While these are generalizations, more than a kernel of truth does exist in them.

Can you think of a person you know with a *warm and dry* temperament? That person that you find attractive because he is a good listener, but at the same time, you do not get that same feeling of attraction *from* him for you that you feel *for* him. His dryness just does not project the same passion you feel.

How about someone you know with a *hot and damp* temperament? She is dominant, controlling, explosive, and things *will* go her way—and if you cannot deal with that . . . well, you'll just *have* to deal with it.

Finally, it should be noted that some people are more temperamental overall, while others are less so. In other words, in some individuals' temperament, regardless of what particular temperament it is, is a more pronounced part of their personality, while in others it plays a less central role. The same is true of foods.

18
A Basic Food Character Chart

The four headings that follow describe various properties of numerous foods, each relative to the category into which it fits. The categorizations given here are highly relative and do not take into account possibilities of variation within each particular species, nor the effects of food combination and preparation, seasoning, and so forth. They are not given as absolute classifications but as guidelines for your continued observation of individual foods' uniqueness.

Food
This heading gives examples of foods and the groups to which they belong.

Temperament
This describes the basic nature of each particular food relative to the group to which it belongs. Keep in mind that these inherent natures are susceptible to change, depending on how the food is prepared and with what other foods it is combined.

Direction
This describes the direction the food will travel when eaten, in other words, the plane or level it seeks as a result of the way it grows and interacts in its own environment.

Body Position

This describes the area of the body where the food resonates.

- Upper: the chest area, lungs, heart, and throat
- Middle: liver, gallbladder, spleen, pancreas, stomach, and kidneys (Note: Some foods may resonate more strongly than others with a specific organ in a particular position. Also, some foods may resonate in more than one area of the body.)
- Lower: intestines, bladder, and reproductive organs

Rhythm

This describes the combination of speed and regularity or irregularity of the food's temperament.

FOOD	TEMPERAMENT	DIRECTION	BODY POSITION	RHYTHM
Whole Grains and Grain Products				
millet	warm and dry	down and in	middle	fast / regular
rice (short grain)	warm and damp	up and in	upper	slow / regular
rice (medium grain)	cool and damp	up and in	upper	slow / regular
rice (long grain)	cold and dry	up and out	upper	fast / regular
sweet rice	warm and damp	up and out	upper	slow / regular
wild rice	cool and dry	up and in	middle	fast / regular
barley	cool and damp	up and out	middle	slow / regular
corn	cool and dry	up and in	upper	fast / irregular
buckwheat	hot and dry	down and in	lower	fast / regular
oats	warm and damp	down and out	middle	slow / regular
quinoa	warm and dry	down and in	middle	fast / regular
amaranth	warm and dry	down and out	middle	fast / regular
teff	cool and dry	down and out	middle	fast / irregular
rye	warm and dry	up and in	middle	fast / irregular
wheat	warm and dry	up and out	middle	slow / regular
wheat gluten (seitan)	warm and damp	down and in	middle	slow / regular
yeasted bread	cool and dry	up and out	middle	fast / irregular
unleavened bread	warm and dry	up and in	middle	slow / irregular
pasta	warm and damp	up and out	middle	slow / regular

FOOD	TEMPERAMENT	DIRECTION	BODY POSITION	RHYTHM
bulgur	cool and dry	up and out	middle	fast / irregular
couscous	cool and dry	up and out	middle	fast / irregular

Beans and Bean Products

FOOD	TEMPERAMENT	DIRECTION	BODY POSITION	RHYTHM
black-eyed peas	warm and damp	up and out	middle	slow / regular
chickpeas	warm and dry	down and out	middle	fast / irregular
soybeans	warm and damp	down and out	middle	slow / irregular
lentils	warm and dry	down and in	middle	fast / irregular
lima beans	warm and damp	up and out	middle	slow / irregular
scarlet runners	warm and damp	up and out	middle	fast / irregular
kidney beans	warm and damp	up and out	middle	fast / regular
pinto beans	warm and damp	up and out	middle	slow / regular
navy beans	warm and damp	up and out	middle	slow / regular
red peas	warm and damp	up and out	middle	fast / irregular
northern beans	warm and damp	up and out	middle	slow / regular
haricots	warm and damp	up and out	middle	slow / regular
green peas	warm and damp	up and out	middle	fast / irregular
broad beans	warm and damp	down and out	middle	slow / regular
mung bean	cool and dry	down and in	middle	slow / irregular
adzuki bean	warm and dry	down and in	middle	fast / irregular
bolita beans	warm and damp	up and out	middle	slow / regular
tofu	cold and damp	up and out	middle	slow / irregular
tempeh	cool and damp	up and out	middle	slow / irregular
natto	cold and damp	up and out	upper	slow / regular
soy milk	cold and damp	up and out	upper	slow / irregular

Leafy Vegetables

FOOD	TEMPERAMENT	DIRECTION	BODY POSITION	RHYTHM
bok choy	cold and damp	up and out	upper	fast / irregular
kale	cool and dry	up and in	upper	slow / irregular
collard greens	cool and damp	up and out	upper	slow / regular
mustard greens	cool and dry	up and in	upper	fast / irregular
broccoli rabe	cool and dry	up and in	upper	fast / irregular
dandelions	cool and dry	up and in	upper	fast / irregular
escarole	cool and damp	up and out	upper	fast / irregular
chicory	cool and dry	up and in	upper	fast / irregular
carrot leaves	cool and dry	up and in	upper	fast / irregular
turnip leaves	cool and dry	up and in	upper	fast / irregular

FOOD	TEMPERAMENT	DIRECTION	BODY POSITION	RHYTHM
radish leaves	cool and dry	up and in	upper	fast / irregular
daikon leaves	cool and dry	up and in	upper	fast / irregular
chives	cold and dry	up and out	upper	fast / regular
scallion	cold and damp	up and out	upper	fast / regular
parsley	cold and dry	up and in	upper	fast / irregular
cilantro	cold and dry	up and in	upper	fast / irregular
leeks	cool and dry	up and out	upper	fast / regular
basil	cold and dry	up and out	upper	fast / irregular
arugula	cool and dry	up and in	upper	fast / irregular
watercress	cold and damp	up and in	middle	fast / irregular
leaf lettuces	cold and damp	up and out	upper	slow / irregular
chard	cold and damp	up and out	upper	fast / irregular
spinach	cold and damp	up and in	upper	fast / irregular
dock leaves	cold and dry	up and out	upper	fast / irregular
Flowers				
all types	cold and damp	up and out	upper	fast / regular
Root Vegetables				
burdock	warm and dry	down and in	lower	slow / regular
carrot	warm and damp	down and in	lower	slow / regular
dandelion	warm and dry	down and in	lower	fast / irregular
parsnip	warm and dry	down and in	lower	slow / regular
celery root	warm and damp	down and out	lower	fast / irregular
turnip	warm and damp	down and out	lower	slow / regular
rutabaga	warm and damp	down and out	lower	slow / regular
daikon	cool and damp	down and out	lower	slow / regular
salsify	warm and damp	down and in	lower	slow / irregular
chicory root	warm and dry	down and in	lower	fast / irregular
lotus root	cold and damp	down and out	lower	slow / regular
onion	warm and damp	down and out	lower	slow / regular
beets	cold and damp	down and out	lower	fast / regular
taro	cool and damp	down and out	lower	slow / regular
jinenjo	warm and damp	down and in	lower	slow / regular
Other Vegetables				
cabbage	warm and damp	down and out	middle	slow / regular
brussels sprouts	warm and dry	up and in	middle	slow / regular
winter squash	warm and dry	down and out	middle	slow / regular

FOOD	TEMPERAMENT	DIRECTION	BODY POSITION	RHYTHM
pumpkin	warm and dry	down and out	middle	slow / regular
potato	cold and damp	down and out	lower	slow / irregular
tomato	cold and damp	down and out	middle	fast / irregular
summer squash	cool and damp	down and out	middle	fast / regular
zucchini	cool and damp	down and out	middle	fast / regular
cucumber	cold and damp	down and out	middle	fast / regular
cauliflower	cool and damp	up and out	middle	slow / regular
broccoli	cool and damp	up and out	middle	slow / regular
celery	cool and damp	up and in	middle	fast / irregular
mushrooms	cold and damp	up and out	middle	fast / irregular
bean sprouts	cold and damp	up and out	middle	fast / irregular
Jerusalem artichoke	cool and damp	down and out	lower	slow / irregular
bell peppers	cold and damp	down and out	middle	fast / irregular
artichoke	cold and damp	up and out	middle	fast / irregular
asparagus	cold and damp	up and in	middle	fast / irregular
okra	cold and damp	up and in	middle	fast / irregular
sweet potato	cool and damp	down and out	lower	slow / irregular
yam	cool and damp	down and out	lower	slow / irregular
garlic	warm and dry	down and out	lower	slow / irregular

Sea Vegetables

FOOD	TEMPERAMENT	DIRECTION	BODY POSITION	RHYTHM
wakame	cold and damp	up and out	upper	fast / irregular
kombu	cold and damp	up and out	upper	slow / regular
hiziki	cold and dry	down and in	lower	slow / regular
arame	cold and dry	down and out	middle	slow / regular
dulse	cold and damp	up and out	upper	fast / irregular
nori	cold and dry	up and out	upper	fast / irregular
agar agar	cold and damp	up and in	upper	slow / regular
alaria	cold and damp	up and out	upper	fast / irregular
sea palm	cold and damp	down and out	middle	slow / regular

Seeds and Nuts

FOOD	TEMPERAMENT	DIRECTION	BODY POSITION	RHYTHM
cashew	warm and damp	up and out	upper	fast / irregular
peanut	warm and damp	down and out	lower	fast / irregular
almond	warm and damp	up and out	upper	fast / regular
filbert	warm and damp	up and out	upper	fast / regular
pecan	warm and damp	up and out	upper	fast / regular

FOOD	TEMPERAMENT	DIRECTION	BODY POSITION	RHYTHM
walnut	warm and damp	up and out	upper	fast / irregular
sesame seed	warm and dry	up and in	middle	fast / regular
sunflower	warm and dry	up and in	middle	fast / regular
pumpkin seed	warm and dry	down and out	middle	slow / regular
Freshwater and Saltwater Animals				
halibut	cold and damp	down and out	lower	slow / regular
flounder	cold and damp	down and out	lower	slow / regular
scrod	cool and damp	up and out	middle	slow / irregular
haddock	cold and damp	down and out	lower	slow / irregular
trout	cool and damp	down and out	middle	fast / irregular
smelt	cool and damp	up and in	middle	fast / irregular
red snapper	cool and damp	up and out	middle	fast / irregular
pike	cool and damp	up and in	middle	fast / irregular
perch	cold and damp	up and out	middle	fast / irregular
mackerel	warm and damp	up and in	middle	fast / irregular
tuna	warm and dry	up and in	middle	fast / irregular
swordfish	warm and dry	up and in	middle	fast / irregular
bluefish	warm and damp	up and in	middle	fast / irregular
clam	cold and damp	down and out	middle	slow / regular
oyster	cold and damp	down and out	lower	slow / regular
mussel	cold and damp	up and out	middle	slow / regular
scallop	cold and damp	down and out	middle	slow / irregular
squid	cool and damp	up and out	upper	fast / irregular
octopus	cool and damp	up and out	upper	fast / irregular
shrimp	cold and damp	down and in	lower	slow / irregular
lobster	cold and damp	down and in	lower	slow / irregular
crab	cold and damp	down and in	lower	slow / irregular
conch	cold and damp	down and out	lower	slow / regular
Land Animals				
cow (beef)	hot and damp	down and out	lower	slow / regular
lamb	warm and damp	down and out	middle	slow / regular
pork	hot and dry	down and out	lower	slow / regular
goat	warm and dry	down and out	middle	fast / irregular
deer	warm and dry	up and in	middle	fast / regular
rabbit	warm and dry	down and in	lower	fast / irregular
chicken	warm and dry	down and in	middle	fast / irregular

FOOD	TEMPERAMENT	DIRECTION	BODY POSITION	RHYTHM
duck	warm and damp	up and in	middle	fast / regular
pheasant	warm and dry	up and in	middle	fast / irregular
eggs	hot and damp	down and in	lower	slow / regular
		Fruit		
strawberries	cool and dry	down and in	lower	fast / irregular
raspberries	cool and dry	down and in	middle	fast / irregular
blackberries	cool and dry	down and in	middle	fast / irregular
melons	cold and damp	down and out	lower	slow / regular
blueberries	cool and damp	down and in	middle	fast / regular
grapes	cool and damp	up and out	upper	slow / regular
plums	cool and damp	up and out	upper	fast / regular
peaches	cool and damp	up and out	upper	fast / regular
pears	cool and damp	up and in	upper	slow / regular
apples	cool and damp	up and in	upper	slow / regular
cherries	cool and damp	up and in	upper	fast / irregular
apricots	cool and damp	up and in	upper	fast / regular
orange	cold and damp	up and out	upper	fast / irregular
grapefruit	cold and damp	up and out	upper	fast / irregular
banana	cold and damp	up and out	upper	fast / irregular
lemon	cold and dry	up and out	upper	fast / irregular
mango	cold and damp	up and out	upper	fast / regular
papaya	cold and damp	up and out	middle	fast / regular
		Dairy Products		
hard cheese	warm and dry	down and in	lower	slow / regular
soft cheese	cool and damp	up and in	middle	slow / irregular
butter	warm and damp	down and in	middle	slow / regular
milk	cold and damp	up and out	upper	fast / irregular
ice cream	cold and damp	up and out	upper	fast / irregular
yogurt	cold and damp	up and out	upper	fast / irregular
cream	cool and damp	up and in	upper	slow / irregular

19
Shaping Characters

So far, we've been referring to character and temperament in terms of what is inherently born to a food. However, after a plant is picked or an animal is prepared, the process of change continues to color the life of food.

Like anything in life, foods constantly experience actions and reactions of compliant and dominant food combinations and of the interplay of contrasts in food on different levels.

When you take an active role in bringing different foods together— whether combined in one recipe or organized into a complete meal—you are the director of what will happen and how, on an energetic level.

Learned Temperament

The inherent temperaments of a particular food may be altered conditionally in such a way that it acquires a new set of characteristics. I call this a food's *learned temperament*.

A food's learned temperament will contribute different effects than the food originally would produce in and of itself. A food's learned temperament is affected by a number of variables, including the combining with other foods and the methods of preparation you choose for it.

Like a particular food, your human constitution is largely determined at birth, with various alterations occurring during your growth process, and these acquired or conditional alterations tend to color your constitution—your inherent nature. These alterations or conditions go through many changes during your lifetime, yet the basic foundation of your constitution remains the same.

For example, if you are out of shape and decide to exercise, your condition will change, and this will add a different dimension or color to your constitution. If you are hungry and eat, your condition will change; if you become seriously ill and receive medical treatment, your condition will change. Through all of these changes, your constitution, which you are born with, will remain the same.

Altering Temperaments

The inherent temperament of a food can be altered by the addition of other foods. When this happens, the inherent temperament of the original food takes on and learns some of the qualities of the other foods, sometimes to a great degree and other times to a lesser degree. The degree to which a food acquires a different temperament than its original one can be determined by how strong or dominant are the foods with which it is combined and the method of preparation.

For example, the essential character of dandelion greens is *cool and dry*. When you cook them with garlic and olive oil, they acquire a learned temperament that will produce a *warm and damp* effect. The cooked oil adds both the warming and damp qualities to the dry, cool, and bitter dandelions. Dandelions also have an *upward and inward* direction, and the oil and heat of cooking tend to partially reduce the upward nature of the greens while the garlic disperses the inward nature.

The inherent temperament of tofu is *cold and damp,* yet if you deep fry tofu, the acquired effect becomes *warm and damp*. (Although not much: it takes a lot to warm tofu!) Seaweeds have inherently *cold and dry* temperaments. These can be enhanced by soaking the sea vegetable and using it in a salad, which maintains its cold, dry temperament. Hiziki (a sea algae) prepared this way is very different from when soaked and rinsed, then cooked for an hour or more with added fat and more warming vegetables, such as carrots and onions. The acquired effect would then be *warm and damp*.

When you acquire a taste for a particular food, you also acquire the energetic properties of that food; likewise, a particular food can acquire and thus be influenced by—even dominated by—the energetics of another food or method of preparation.

Food temperaments can be expressed by a single food or by a prepared combination of foods. They can also be expressed in a particular diet overall.

The Five Energies

Another important working model, originating in the ancient healing model of traditional Chinese medicine, and one that will help renew your knowledge of food energetics is the nature of the five flavors. The five flavors or tastes include: *sweet, bitter, sour, pungent (spicy),* and *salty.*

The qualities of each of these five flavors vary in their degree of intensity. For example, one food may taste very sweet and sugary, and another may taste subtly sweet as well as slightly sour. Each food has a predominant flavor and often one or more subtle flavors.

Each flavor has a tendency to enter one or more specific organs of the body, where it creates a particular condition in that organ. Some of the ancient works on Chinese medicine and healing contain detailed explanations of the five flavors and their relevance to health and sickness. It is in these translated works where we find the clearly expressed— yet often misinterpreted—explanation of the potential energetics of the five flavors.

In the classic texts of Chinese medicine there is mention of how each of the five flavors enters and resonates with an associated organ. The flavors of *sweet, sour, bitter, pungent, and salty* enter their respective organs: *spleen and pancreas, liver, heart, lungs, and kidneys.* The energetic potentials and associated organs of the five flavors are listed as follows:

• Sour: astringent, centrifugal, upward effect, wrinkling, shriveling, tendency to empty fullness, and cool. The sour flavor enters the *liver,* which is associated with the *gallbladder.*

- Sweet: calming, soothing, relaxing, sinking effect, rounding, settling, tendency to fill emptiness, and warm. The sweet flavor enters the *spleen and pancreas,* which are associated with the *stomach.*
- Pungent (spicy): dispersing, releasing, outward effect, stimulating, exciting, tendency to rapidly empty fullness, warming at first yet later cooling. The pungent flavor enters the *lungs,* which are associated with the *large intestine.*
- Bitter: drying, purging, evaporating, inward effect, tightening, tendency to create both full and empty. The bitter flavor enters the *heart,* which is associated with the *small intestine.*
- Salty (mineral): softening, pliable, flexible, energizing, holding, storing, tendency to create both empty and full. The salty flavor enters the *kidneys,* which are associated with the *bladder.*

These corresponding relationships between flavors and organs are often mistakenly described as the flavors being "good for" those organs. In actuality, the flavors are neither "good" nor "bad" for those organs. Rather, they produce an energetic effect that results in a quality of *emptying out or filling.* (It is also important to note that the many other associated phenomena—other than five flavors, that is—described in Chinese medicine to a particular organ are not necessarily always beneficial to that organ.)

Each of the five organs can have one of the three following conditions: *empty, full, or balanced.* Using the liver as an example, let's describe two conditions of the liver to get an idea as to how a flavor (in this case, the sour flavor) can influence an organ.

The sour flavor enters the liver, regardless of whether it is empty or full. However, the sour, tart flavor has an astringent quality, which has an *emptying* tendency. Think of the sour flavor as having the ability to shrivel and cool, not unlike a wet sponge that is being squeezed and its liquid released. Or, imagine biting into a fresh lemon and how the astringent quality of the sour juice causes you to pucker up.

When you apply these qualities to a *full* condition in the liver—a condition where one's liver tends to be overheated and congested, where one's temperament is hot and angry—the sour flavor likely will have a beneficial effect. But if the liver's condition is empty to start with—as in the disease of cirrhosis, where the liver cells are replaced with inactive scar tissue—and the liver is weak and depleted, the sour flavor may create further weakness and not benefit the organ.

The five flavors are relative to each situation to which they are applied.

Another common misinterpretation and misrepresentation of the five flavors is a strict categorizing of foods within a particular flavor or element. For example, the spicy or pungent flavor corresponds to the "metal" phase of energy, which includes the corresponding organs of the lungs and large intestine. This is often interpreted as meaning that "spicy foods are good for the lungs and large intestines," and numerous spicy foods are often listed as aiding the lungs and large intestines.

As you already know, spicy foods enter, yet are not *necessarily* beneficial for, the lungs and large intestines. What's more, each spicy food has *its own unique energetic effect*. Spices are dispersing, with the ability to release stored energy. If one's lungs are filled with accumulated energy, the spicy flavor can support a dispersal of that condensed energy. On the other hand, if the lungs are depleted of energy, the spicy flavor may not be supportive, but may even be injurious.

Raw daikon (long white radish) has a spicy flavor and therefore enters the lungs. However, boiled daikon has a sweet flavor, and thus enters more the spleen/pancreas or "soil" category. Fried daikon has a bitter flavor, and thus enters the heart/small intestine and "fire" category.

When used to determine the energetics of foods, the five flavors cannot be thought of as static or fixed categories of foods, each with its single purpose.

A practical application of the five flavors for daily use would be to make sure you have all five flavors present in your main meal. Whether it is lunch or dinner that is your main meal of the day, try to have each flavor present. Below are some examples of how to find these flavors.

Sour

Lemon, lime, green apple, and other fruits with a sour flavor, vinegar, wine, fermented foods (pickles, olives, sauerkraut, etc.). The sour flavor is usually used in small quantities as seasoning or a side dish of fermented foods. However, there are those of us who may enjoy a glass of wine or two on occasion with nice meals.

Sweet

Winter squashes, pumpkins, carrots, beets, many whole grains and grain products, many fruits (dried and fresh), natural sweeteners (grain malts, maple syrup, agave syrup, honey). Natural sweet foods have long played a major role in traditional diets; in agricultural diets, in the form of whole grains, and in hunter-gatherer diets, in the form of roots and tubers. The quantity of sweet flavor in a meal is usually higher than other flavors; when it is not, one will tend to crave additional sweets (often in the form of unhealthier, refined sweet foods).

Pungent (Spicy)

Onions, garlic, ginger, chives, peppers, curry seasoning, spices. Like the sour flavor, traditional diets tend to use small quantities of spicy foods to enhance the flavors of a meal, as well as for other, equally important reasons, which we will discuss later.

Bitter

Some leafy green vegetables, some root vegetables, some herbs, grilled foods, roasted or toasted foods, including seeds and nuts, chocolate, coffee, tea. Traditional diets usually incorporate small amounts of bitter foods. You can see how more extreme bitter foods, such as coffee and chocolate, are often consumed in large quantities by those not consuming quality vegetables, seeds, and other quality bitter foods. Not that chocolate is necessarily a poor-quality substitute for the bitter flavor, but one who eats bitter greens, grilled foods, and toasted seeds and nuts will have significantly less desire for large amounts of chocolate and coffee.

Salty

Sea salt, marine algae (sea vegetables), salt water fish, some dried and smoked foods. Traditional diets include regular amounts of mineral-based foods or foods with high mineral content in reasonable quantities. Salts of varying types were also used to concentrate flavors of foods.

Quality is an important factor in determining how you support your health with the five flavors. When a flavor is not present in one's daily diet, one will inevitably experience a craving for it and more than likely compensate by indulging in poor-quality substitutes, especially what is familiar. Therefore, it is important to introduce additional foods with different flavors that may be unfamiliar yet highly supportive to your health.

Here is a simple rule of thumb. As much as possible, get all five flavors in your main meal and you will notice a marked difference in how you feel and what you crave.

20
Preparations

The art of food preparation includes—but is not limited to—boiling, steaming, baking, grilling, sautéing, stir-frying, marinating, deep frying, drying, and pickling.

Peoples throughout the world have practiced these methods of preparing foods for generations. Many traditional cultures incorporated various methods of food preparation for flavor and visual appeal, as well as for improving digestion and many other health purposes. Many of these traditions along with other new methods continue to be creatively explored in the cuisine of today.

The art of food preparation ranks as one of our highest art forms, if not *the* highest. There are "technical chefs" and "intuitive chefs," and if you do enough experimenting with food preparations, you can easily become both.

What technical and intuitive chefs have in common is a willingness to have a deeply personal relationship with the food they prepare. These artists know the essences of foods and how to establish harmonious relationships among them through creative and flavorful combinations. They not only know the characteristics of foods, they also know intuitively (if not always consciously) that the food will, in some magical way, *become* the person eating it. Their goal is to create balanced preparations and meals that are satisfying to the palate.

The artist knows that well-cooked beans and rice constitute the beginning of a harmonious relationship, whereas boiled tofu with tomatoes is the beginning of dissent.

True artists in this field explore the unlimited possibilities of their imagination and create preparations based on the principles of natural law. They do not operate strictly from man-made rules and regulations. They simply do what must be done in order to nourish those who will partake of their talents and skills.

By observing what occurs during preparation, you can get an idea of what happens energetically to foods. For example, cooking can affect the texture of a plant or animal food by altering the structure of cell walls and the water pressure in a food's tissue. Through the application of heat, the cell walls of a food soften and the tissue becomes tender. This results in the food becoming moist due to the absorption of added water, or drier from heat with little or no water.

The examples of food preparation that follow focus on vegetable quality foods, but the principles can be applied to most animal foods as well.

Boiling

With this method of preparation, a food is submerged in boiling water. Using kale as an example, first note the energetics of kale as a vegetable that grows upward. Like other leafy greens, kale is also an oxygen enhancer because of its chlorophyll content, and this gives kale a tendency to affect the upper part of the body (lungs and heart).

Once submerged in the boiling water, the kale begins to relax. The cellulose fibers soften and the constituents of the plant (its vitamins, minerals, etc.) enter the water. The boiling water sets up an exchange with the plant: the kale begins to release its essence into the water even as the water enters the fibers and cells of the kale. The result: the kale becomes more dense and heavier from the water it has absorbed, and the water becomes green and mineral-tasting from the kale.

Kale prepared in this manner now has the potential to bring its original energetic qualities, combined with the addition of accumulated water, to the upper part of the body. This can be supportive for a dry condition in the heart or lungs.

However, for a wet condition in this area of the body, this style of preparing greens may not be as supportive. People who tend to retain water or who are full with a damp condition may feel uncomfortable after eating boiled foods. Therefore, boiling foods may not be the best method of preparation to use on a regular basis for individuals with these problems. Excessive water in your food can also dilute nutritional factors of the food.

Adding excessive amounts of water to food can contribute to other problems, too. For instance, you might feel less satisfied with your food and seek stronger or dryer foods with more substance. Psychologically, an excess of wet, heavy, boiled food may contribute to frustration, insecurity, and a lack of mental clarity. Watery foods can also contribute to an inability to express oneself clearly or precisely.

Boiling food tends to make the food heavier and denser, as well as more watery. Boiled foods add extra water to the body and can be helpful for dry and tight conditions.

Steaming

This style of cooking involves using a steamer to separate the boiling water from the food. The food comes in contact only with the steam from boiling water, and not with the boiling water itself.

Steaming food has an opposite effect of boiling: the food becomes *lighter* in weight and density. (If you weigh two equal portions of a food, one boiled and the other steamed, you'll see the palpable difference.)

Have you ever been in a steam room? The steam adds warm moisture to your lungs and opens the pores of your skin, and you begin to perspire. The rising steam then makes you feel warmer and lighter. Deep internal heat is brought to the surface of the body and released as perspiration. Once out of the steam room, for an hour or more, you will start to feel cool, and soon begin to crave rich foods containing fat and salt, both of which were reduced through the excess perspiration.

Steam is hotter than boiling water. When food is steamed, the hot steam loosens the fiber of food causing an exchange of moisture between the steam and the essence of the food. Steamed food becomes cooler more rapidly at room temperature than boiled food. Therefore, steaming, in addition to making food lighter, has a more cooling effect.

This method of cooking (especially when applied to green vegetables) has the potential to create a damp, cool condition in the upper part of the body. This may be beneficial for an overheated, dry condition, yet not so beneficial for a cool, damp condition. Steaming has an upward tendency and acts more on the upper part of the body in general, while at the same time it draws from and cools the energy in the lower body. This form of preparation, if used exclusively, can contribute to a lack of confidence, loss of weight and physical stamina, and poor circulation in the feet and hands.

Keep in mind that we are using only one vegetable (kale) as an example. The principles of these cooking methods are applicable to all vegetables (and animal products, for that matter), yet all vegetables are different. For example, a carrot grows downward, centripetally, and therefore it affects the lower body more than the upper, but a boiled carrot is still heavier than a steamed carrot.

Sautéing

In sautéing kale (to stay with the same example), the hot oil acts as a coating on the kale, causing it to contract and locking in its essence. Some of the water from the vegetable is released in the process, yet the vegetable still closes up, and any flavorings that are added tend to adhere to the periphery of the food, as opposed to being absorbed into it, as would happen if the food were boiled. This method of preparation produces a warm and damp effect in the body.

There are different ways one can sauté with oil. One method is to add oil to a pan, add vegetables once the oil is hot, then stir and mix slowly and consistently, adding flavorings in the process. When the vegetables are done to your liking, remove them from the pan and serve.

Another method, commonly called stir-frying, is to add oil to a pan, add your primary foods once the oil is hot, then add seasonings and stir and mix rapidly. With this method, the flame on the stove is usually higher, the cooking time is shorter, and vegetables are still crisp upon completion.

Sautéing and stir-frying both are forms of cooking that use hot oil to embrace the food and lock in its essence. Cooked oil has a warming effect in the body, whereas raw oil (as commonly used in salads) has a cooling effect in the body.

Sautéing or stir-frying when applied to kale creates a warm and damp effect in the *upper* part of the body (upper because we're still dealing with kale). This may be supportive for a dry and cool condition, but for those with a hot and damp mucus condition, it may not be the best cooking method to use on a regular basis.

Excessive use of sautéing, while it does contribute to warmth, can also contribute to feelings of restlessness, dependency, and irritability. Sautéed food tends to remain warm at room temperature longer than steamed or boiled foods.

Pressure Cooking

In this method of cooking one places hardy, more durable foods—most commonly whole cereal grains, dried beans, or meats—into a stainless steel or enamel-coated pressure cooker with added water. (Aluminum vessels are also available, but these are not recommended due to aluminum's toxicity.) The food is then locked into the pressure cooker with a tight-fitting lid, and as the contents are heated, they are brought up to high pressure.

This method of cooking is commonly used for grains and beans because grains, beans, and some meats are foods that can withstand the intensity of pressure and heat produced by a pressure cooker. Most other vegetable foods would collapse under such pressure, so we won't use kale as an example for this cooking method.

The combination of boiling water, steam, and intense pressure causes the grains or beans to burst open and release their hidden potential. The effect of pressure cooking in the human body is one of deep warmth and satisfaction. It also affects one's deep energy reserves, often unlocking hidden physiological and psychological potential, bringing it to the surface. Because of this, people with high stress or excessive emotional problems might refrain from using this method of cooking.

Pressure cooking whole grains and beans can be helpful for those willing to face their seemingly hidden past and suppressed emotions. If you have ever been in an extremely stressful situation ("in a pressure cooker") and felt like you were going to burst, well, this is what pressure cooked food goes through, only it *does* burst, and as a result, it becomes sweeter. It is easy for grains and beans to adapt to this environment and improve from it. Many human beings, when experiencing what they call pressure, tend to resist or retreat, or they hold on to the situation, often making it more difficult to adapt. Pressure cooking certain foods could help some individuals in the process of letting it all out.

Stewing

In stewing, various foods are boiled slowly in water with seasonings to form a thick stew. Stewed foods are sometimes sautéed or braised first and then boiled; or they may simply be chopped and boiled as they are. A thickening agent, such as flour, cornstarch, arrowroot, or kuzu, may be added to the stewed meat and vegetables. The result is a hearty and deeply warming one-pot preparation often eaten with fresh baked bread.

Stewing causes the different foods used to meld their individual essences together into a unified and satisfying flavor. The foods release their essence into the water, and the water is absorbed into the vegetables. Thick, rich stews have a sinking effect that can be especially beneficial for those lacking in strength and stamina, as well as for those who have trouble gaining weight. Overweight people may find regular preparations of stews to be heavy and of little help in losing weight.

Another type of stewing common in Japan is a layering method called *nishime*. The basic difference between layering and stewing, in the conventional sense, is that the layering method uses little water in the cooking, and the finished product has very little or no water left in the pot.

Like many other preparation methods, there are numerous varieties of the layering method. A common method is to place a strip of kombu (a sea vegetable) on the bottom of an oiled heavy pot with enough water to cover the kombu. Large pieces of hardy root or ground vegetables (squash, carrots, sweet potatoes, cabbage, etc.) are layered on top of each other with added seasonings. Cover and bring to a boil, then lower the flame and let simmer until the vegetables are cooked. Remove the lid and gently mix the vegetables. There should be no remaining water in the pot at the end of cooking, and the vegetables will be very sweet tasting. Other methods differ only in that the vegetables may be layered without the kombu.

The small amount of water used in the layering method is brought to a rapid boil with a high flame, and then the flame is reduced to low, which produces a gentle steam heat combined with a small amount of boiling water. The vegetables slowly and gradually release their essence together in such a way as to meld the individual flavors into each other. The overall process can last anywhere from twenty to forty minutes, and the result can create a warm as well as a centered feeling. The layering method of cooking has a very soothing effect on the digestive system, and may be helpful for those who are hyperactive or suffer from anxiety, as it contributes to relaxation and an overall settled feeling. It has a warm and damp effect on the body.

Grilling

There are a number of ways to grill food. The barbecue grill is a common method, and closely resembles the traditional method of spit roasting, which uses a long skewer rather than a grill to hold the food. The effects are similar. One can also grill on a stove equipped with a grill.

Whatever way you grill, you generally begin by using a high heat and then lower it to a medium-high or low flame. This method of cooking tends to sear and blacken the exterior of food. It is a highly energizing method of cooking that can produce a hot and dry condition.

Marinating and Pickling

Marinated foods are soaked in various combinations of oil, vinegar, salt, herbs, and spices, which help break down food tissue through enzymatic action. This is a natural form of food preservation that has been used for thousands of years. Foods are commonly marinated from one or two hours to a number of days.

One form of marinating and pickling is called *pressing.* Sauerkraut is a common, traditional example of pressing: chopped cabbage and salt are combined and placed in a crock with added pressure. The salt and pressure cause the cabbage to release its contained liquid into the crock. The cabbage then sits and ferments in its own brine.

A variation of this approach involves slicing raw vegetables and pressing them between two plates, with a heavy weight placed on top of the upper plate. Another variation is to place the vegetables in a salad press, a container made expressly for this purpose with a screw-down lid that can be manually tightened down onto the vegetables to achieve optimum pressure. In addition to the pressure, a salty flavoring—sea salt, umeboshi plum or vinegar, miso, etc.—is often added to initiate and maintain a mild fermentation.

The health benefits of this method of preparation are well documented in research on *kimchi,* a spicy pickled cabbage preparation that is native to Korea and a famously staple part of Korean cuisine.

Pressed vegetables have a cooling effect in the body and they introduce healthy doses of enzymes and lactic acid into the digestive system. If root vegetables are used, the cooling effect occurs more in the lower part of the body; if leafy vegetables are used, the effect occurs more in the upper area of the body. If spicy vegetables (for example, watercress, scallion, radish, onion) are used, the effect may include a temporary increase in blood circulation.

The pressure on the vegetables through pressing causes the vegetables to contract and release liquid, which rises to the top. The salty flavoring interacts with the pressed vegetables and liquid to create a light, fermenting brine. The longer it sits, the more it ferments. Sometimes, the brine is mixed back into the vegetables; sometimes it is discarded.

In this style of preparation, the force of pressure replaces the force of heat typically used in cooking; this results in the vegetables remaining fresh, crisp, and fermented.

There are many ways to make pickles other than pressing, and pickling may use a wide variety of vegetables (and not just cucumbers). Each vegetable has its own unique quality, and each style of pickling enhances each vegetable with varying qualities of time, pressure, and salt. Vegetables may be pickled in salt brine, vinegar, umeboshi (pickled plum), tamari soy sauce, miso (fermented soybean paste), rice bran, corn meal, and so on. Traditional Italian cuisine features a delicious brine pickle that includes a wide variety of raw vegetables placed in a large jar or crock and left to ferment. Olives are another important fermented food with numerous health benefits.

In general, the pickling or fermenting of foods has a cooling effect in the body; however, certain methods of pickling have a more warming effect, if hardy root or ground vegetables are used and the pickling process lasts for a long time. If leafy, light, or more fragile vegetables are used, and the pickling time is short, the pickles tend to be more cooling.

A few tablespoons daily of some type of fermented food are essential for healthy digestion and for balancing one's diet. In fact, incorporating small amounts of these salty-and-sour pickled foods into your everyday diet helps you feel alive! On the other hand, an excessive amount of fermented foods (or of sour foods in general) can contribute to withered and wrinkled skin, as well as to fatigue.

Deep Frying

In deep frying, a food is typically (though not always) coated in a batter of flour and sometimes other ingredients and then completely immersed in very hot oil or fat. The coating of flour acts as insulation that holds heat in; upon contact with the hot oil, it forces a rapid influx of intense heat into the food. The food cooks rather quickly, as compared to other cooking methods. If done properly, the food contained within the batter absorbs little oil.

For the sake of easier digestion, deep-fried foods are served with a spicy dipping sauce to balance the fat. Fried foods of this nature produce a hot and damp condition that may be supportive to the individual who is tight, dry, and cold. For someone who is hot, sweaty, and heavy, this method of cooking may not be as supportive.

Fried foods can also be beneficial for people who are dry, lack a sense of humor, and lack emotional warmth. When eaten in excess, however, fried foods may produce cravings for stimulants, especially coffee and alcohol. These help to emulsify the excess fat from fried foods. In addition, one's skin may began to look and feel dirty and greasy. These symptoms are often accompanied by feelings of heaviness, depression, and cynicism. For health purposes, when frying, it is suggested to use heat-stable fats such as coconut oil, palm oil, lard, or other animal fats.

Baking

In baking, food is placed in an oven and surrounded by dry heat. When a food is surrounded by heat, it has the tendency to become dry; baked bread, cookies, and other flour products, and baking in general, tend to produce a dry or drying effect.

Most baked foods start out as a moist batter, or have water or oil added for additional moisture, before the baking process. A hot oven encloses the food and begins to evaporate its moisture (even if extra liquid has been added). Imagine sitting in a dry sauna. The longer you sit, the hotter and dryer you become. The peripheral body fluids evaporate almost as quickly as you perspire. Even if you add water to the sauna, the water quickly evaporates. Unlike food in an oven, you will get out of the sauna before you are truly done, but the food baked in an oven remains in the oven until it is *done*—in other words, *dry*. A baked food is "done" when much of the fluid evaporates and its body either softens and dries, or hardens and dries.

The consumption of large quantities of baked foods produces a desire for additional liquid. It seems as though nothing goes better with bread, cookies, or muffins than a cup or two of hot beverage. Baked foods crave moisture, and our internal environment has plenty of it.

Baked foods have a tendency to absorb internal body fluids to compensate for their own dryness, and this often results in digestive troubles and poor circulation.

The occasional use of baked foods for people with a wet condition can be beneficial; however, for people with a dry and wrinkled condition, this type of cooking may not be beneficial. Excessive eating of baked foods may contribute to a warm and dry condition.

Be Creative

There are many other types and styles of food preparation; through common sense and direct experience, you can get to know the potential effects of each one.

When eating a natural foods diet with whole grains, fresh vegetables, and naturally raised animal products, you may have a tendency to limit yourself to the easiest or most convenient forms of food preparation. Don't! Whole foods require you to be creative and imaginative in their preparation in order to appreciate and experience their full potential.

Variety *is* the spice of life! When it comes to how you prepare your food, variety in preparation is equally as important as a wide variety of foods.

PART IV

The Cast of Characters

21
A Symphony of Flora and Fauna

Part of getting to know foods includes knowing the larger families they come from and how those families interact with each other. This is not so different from the way you'd get to know other people.

In the chapters that follow, we'll get to know specific foods by becoming acquainted first with their general families and the personalities shared within those families, starting with the two most general: animals and plants.

The creative tension and interplay between the animal and plant realms is one of the several principal forces that animate the existence of life on earth. Several other major forces include the creative tension between other larger realms:

- plant and animal life as a whole and the simpler life forms of bacteria and viruses
- water (fluids) and minerals
- biological life and air
- matter and light

We human beings contain the creative tension of all these realms and their interactions within us, and they all come into play in our psychophysical selves through the process of nourishing ourselves.

For example, the preparation of food and the process of digestion both employ the rhythmic, balanced interchange of salts and fluids, and of matter and light (heat). Digestion, assimilation, and some forms of preparation (pickling) use the creative tensions of bacteria versus plant or animal, as does the process of digestion and absorption (our "internal cooking"). The oxidation of foods also merges the realms of biological life and air.

Most of our foods come from the larger families of plant and animal, so let's explore some of the correspondences between these two realms and how they relate to us as human beings.

Plant and Animal

The polarized qualities that distinguish plants and animals are expressed through their *opposite structures and functions*. The following examples are only a few of the many ways nature has set the stage for the symbiotic dance between flora and fauna—a dance of life that reveals much about the human species. I will not add any commentary to point this out specifically, but as you read each pair of characteristics, think for a moment about what implications these personality traits have for you and me as we eat these traits in our foods.

Mobility and Immobility

Plants are immobile and centered by their roots, which fix them to their environment. They are nourished through an essentially passive process by taking in their immediate environment: food comes to them and is absorbed through chemical functions (such as photosynthesis and osmosis).

Animals are mobile and centered by their nervous systems. They have a certain degree of freedom to roam and forage within their environment. Unlike a plant, whose particular needs exist within its immediate environment, an animal's life is largely dependent upon its mobility and motivation to function physically and actively, according to its instinctual needs.

Foods' Food Sources

The primary food sources of plants are light, carbon, hydrogen, nitrogen, oxygen, water, and minerals. Plants absorb and use these substances directly from their environment and then record them as nourishment into their tissues and cells. The survival of seeds and growing plants depends both on their individual ability to absorb and record these substances, and on the availability of these substances in the environment.

Animals' principal food sources consist of plants, insects, and other animals. Each animal ingests and records these substances through its nervous system to create its specific character. While animals obviously rely upon oxygen, water, and other basic environmental elements, they utilize and record into their nervous systems—*secondhand*—the first-hand experiences of the plant kingdom.

Growth Patterns

The growth patterns of plants are largely due to an *increase in the size* of their cells. By absorbing water and nutrients from the earth, plant cells increase primarily in size, and the plant develops accordingly. There are more varieties of plants on earth than there are varieties of animals.

Unlike plants, growth in animals (including humans) is largely due to the *multiplication* of cells in their bodies—in other words, by an increase in the *number* of their cells, rather than an increase in the size of each cell.

Material Substance

The basic material substance of plants is *carbohydrate*. This plant fuel is organized primarily by *chlorophyll*. Carbohydrate, a basic substance that energizes our body and cells, acts as fuel when ingested into the human body. The more complex the carbohydrate, the more concentrated the fuel source. Complex carbohydrates, as found in grains and beans, represent the most concentrated source of fuel, whereas simple sugars, as found in fruits and refined sweeteners, represent the most decentrated source of fuel in the world of edible plants.

The basic material substance of animals is *protein*. This substance is organized primarily by *nitrogen*. Protein acts as the prime body-building material and, when ingested into the human body, serves to build tissue and bulk.

Nitrogen, the motivating force of animal protein, is the relatively inert "silent majority" among gasses that make up the atmosphere, yet when contained, nitrogen becomes an explosive element. Thus, the con-centrated containment of nitrogen in animal tissue gives it a somewhat explosive tendency, making it highly energizing and stimulating to our metabolism through what is called thermogenesis.

Reproduction

The plant's reproductive process is external and unfolding. Once the seed of a plant sprouts, the plant reveals its whole sexual process: noth-ing is hidden except for the root of the plant.

The animal cycle of reproduction is a very private affair and takes place in the dark recesses of the animal's womb, in the case of mam-mals, and in an enclosed compartment of a shell, in the case of birds and reptiles.

Temperaments

Plants are *autotrophic* or self-nourishing organisms. Given the right materials by their environment, they can survive and flourish indepen-dent of other organisms.

Animals, on the other hand, are *heterotrophic,* meaning that they are nourished by and dependent on other organisms in order to survive.

22
A Matter of Meat

Throughout history, animal meats and animal organs have been used as an important part of quality-conscious approaches to food energetics. People have eaten animal flesh in varying proportions throughout the world for ages, and though there are large populations of both agrarian and hunter-gather peoples who have subsisted on high percentages of plant foods, when animal protein is in short supply many suffer from some form of malnutrition.

Whether you eat meats wild, free-range, factory-farmed (or none at all) is a choice you must make for yourself—a choice I trust you will make based on numerous considerations, and not by sentiment alone.

Historically, animal meats were prepared through the mediation of fire, dried, smoked, fermented, or consumed raw, among other traditional ways.

The most compliant of these methods are marinating, raw, steaming, and boiling. These methods served to impart a mild flavor to meats. On the other hand, the more dominant methods, often preferred because they bring out the strong flavors of meats, are grilling, broiling, frying, and roasting.

White meats, including pork, fish, and poultry, were thought to have activating qualities and were often suggested for those recovering from illness. On the other hand, red meats (beef, lamb, venison) were considered masculine and fit for robust heroes and warriors. In some chapters of history, they were considered one of the few foods fit for the gods.

While the most commonly consumed meat animals are cattle, chicken, turkey, goat, duck, pig, lamb, and fish, traditional cultures throughout the world also consume as staple foods alpaca, guinea pig, monkey, and many other animals that might seem exotic to those uninitiated to such traditional practices.

The actual meat, or muscle tissue, of animals serves two major functions for the animal: to move various parts of the animal's body, and to supply it with bulk.

Structural Variety

Meats of all types, compared to plant foods, are highly concentrated foods that pack their nutrition into small volumes. The three basic material substances of meat are water, protein, and fat, all of which vary in content depending on the cut, type, and animal. Contrary to popular belief, the protein and fat components from different animals are not all alike, nor do they act alike when absorbed and assimilated in the human body. A protein is *not* simply a protein—each animal has its own unique character, and this uniqueness permeates every part of the animal, including the quality of its protein and fat.

The structure of meat consists of long, thin cells of muscle tissue that are grouped in bundles and bound by thin, tough sheets of connective tissue that serve to hold them together.

Muscle fibers contain *actin* and *myosin,* two proteins called the "proteins of motion." When these two proteins receive the appropriate message from an animal's nervous system, they cause constriction or expansion in the muscles of the moving animal.

The textures of different meats—tough, flaky, chewy, etc.—are determined both by the length of fibers contained in the muscle tissue and by the thickness of the connective tissue. Mammals have muscles composed of very long fibers arranged in longitudinal bundles with thick connective tissue. These qualities make mammals' muscle fibers and connective tissue both longer and thicker than those of fish or chicken. Fish muscle has shorter fibers, separated by sheets of very thin connective tissue. This is why fish meat is more delicate than cow or chicken meat, and why chicken meat has a more delicate texture than cow meat but not as delicate as fish. Chicken muscle has medium length tissue relative to cow and fish.

The different textures of meats determine how a particular type of meat will energetically affect your muscular tissue when consumed. Beef will contribute to hotter, fuller, harder, and denser tissue in your body than the meat of chicken. Chicken, however, contributes to a tight, dry, warm, and spastic effect on your body tissue. Fish meat contributes to a weak, flaccid, and cool tissue condition compared to that produced by meat or chicken. However, red-fleshed fish, tuna, salmon, etc. have a warming and full effect on human tissue and muscle.

Color Variety

Animals have white meat, dark meat, or both, and the lightness or darkness affects the circulation of blood and body fluids in our muscles. As with humans, the blood of animals contains oxygen-carrying *hemoglobin,* the substance that gives blood its red color. Muscle cells also contain a substance called *myoglobin.* Unlike hemoglobin, which carries oxygen, myoglobin *stores* oxygen brought to it by the blood, and then supplies cells with oxygen when needed.

Meats with different colors vary with their concentrations of oxygen-carrying myoglobin. Animals whose muscles need a large quantity of oxygen have a greater storage capacity of oxygen than animals whose muscles need little. Therefore, animals with a greater storage capacity of oxygen (myoglobin) in their muscles have darker meat.

Muscles that are exercised regularly and strenuously need more oxygen than less active muscles. Chickens and turkeys use their legs more than their wings (some cannot even fly) and, as a result, their leg meat is dark and their breast meat, being less active muscle with less oxygen-storing myoglobin, is white. On the other hand, duck, pheasant, quail, and other more active birds generally have darker meat. Lamb and cow, both naturally grazing animals that tend to roam, have more oxygen-rich dark meat.

Dark and light meat also differ in the characteristics of their cellular makeup. This is largely due to the many forms of myosin, one of the basic muscle proteins existing in meat. Rather than get into a lengthy discussion about amino acids, proteins, and so on, suffice it is to say that the quantities and varieties of myosin, along with levels of hemoglobin found in different meats, determines the red or white of meat.

The basic characteristics of red and white cells found in dark and light meat are as follows:

Red Cells /Dark or Red Meat

Red cells are designed to meet the need for slower and more regulated muscle activity and are referred to as slow-twitch fibers. They specialize in burning fat as fuel, a process that requires large quantities of oxygen. These cells also contain more myoglobin and are well supplied with circulating blood.

Beef, lamb, venison, duck, goose, and the legs and wings of chicken are examples of dark meat.

Grass-fed beef ordinarily is a dark red color. However, due to the inactivity of many domesticated cattle through factory farming, their meat is typically quite pale in comparison to their more active natural counterparts. Consequently, commercial beef is often tainted with chemical dyes to give it a deeper color. Veal's meat is light pink to white, because veal calves are usually bred to be anemic.

White Cells/Light or White Meat

White cells are designed for quick, intermittent bursts of activity with long periods of rest. They are often called fast-twitch fibers. They specialize in burning carbohydrates and are capable of doing this in the absence of oxygen. They therefore contain less myoglobin than red cells and have a reduced supply of circulating blood, as compared to red cells.

Pork, domestic rabbit, frogs, chicken breasts, and turkey breasts are examples of white meat. However, natural free-ranging chickens and turkeys, as well as wild rabbit, have darker meat overall and are more active than their domestic counterparts. Modern pork is a good example of how factory farming has affected the quality of meat. Wild boar, the ancestor of the modern pig, is a very active animal and the meat of the boar is darker than its commercial counterpart, the pig.

Though white cells tend to burn the carbohydrate *glycogen* (often without the assistance of oxygen) as opposed to fat, this process often produces a residue of *lactic acid*. Lactic acid is a waste product that can accumulate and limit a cell's endurance. This is why white cells tend to work only in short and quick spurts. Animals that function in short spurts tend to have paler white meat.

Among fishes, the bottom feeders, along with less continuously active fish, have whiter meat and function with sudden, intermittent bursts of speed. On the other hand, aggressive and continuously active fish have darker meat.

Since white meats tend to burn and utilize carbohydrate (sugar) as fuel when metabolized, an excessive consumption of white meat can lead to strong sugar cravings in the person who eats it. On the other hand, an excessive consumption of fat-burning red meats can lead to strong fat cravings.

Light or Dark?

Many people still believe it is better to eat white meats rather than dark meats because of the proliferation of nutritional propaganda claiming that consuming saturated animal fats is harmful. Eating one and not the other because of fat content is not the issue; rather, you need to consider the energetic effects of different types of meat and how they will affect *you*.

Perhaps a more relevant matter, in terms of physical health, is the fact that consuming meats of *any* type is an issue of some qualitative concern, especially when considering the health of most commercially raised animals. Most food animals today are raised with their flesh drenched in obscene quantities of chemicals and preservatives. Nearly half the antibiotics manufactured in this country are poured into factory-farmed animals. Among mammals, especially beef and lamb, grass-fed and not grain-fed (grain is not a natural food for ruminants) are the best, along with free-range poultry, and have long proven to be healthy for humans.

Darker meats tend to have more fat and to utilize and store more oxygen. This gives dark meat the energetic properties of being more heat-producing and to generate a more consistent quality of energy than white meats as they metabolize in the human body. For a hot-natured personality, dark meat is obviously not a wise choice of meats to eat in large quantities.

Light meats, while lacking in oxygen, can yield a sudden spurt of energy—yet this sudden spurt may occur when you least expect it. When that spurt of energy does occur, respiration increases and the heart beats faster. This can lead to nervousness and strong or overly reactive impulses, as well as an increased need for oxygen intake.

Neither type of meat is "better" than the other; they produce different effects, including benefits and drawbacks, depending on one's individual temperament. The matter of meat, what kind, and how much is a matter of choice—yours.

EFFECTS OF DIFFERENT ANIMAL FOODS ON HUMAN BODY TISSUE AND MUSCLE

	Mammals	Poultry	Fish
Tissue Structure	long	medium	short
Temperament	hot	warm	cool
Excess Condition	full and firm	tight and inflexible	delicate and flaccid

	Red Meat	White Meat
Blood Cells	more red blood cells	more white blood cells
Oxygen Content	more oxygen	less oxygen
Type of Motion	slow-twitch fibers	fast-twitch fibers
Fuel	burns fat as fuel	burns carbohydrates as fuel

The Essence of Protein

Protein is the essential building material for the body. It is needed for growth, for tissue repair, to help heal wounds and fight infections, and for muscle definition.

Thermogenesis is a process that occurs when body cells increase their activities to facilitate digestion and assimilation. It is also the process of the production of heat in a human or animal body by physiological processes.

Protein-rich foods increase thermogenesis and thus create an energizing, stimulating, and warming effect in the body. Of the many possible sources of protein, red meat has the strongest thermogenic properties. Fats, especially saturated fats, also have strong thermogenic properties. Animal sources of fat also contain fat-soluble vitamins A and D, which are essential for assisting in the digestion and assimilation process of animal protein.

Some important components of animal protein include: fat, omega-3 fatty acids, CoQ_{10}, vitamin A, the entire B complex, B_{12}, B_6, zinc, iron, copper, and iodine.

Amino Acids

The building blocks of protein are called *amino acids* and are made up of carbon, hydrogen, nitrogen, and oxygen. There are twenty-two amino acids, twelve of which can be made by a healthy body; the other ten must be supplied by diet and therefore called essential. (They are actually *all* essential to health; strictly speaking, this term really means "essential to get in one's diet" or "dietarily essential.")

If one lacks a single essential amino acid, or if that essential amino acid is low in a particular food that is your only source for that amino acid, then your body will begin to break down its own muscle tissue, harvesting it to compensate for the deficiency. If it continues for extended periods, this compensation process can result in several deficiency problems, along with severe loss of muscle tone. This is why it is so important to be careful with diets low in complete sources of protein.

Amino acids also serve as a buffer for maintaining a normal pH of the intracellular fluid, so an imbalance in amino acids can easily lead to fatigue and overacidity.

Every source of protein has its own unique profile of amino acids that determines its nutritional value and individual identity. Many plant and animal sources contain all ten essential amino acids, but the precise ratios differ among plant and animal sources.

Unlike the amino acid profile of animal protein, which generally match or are fairly similar to human ratios, those occurring in plants are quite different from those in humans. Because of this, most plant proteins are considered "incomplete proteins" and need to be balanced with additional support from other plant protein sources having complementary amino acids or animal sources. One common traditional example of such complementing protein-source pairings is that of grains and beans. Animal protein, often considered "complete protein," has also served as a traditional accompaniment to grains and beans. When consumed together, these three sources of food make up the ideal balance of amino acids.

Amino Acid Cycle

The amino acid cycle represents how our human body transforms an alien (nonhuman) identity, through digestion and assimilation, into human tissue.

For example, a chicken is a form of protein with a very specific identity based on its amino acid profile that differs from a cow or any other animal or plant protein source. It is also different from our human tissue, yet when we choose to eat the chicken, our biochemistry has to remove the foreign character of the chicken (*substrate*) and transform it into human tissue. This is accomplished through several stages, through which the animal tissue is broken down and transformed.

The following steps are meant to show the basic process of this breakdown. Naturally, it is far more complex than this, but this will suffice to get the point across.

Disassembling the Protein's Identity
- A protein (substrate) is chewed and consumed.
- Our stomach's hydrochloric acid breaks down the protein into bonded chains of amino acids called *peptides*. When animal protein is consumed, the fibers are first broken down by an enzyme secreted by the pancreas called *elastase*.
- Further digestion, involving digestive enzymes in the small intestine, breaks down peptide bonds into singular chains of amino acids called *oligopeptides* that can then be absorbed into the system.

Configuring Stage

- After being absorbed, amino acids are distributed throughout the body to wherever they are needed; others form a pool for cells of organs and tissue to draw from.
- The pool must be well stocked with the ten essential amino acids. If one is missing or is used up before the others, certain proteins will not be formed properly; the process of configuring amino acids into the human blueprint will be incomplete and therefore will cease until the pool can be properly restocked.
- Unused amino acids are converted into energy and burned up or stored as fat.

We humans must be able to disassemble the protein identity of a plant or animal and then reassemble it into our own tissue's blueprint. This is done by the protein source giving up the form given it by nature.

For example, in the African savanna, when a lion hunts and consumes an antelope, the antelope is digested and assimilated into the lion. The lion does not *become* the antelope, because the lion instead transforms the identity of the antelope into that of the lion. Does the lion take on some of the essence and qualities of the antelope? Of course, just as the antelope has now become the lion's flesh. The antelope is the essence of the lion's flesh.

When you eat that free-range healthy chicken, it too becomes you—and to some degree, you become it: you take on qualities of that chicken. Like the lion's antelope, your chicken is something the human digestive tract has been transforming into vital human tissue for thousands of years, and the same goes for other naturally raised or wild animal sources. However, when you eat that factory-farmed chicken that is riddled with bone disease and laden with antibiotics, hormones, and other toxic substances, you also transform *that* animal—and all that it is—into your flesh and blood. This foreign invader is *not* something that has been supporting the integrity of the human species for very long—and it will have a very different effect on your blood and tissue than a healthy version of the same animal.

Since proteins differ in nutritional value based on their amino acid composition and other factors, it is extremely important that you choose the best quality with which to nourish yourself. Also, the transformation of food into human tissue is largely dependent on your personal digestive fire. Therefore, both vital digestion and a healthy, varied diet help to remove a protein's foreign character and assemble it into our likeness.

Because of a lack of adequate digestive fire, people really *are* becoming what they eat. Toxic chemicals, trans fats, and other nonfood substances have a way of putting out the fire of life.

The Wild and the Domestic

There are two categories of land animals humans have traditionally eaten: animals existing in their natural habitant (*wild animals*) and *domesticated food animals*.

The wild varieties of fowl, deer, rabbit, and other creatures have a distinct advantage that sets them apart qualitatively from their domestic counterparts: they are *free to choose and adapt to their environment,* an environment naturally suited for them, where nature supplies all the raw materials for their survival.

Survival and the will to live are the strongest energetic factors available to humans through the embodiment of these particular animals. Adaptability to nature, instinct, and keen senses are additional energetic properties reinforced and imprinted on our nervous systems through our food relationships with wild animal foods.

Each wild animal embodies the total sum of its surroundings. When you eat a wild animal, you too embody the total sum essence of the animal's character and environment. These qualities are recorded into your human nervous tissue and cells. If you choose to consume these animals, the natural law of balance requires active physical interaction with the natural environment through some form of exercise or work.

The second category of animals traditionally consumed for thousands of years is pastured, naturally raised animals. These animals are superior as a food source as compared to the toxin-laden flesh of factory-farmed animals, a class of animals that should be minimized or eliminated from any healthy diet. Just as your plant foods should ideally be organically or biodynamically grown, so too should your animal products be raised in a natural, traditional way.

These days, followers of exclusively plant diets often preach about the association of eating the flesh of animals with anger, irritability, and elevated sensual passions. However, among traditional peoples, meat has been associated with strength, courage, bravery, and a psychological sense of earthly realism.

Followers of meatless diets also unjustly claim superiority above meat eaters in their cleanliness, devotion, compassion, and spiritual idealism. But realistically, while a diet heavy in meat has its share of drawbacks, so, too, can a meatless diet. For many, a meatless diet can result in various forms of malnourishment as well as feelings of instability, fanaticism, and unrealistic idealism. (Not to put too fine a point on it, but Adolph Hitler was, after all, a vegetarian.)

While there may very well be a human predisposition toward consuming plant foods, animal flesh has historically been consumed throughout the world in moderate quantities. In modern times, many people following experimental nonanimal diets for any length of time have found they are unable to process their food completely without some form of animal protein.

Meat takes longer to digest and is digested more slowly than carbohydrates, yet contrary to the claims of some, it is not *harder* to digest than plant foods. If it is of good quality, meat can be digested completely, with a minimum of waste. Alone, meat is not a complete food, but then neither is any other food "complete," in terms of fulfilling all of your nutritional requirements.

Like any other food, meat is complete only in the sense of what it is, which is simply a choice—yours—and one that requires the responsibility of making additional choices of foods and activities that will balance it.

By the Hand of Man

A third category of land-animal foods with a brief history includes those of the factory-farmed domesticated order: cows, chickens, turkeys, ducks, sheep, and pigs, etc.

The *quality* of these industrialized, often genetically manipulated creatures differs greatly from both their ancestors of wild descent and the original, naturally raised domesticated species of millennia past. Not only are these inactive creatures 20 to 30 percent higher in fat than their naturally raised counterparts, but these poor souls have also lost much of their survival instincts and will to live. Their environment is chosen and constructed by man for his own convenience and indulgence. The energetic properties of these mutants are but troubled ghosts of the animals that once were.

Another qualitative difference between naturally raised and factory-farmed animals can be found in the important nutritional component of omega-3 fatty acids. For example, grass-fed beef has a fatty acid profile similar to that of wild game. The body fat of an animal is a reflection of its food, just as it is with us. Grain is not a natural food for cattle; therefore, grain-fed cattle tend to be higher in fat and less active than pastured cattle. Some feedlot cattle have been found to have little to no omega-3 fatty acids. It is said that the ideal ratio of omega-6 to omega-3 fatty acids is about 4:1. While pastured beef is close to this, factory-farmed cattle can be anywhere from 17:1 to 25:1.

Through overcrowding, deprivation of proper food, improper sanitation, inadequate ventilation, and drug dependency—all components of modern agribusiness—humans have produced mutated strains of livestock with energetic qualities that can only be compared to the insensitive people who created them and those who support the continuation of this madness.

The Cartesian principle, when applied to farm animals, implies that animals are not aware of their emotions and feelings, and therefore are not actual beings—only dumb nutrient sources. This attitude prevails in much of the livestock industry, and it is this very thinking that continues to inspire the distorted minds of the scientists and farmers who indulge in the tortuous and unspeakable acts of physical and genetic manipulation of modern livestock.

Most people tend to view animal foods as sources of protein and other nutritional factors. But there is much more to these creatures than meets the analytical mind's eye. The hidden *qualities* of these creatures, which cannot be seen but can be *known,* include all the experiences of each animal in its environment. Every experience, from birth to slaughter, is recorded in each and every animal's nervous system and cells to produce the *quantity* we see in domesticated chickens, cows, pigs, and the rest.

Support natural agriculture and pastured animals as our traditional food sources and avoid, as much as possible, the alternatives—for they truly are poor excuses for food.

23
A Chicken in Every Pot

King Henry IV of France first coined this familiar phrase in the sixteenth century, a time when chicken was a luxury available only to the rich. Hank claimed he would make France so prosperous that on Sundays, the food of the rich would appear in *everyone's* kitchen. In 1928, America's Republican party adopted "A chicken in every pot" as their slogan. And sure enough, since then, the chicken has become the most widely eaten meat in America.

The human/chicken relationship goes back thousands of years, with origins reportedly in India or China. It all began with a feisty wild red jungle fowl, the ancestor of the Brahman, the Leghorn, the Jersey, the Rhode Island Red, and all the other modern varieties of chickens.

The wild red was originally found in forests gathered in groups of five to twelve birds. They lived in trees and ate small animals and various seed plants. At first, eating the wild red was thought barely worth the effort because the little bird had so little flesh, and what there was of it was tough and dry.

The domestication of this variety of chicken began about five thousand years ago. The wild red was first raised as a source of meat and only later for its eggs. Some contemporary varieties of chicken are exclusively meat birds, while others make superior egg layers. It is interesting to note that only two hundred years ago, domestic chickens would lay from six to twelve eggs per year! By 1870 farmers had managed to increase production to eighty per year, and by 1950, to 120. Today, with modern methods, this figure has doubled.

Many people accustomed to eating factory-farmed chickens find the meat of natural free-running chickens lean and not very succulent. However, those who prefer to eat the real thing find the lean earthy flavor unmatched by any commercial wannabe.

When a food becomes as universally popular as the chicken has, it inevitably goes through some serious changes—and the chicken is no exception. The present-day, genetically altered, mass-produced version of the chicken has got to be one of the most lethal foods one can consume—in many ways, more lethal than factory-raised beef (its runner-up in the animal food popularity contest). Let's take a closer look at this most unusual creature's energetic qualities and its connections to human psychology and physiology. Please note that while some of the descriptions that follow apply to the nature of chickens in general, most are specifically describing the genetically altered, factory-farmed, and confined chicken that graces our supermarkets and fast-food chains.

A New Breed of Bird

Chickens have vastly different eating patterns than humans and other animals, for a number of reasons. For one thing, they have a different digestive structure. They do not have teeth, nor do they have compartmentalized stomachs in which to digest their food. When they eat, food passes down into a narrow gizzard, where it is ground up for digestion.

Also, the majority of chickens in America are housed in total confinement, and this results in boredom eating. These birds are generally incapable of making major distinctions concerning food, and will eat just about anything they come across, much like many humans who consume excessive quantities of this mutated version of a chicken.

Factory-farmed chickens spend 75 percent (or more) of their time eating and drinking. Such an obsessive need to satisfy an oral fixation is often the result of malnutrition and lack of exercise, and can energetically manifest in humans who eat these birds as hypoglycemia, overeating, hypermetabolism, and constriction of the stomach, which in turn can show up emotionally as irritability and anger. Chickens tend to be noisy and nervous animals, especially when their food supply is limited.

Chickens will peck instinctively at anything and are particularly fond of shiny and shimmering objects like gold and silver. Chickens also have a habit of scratching and clawing the ground in search of food. These traits can manifest in humans as agitation and obsession.

Confined chickens become carnivorous animals; when overcrowded or bored, they frequently resort to cannibalism. They have a strong attraction to blood and when blood is drawn from one bird (which often results, for example, from feather-picking by one or more chickens), the whole flock will often pick each other apart in a frenzy. This alarmingly aggressive behavior has become so common in factory-raised chickens that it has led to debeaking, a process of trimming the beaks with machines.

Chickens also have a tendency to eat their own eggs or the eggs of other unwitting brood hens. In fact, self-mutilation is common among confined chickens: they often pick at themselves aggressively and then, at the sight of their own blood, begin literally to destroy themselves.

These cannibalistic qualities manifest in humans as food indulgences and compulsive eating disorders, where anything and everything in sight is gobbled down in a vain attempt to satisfy emotional needs or physical malnutrition. Cannibalism and self-mutilation also energetically manifest in human emotions and can show up in behavior when a person avoids intimate relationships for lack of self-trust and fear of being abused, or in the opposite case, when a person willingly indulges in abusive relationships in which he or she dominates or is dominated by another.

Other qualities derived from these captive pseudobirds' bizarre behavioral patterns can include poor self-image, anorexia, emotional instability, and utter disregard for taking care of one's appearance and health. These can in turn lead to further self-destructive patterns on many levels.

Isn't it amazing how one food, altered from its original form, can so strongly affect our psychophysical nature? And here is the really fascinating part of it all: for the most part, psychologists don't even *consider* our daily food an influential factor in our psychology!

With mass production comes the need for rapid growth. Through modern technology, commercial chickens are forced to grow so fast that their heart muscles cannot keep up with the growth of their body tissue. This results in something called ascites: the resulting heart failure is preceded by dehydration and respiratory failure and ends up costing the poultry industry up to $500 billion a year.

These industrial hybrid chickens reach adulthood and are ready for processing at between forty and fifty days from birth; they are the most processed of all animals bred. A free-range chicken, on the other hand, takes five to six months to reach adulthood.

Again, I want to emphasize the point that these extreme influences are from mutant chickens resulting from an extremely tampered-with environment, and not from free-ranging, naturally raised chickens. These latter, by the way, derive up to 30 percent of their nourishment from grass, and they are rarely sick. They do not produce this bizarre range of negative and even destructive effects.

Why such a drastic difference between the two types of chicken?

Animals, like people, are at their best when free to enjoy a natural life. While most modern humans have a tendency to be detached from their relationship with nature, animals harbor no such illusion. It is only through humans that animals are cut off from their natural lifestyles; when removed from their natural environment, they become physically and mentally ill.

Consuming unhealthy animals raised in suppressive environments results in the human nervous system recording all those negative qualities of those animals. Because factory-farmed chickens, loaded with antibiotics and suffering from numerous diseases, are among the most popularly and quantitatively consumed foods today, the effects of this "food" on consumers are also among the most obvious.

A Class Act: The Pecking Order

Chickens have a "pecking order" wherein the stronger dominates the weaker. The cock or rooster represents the stronger, the family man endowed with sexual vitality and pride.

The cock is an alarmist. He is very suspicious and paranoid, qualities also shared by hens.

A single cock usually has many partners and will vigorously impose his authority over them at any time. At his convenience, a cock can grip any one of his submissive hens by the neck, hold her down and proceed to have intercourse with her until he is satisfied, which doesn't take very long. If male chauvinism is a learned behavior, perhaps it is learned by human males from their dinners-in-a-bucket.

Roosters have been known to attack humans, especially if the human interferes with the rooster's harem of hens. Even then, the rooster generally will not attack the human head on, but will wait until the person's back is turned.

The cockfight, where two cocks are placed together to do battle until one or the other drops dead, is one of man's oldest extant sports. Cocks are naturally aggressive and love to fight. But cocks-as-jocks may be a dwindling resource. In large hatcheries, about 99 percent of newborn cocks are either crushed or suffocated and then fed to other livestock. I guess roosters become dispensable when we have men to do their job.

The hen also has her own pecking order. One of her basic priorities is to develop a sense of social order and her individual place within it. However, when chickens are factory farmed, the resultant overcrowding prevents them from exercising this tendency. This leads to claustrophobia and often to madness.

While she can be very motherly to her flock of chicks—who incidentally have no use for fathers—mother hen can be very bossy and domineering to her young, which she begins laying when she reaches the age of about six months. Like the rooster, she too is promiscuous and indiscriminate in her sex life. Within her pecking order, the stronger hen can dominate and demand submission from the rest of the flock.

This process works its way down the line, with the slightly weaker hens dominating the even weaker, all the way down to the frail and weakest. When newcomers are introduced into the pecking order, it can result in violent battles with much bloodshed. The stronger of the pecking order are the first to get food, and the weaker often die of starvation—or are eaten by the stronger.

Such a pecking order exists among other farm animals as well, but nowhere does it exist as strongly as it does among chickens—except perhaps among humans.

Racism, prejudice, inferiority and superiority complexes, and war-mongering are some of the attitudes that sprout from the human pecking order. Lower class, middle class, upper class, high school cliques . . . all have their pecking orders, and they have been around for a long time. It is a learned behavior that most of us were brought up with and that too many have learned to accept.

Were Darwin alive today, he might say that this is "normal behavior" and not learned. But witness the young child who has not been taught prejudice and racism; that child easily enjoys the company of black, white, Asian, or Hispanic children as playmates. Obviously, this is a sociological issue that has been debated for years. Suffice it to say that through the years, the human pecking order has become increasingly more aggressive and violent. So have the pecking orders of factory-farmed chickens and other farm animals.

Coincidence?

Or is it possible that the increased consumption and poor quality of modern, domesticated animal foods may be having a deeper influence on human social behavior than most people realize?

A Nation Cooped Up

My observation is that the social structure of man-woman relationships, especially in America, is strongly influenced, if not actually based upon, the social and pecking order of chickens. The man represents the stronger of the sexes, the provider, the authoritarian, and the head of the household. The woman is supposed to represent purity, to be submissive and hardworking at her tasks at home . . . the stereotypical feminine path to righteousness. While there are exceptions among individuals and families, the fowl air of a poultriarchal society still forms a blanket that covers and permeates the nervous tissue of many relationships.

The family unity that once existed at the dinner table, when a free-range whole roast chicken, turkey, or goose was carved and served, has gradually been replaced by the serving of an inferior product consisting of precarved parts or frozen and processed bits of something that vaguely resembles—yet is not even close to being—a real chicken.

The care and attention given to the preparation of chicken as a main course by great-grandma certainly did impart, in those who participated in her feast of fowl and fixin's, the energetics of a healthy, free-running animal that seasoned lively conversation with humorous anecdotes.

Now, however, the fast-food industry offers their fare of chicken fragments, seasoned with hormones and chemicals, to dismembered families. Mealtime communication—devoid of any listening—revolves around the plague of disease spiced and garnished with arguments about being right.

Light and cool air make for lively chickens. The lack of these, along with numerous antibiotics used to control disease, has served to weaken chickens and increase the strength of pathogenic bacteria. In poultry, as in humans, bacteria and viruses are having a field day in modern society. Indeed, they are just about the only species getting stronger, instead of weaker. They build up resistance to the antibiotics, and this creates the need for more research into disease control by those specialists who have fallen prey to their own beliefs. Finally, people ingest all of these disease-related factors. The result of consuming this mutated, medicated life form has further resulted in nonthinking beings with immunological weaknesses and the inability to resist the social disease of control and domination.

A far cry from Grandma's Sunday dinner!

Hen House or Nut House?

Like other birds, chickens have a natural tendency to preen themselves. However, among modern chickens this becomes an obsession rather than a natural act. It can manifest in humans as an obsession with looking good, the kind of pattern where you take extensive care of your outward appearance, yet pay little attention to the inner quality of health. The "lookin'-good" obsession has people attempting to mask or cover up their true feelings and appearance with the heavy use of cosmetics, clothes shopping, and compulsive washing, cleaning, deodorizing, and disguising.

Confined chickens tend to be hysterical. The reactions of one or two birds, when many are housed together, can be magnified to create a chain reaction that results in mass hysteria. They cannot adapt to spontaneous or sudden changes in their environment and when these occur, they can evoke mass panic, leading to feather picking, piling, and cannibalism. These hysterical and panicky reactions manifest in humans as the inability to withstand criticism, loud emotional outbursts, nervous breakdowns, hyperactivity, emotional instability, lack of self-control, stubbornness, verbal rambling, and an obsession with details.

Chickens are normally very active and alert. They need room to move. When given the opportunity to stay together in groups or enjoy an open run, most prefer the latter. This kinetic energy manifests in humans as the constant need to be doing something, usually away from their immediate environment, where they find difficulty relaxing. In relationships, it can manifest as one not wanting to settle down until everything in the relationship meets one's ideal of perfection.

Factory chickens have a rather funny way of shaking their heads from side to side while pacing back and forth with a look of intense frustration. This—along with the sudden death syndrome (also called the "flip over syndrome"), where a chicken will suddenly flip over onto its back and expire from an acute cardiac arrest—is a sign of extreme stress and a frayed nervous system. These traits are manifested in humans as rapid heart palpitations; an inability to cope with work or stressful situations; sexual frustration; severe premenstrual difficulties; and feelings of hopelessness, defeat, and despair.

Fowl Play

Some common physical problems associated with caged chickens are breast blisters, foot problems, osteoporosis (bone weakness) and especially viral diseases. These manifest in human physiology the same way they do in chickens.

Studies have shown that chickens lacking in adequate nutrition, particularly minerals, are prone to osteoporosis, which results in fragile bones. If they have this problem and you eat them regularly, it becomes your problem. The problem of osteoporosis has a deeper origin than being solely a deficiency of calcium, and the remedy for this rapidly growing problem does not lie in simple calcium supplementation.

Hens begin their lives with paired ovaries—but as the bird ages, its right ovary withers away. Interestingly, this has shown up as a characteristic among women who routinely indulge in chicken as their primary animal food.

People who consume large quantities of commercial chicken usually have pale, white skin with red or pink blotches on the face and around the neck. Their facial features appear pinched and their eyes have an intense and often a scowling appearance.

At this point you might be saying to yourself, "Doesn't he have anything nice to say about these poor creatures?" No, I do not have anything nice to say about factory-farmed chickens—and I haven't even mentioned half of their negative traits, such as: they are almost all drug addicts, and many carry the deadly salmonella bacteria as well as various viruses.

However, again, all of the above applies primarily to the modern, thoroughly colonized, and brutalized factory-farmed chicken—a distorted caricature of the real, normal chicken—indeed the product of modern foul play.

Real chickens share some of these basic personality traits and have their nobler compensating traits as well.

A real chicken, as I mentioned above, is quite a bit leaner (and in fact *not* meaner) than the poor inmate chicken.

This real chicken has a warm and dry effect on the body and can be beneficial for those lacking in energy and motivation. Like other animal foods, it offers many health benefits; its negative traits are so commonly pronounced primarily because it is one of the animal foods most commonly eaten repetitiously, often to the exclusion of all others.

If you should notice in yourself or in someone else the qualities of control freak, panic attacks, OCD, loud emotional outbursts . . . you will most likely find an ample consumption of factory-farmed chicken, too.

Fortunately, there are conscious farmers who feed their chickens organic quality food and let them run free to forage for insects. And in the world of chickens, that makes all the difference.

24
Birds of Another Feather

While chicken is by far the most popular type of poultry consumed today, there are many other birds that are commonly eaten throughout the world, including those that live on land and those that are adapted to water.

Turkey

Turkey was a traditional food of the ancient Mayan civilization going back at least three thousand years. Today Mayan descendants still enjoy the meat of this large bird in preparations that utilize many of the same herbs and spices handed down from their ancestors. In Guatemala and throughout South and Central America, one can still see wild turkeys roaming freely among the ancient Mayan ruins.

Many of the characteristics of factory-farmed turkeys are equivalent to those of chickens. They tend toward cannibalism, when nervous they scratch themselves until they bleed, and so on. Turkeys are very paranoid (more easily frightened than chickens) and, as turkey farmers will readily attest, they are incredibly stupid. Turkeys tend to pile (stack themselves on top of each other when frightened or nervous) and, like chickens, are prone to panic attacks. Older birds, especially, tend to panic and suffocate themselves by pressing themselves together out of fear.

In the recent past, turkeys were bred to have larger breasts so as to meet the demand of consumers. But this experiment didn't work so well: they had such large breasts that they toppled over when they tried to walk—so it was back to the drawing board.

Modern turkeys are not exactly sexual acrobats. In fact, the large commercial brand of turkeys have such little sexual prowess that coition has to be replaced by human intervention.

Turkeys are very sensitive to drafts and dampness and will catch cold easily if their feet get wet. They are large birds and do not have much endurance when it comes to long-distance flying, usually traveling in short spurts before landing to rest. They also tend to have visual problems, which makes it difficult for them to find feed and water. Apparently, turkeys are the hardest poultry to raise: not only do they need plenty of space in which to run, but wild turkeys also spend a good amount of time in the woods.

While they are similar in many ways, turkeys and chickens do not get along together.

Energetically, like chicken but even more so, turkey may contribute to claustrophobia, nervousness, and eye problems, especially twitching, redness, and an imbalance between the two eyes that can affect one's depth perception.

Because factory-farmed turkeys have a difficult time finding food and water, they become very dependent upon their caretakers. This may manifest in humans as emotional dependency, memory loss, and difficulty in understanding and meeting one's nutritional requirements. Contrast this with naturally raised free-range turkeys. They are self-sufficient, powerful birds that can derive up to 40 percent of their food from foraging.

Turkey meat tends to be dry (though less so in factory-farmed turkeys) and the darker meat can be sinewy. Turkey has a warm and dry nature, and wild or free-range turkey can be beneficial for those who suffer from hyperactivity, loose muscle tone, body heaviness, and racing thoughts that interfere with one's ability to concentrate.

Once a traditional and regular source of protein for Native Americans, free-range turkey is now consumed less often and in far smaller quantity than most other domestic fowl. And while there are no valid reasons for this, it has become an occasional food for most people, relegated to holidays and special occasions.

Ostrich

Now gaining in popularity as a food source, ostrich actually has a long history as a food source in parts of Africa and other parts of the world. It was a symbol of virility among the Egyptians and Romans. Like most other fowl, ostrich is now raised for both meat and eggs.

As a source of meat, ostrich is about halfway between beef and poultry: dark but tender due to short muscle fibers. It is easy to digest, low in fat, and high in minerals, especially iron and phosphorus. Ostrich eggs are an excellent source of protein but if serving one, it would be wise to have several guests to join you, as one ostrich egg is equal to twenty-four hen eggs.

The ostrich is the largest living bird, and though it cannot fly it can run up to forty-five miles per hour with great endurance. One might think the ostrich would be shortsighted due its brain being the size of a pea, but it has perfect eyesight with a cornea that is similar in size and shape to a human's.

Its natural habitat is deserts and savannas and it is strong enough to endure cold and snow, but they dislike rain and high humidity. Ostrich is a superb warming food beneficial for increasing strength and stamina.

Waterfowl: Ducks and Geese

Almost all ducks are descended from the mallard of the northern hemisphere. Asian peoples, particularly the Chinese, Thais, and Japanese, kept ducks in their wild state for thousands of years. Ducks provide these people with superb table fare, eggs, and down (fluffy feathers used for pillow stuffing).

Ducks also offer entertainment and friendship: they make good pets. In fact, the most pronounced distinction between waterfowl and chickens and turkeys is that waterfowl have much more lively, distinct personalities.

Ducks and geese are more hardy, less disease-prone, and much more alert and intelligent than chickens and turkeys. Most wild ducks carry only about half the weight of domestic varieties. When properly cared for, ducks can live up to twenty years, and geese up to forty years. They can easily forage for much of their own food, are more adaptable, and, unless disturbed (for they are a bit high-strung), are quieter than chickens and turkeys. Females honk with a harsh, loud quack, and the males tend to belch with a soft throaty quack.

Geese are the hardiest of all poultry, as well as the most disease-resistant. They are excellent foragers and can pretty much take care of themselves. In Scotland, the famous Ballantine distillery is guarded and patrolled nightly not by dogs, but by geese; according to the owners, the birds are very effective in their role as watch geese.

Domestic geese have about 50 percent more meat and fat on them than wild ones. This, of course, is due to confinement, quality of feed, and a lack of activity.

Both ducks and geese demonstrate some selectivity in mating. Ducks are basically polygamous, while geese tend to be monogamous and mate for life, though this does not always hold true. Mating may take place every year, or it may occur once and last the lifetime of the bird. The ratio of drakes (male ducks) to ducks can average one to six. Among ducks, it is the female who decides and chooses who her mate will be. Among geese, the mating and the sexual act are community affairs that include the entire flock in a noisy honking celebration. Flocks of geese are very tight-knit and do not like newcomers. Like those of chickens, their one working left ovary generates the eggs of waterfowl.

Female ducks tend to be good mothers, while drakes prefer to be anonymous when it comes to family life. On the other hand, ganders (male geese) are especially proud and protective of their young.

Within hours after hatching, a learning behavior called "imprinting" occurs among waterfowl. Imprinting is sort of an absolute form of what humans call "bonding"—the first moving object they see automatically becomes Mom to the youngsters. Whatever or whoever it is, it is imprinted in young waterfowl and becomes the object of their affection until the day they die. Because of this it is not unusual for waterfowl to form strong friendship bonds to dogs, cows, and other animals they are raised around.

Waterfowl do not peck like chickens. They do establish themselves in a sort of pecking order, but it is more dignified and peaceful than chickens. Ducks and particularly geese can be aggressive, though not usually among their own kind, except when it comes to protecting their mates or young, or if they are overcrowded. They can be intimidated easily and when firmly confronted, are well prepared to retreat. Being quite a bit more intelligent than other fowl, ducks and geese know how to carry a grudge and will let their owners know it, especially if their living conditions are not up to par.

Waterfowl tend to be restless at night. They sleep when they are tired and are active when they're not. When confined, they are prone to nervous breakdowns, which can occur from sudden disturbances that overstimulate them. Both ducks and geese prefer to lay their eggs at night or early morning hours, and they prefer seclusion when doing so. Ducks can go without water overnight, provided they do not eat. If they eat without a supply of water, they can easily choke to death on their feed.

Unlike turkeys and chickens, ducks do not pile and suffocate each other when frightened or suddenly startled; rather, they will either huddle or run around in circles. They also are very sensitive to changes in weather and become especially noisy and nervous well before most humans might sense a storm is brewing. They prefer to be outside in their natural environment, even in severe weather. They love water, yet are just as comfortable on land, and this gives them the edge of being more flexible and adaptable than other fowl. If deprived of water in which to swim and play, they will stand around looking depressed and sullen. Being naturally adapted to a water environment, they tend to eat their food (which is primarily composed of vegetable matter with a small percent of animal matter) moistened. They are proud creatures and preening, usually after a swim, is very important to them. They enjoy looking good, yet unlike chickens, do not get obsessive about it.

Energetically, these creatures can produce some unusual qualities in the human condition. Their tendency to huddle when frightened can contribute to a seeking of like minds, sympathetic and understanding to one's problems or troubles. However, this can also result in recruiting friends or relatives to rationalize one's beliefs or sense of self-righteousness and pride.

When confused or disturbed, waterfowl tend to run frantically in circles, and as the danger subsides so do they, with a gradual slowing down in order to calm down. Energetically, this can manifest in strong outward emotional reactions, where one gradually comes to his senses with feelings of embarrassment and wonder concerning his own reaction and how other people might have perceived it. A waterfowl's sense of pride and family manifests as commitment to friends and family, yet in the extreme, it may result in prejudice toward anyone outside of one's chosen clique or group.

People who eat excessive quantities of waterfowl have a strong sense of pride and posture, often holding their bodies in a poised stance, standing or sitting very straight with heads held high. Many have thick protruding lips, which they continuously moisten with their tongues. They usually have lean bodies with slightly oily skin.

Ducks and geese have dark meat and their meat has the warmest effect on the human body of all fowl. Its nature is warm and damp. Duck or goose can be supportive for people who suffer from depression, inactivity, or water retention.

There are many other types of fowl used as traditional foods throughout the world, all of them highly nutritious and each with its own unique energetic qualities. The hearty pheasant and the tiny quail, the partridge, grouse, and pigeon have long been part of traditional cuisines where they have supported robust health for generations.

Pheasant, Quail, and Other Game Birds

Wild birds are also popular foods throughout the world. Though quail have an aversion to flying, when in their natural environment they are migratory birds, muscular in stature and capable of rapid flight for short bursts.

Quail are often compared to pheasant because, while they both are able to fly, they also share a suicidal habit of running instead of flying when trying to flee danger. It takes much energy to fly in quick short spurts, so much so that hunters know that if they can startle a group of quail two to three times, the birds will be so exhausted that the hunter can literally walk over to them and pick them up by hand.

Quail are one of the most monogamous of feathered game. They are also belligerent little creatures, and this is probably why quail fighting has been a popular sport for centuries. Being small birds with delicate and tender meat, they are often served in pairs in many restaurants that carry such fare.

In the Middle Ages, the pheasant was a bird of nobility, a royal bird crowned the king of feathered game and considered by the upper classes too good a food for commoners. Pheasant is a beautiful bird with brilliant plumage that somewhat resembles that of the peacock (a member of the same family). The male and the female have similar plumage; however, the female has drab camouflage feathers until after her incubation period is over, and only then develops her brilliant plumage. Needless to say, she ages gracefully (unless caught and eaten).

Pheasant is the most widely eaten and considered by many the finest-flavored game bird. It is also the most digestible, with a distinctly delicious flavor to its flesh. The hen is slightly smaller than the cock and has a more delicate yet equally delicious flavor.

The grouse is pretty much a ground bird, but can fly very fast for short distances.

The guinea fowl, though mostly raised on farms, still retain much of its dark flesh and gamey taste. They prefer to perch themselves on the uppermost branches of tall trees and come down only to forage food. While many wild game birds lay one clutch a year, guinea fowl will often lay their eggs, which they hide in the ground, continuously from spring through to cold weather. They are noisy birds and remarkably free of disease.

Other game birds include numerous varieties of water and marsh fowl. Game birds offer unique energetic qualities according to the type and character of bird, but in general, all are highly energizing, uplifting foods that assist in stimulating metabolism and motivating anyone feeling down, sluggish, or recovering from debilitating illness.

25
Living on the Egg

Eggs are the counterpart of seeds and are designed to support the survival and continuity of their species, whether of birds, reptiles, or fish. Eggs represent the as yet unfulfilled potential of a living, breathing creature with a nervous system. An egg is the whole animal concentrated to its maximum potential. It is the female reproductive cell awaiting fertilization by the male of the species.

While eggs from various animals are eaten throughout the world, the chicken egg is almost without competition. Chicken eggs are widely considered one of the most versatile foods available. They have the unique ability to bind with other ingredients; they can be used to form light, delicate foam for meringues; they can be used in baked products of many varieties, and dressings and batters; and are without a doubt the most popular breakfast food for many in the modern world.

Hens are born with several thousand immature egg cells in their single functioning ovary. Some will lay only a small number of eggs in their lifetime, but if their eggs are removed from the nest, many hens will continue to lay indefinitely. A rooster does not determine how many eggs a hen will lay—hens don't need roosters to lay eggs. A rooster only determines whether or not a hen's eggs will be fertile.

The shell of a hen egg contains about 95 percent calcium carbonate, with about 4 percent protein. The calcium contained in the shell is concentrated into the shell through extraction from the hen's bones. The yolk contains about 50 percent water, 34 percent fats and related substances, and 16 percent protein. The yolk contains most of the egg's cholesterol, vitamin A, omega-3, and iron. The egg white consists mostly of water with about 10 percent albumin, a protein used as a standard to measure the value of other protein sources. Eggs can be a good source of omega-3 fatty acids, if the hens that lay them are free-range. The ideal ratio of omega-6 to omega-3 fatty acids is 4:1; eggs from free-range chickens can average 3:1, while those of factory-farmed chickens average much higher in omega-6, often with ratios as high as 20:1.

Duck eggs are the second most widely consumed egg. They have a rather strong, robust flavor along with a slightly oily taste. Duck eggs have been an essential part of the traditional Chinese diet for so long that carbonized pickled duck eggs have been found in archaeological sites dated at thousands of years old.

Duck and goose eggs have different incubation periods than those of chickens. Mallard-derived ducks hatch at the end of twenty-eight days (as do turkeys), Muscovy ducks at the end of thirty-five days, and geese at the end of thirty days. Ducks and geese lay larger eggs (with proportionately bigger yolks) than chickens, and they normally produce more eggs in a year. They also have a heavier effect on the body than do chicken eggs. Several other eggs have long been consumed throughout history. For example, the tiny quail egg is a popular food in some parts of the world, as is the giant ostrich egg.

Fish eggs of numerous types have served as an essential and nutritious part of creative Japanese cuisine, and are consumed by every other coastal culture throughout the world. Varieties of caviar have long been thought to have aphrodisiac qualities; this is not surprising, when one considers that each of those rich, salty, and tiny eggs, usually eaten by the spoonfuls, has the potential to become a whole fish. During breeding, high quantities of fish eggs are hatched in the wild; it is estimated that less than a third survive the predation they face.

When wild or raised naturally, all types of edible eggs are great sources of omega-3 fatty acids. When raised in artificial conditions, however, the omega-3 factor in eggs can become negligible or even nonexistent, due to the quality of food fed to the animal in question.

The Energetics of Eggs

Eggs have a strong ability to store energy. Energetically, they supply the body with concentrated heat reserve (protein) and at the same time create a damp condition. The experience of extreme weight loss with body coldness is often the result of a lack of inner heat reserve (one form of malnourishment). In this situation, eggs have the potential to quickly supply an individual with the needed nourishment and reserve to reestablish strength and vitality.

Being one of the most concentrated forms of animal food and one that is consumed often to the point of excess, eggs can produce extreme reactions that often manifest as cravings for sweets, coffee, carbonated beverages, and spicy foods (foods that empty and cool) in the person who consumes them. This strong reaction-driven cravings for these foods, stemming from eating an excessive amount of eggs, can easily become excessive to the point where the person defeats the very purpose of eating the eggs in the first place (i.e., to build up strength and reserve).

In addition to their being a primitive food, eggs have a tremendous ability to bind and hold. Psychologically, this can affect a person's thinking. Eggs have a powerful effect on the reptilian section of the human brain, where many memories are stored, and the individual who eats a preponderance of eggs can easily get locked into old habits and modes of thinking that can be difficult to change. The combined qualities of tenacious binding and constriction also can manifest in such traits as lying, deviousness, the need for control and power, domination over others, and any other of the fine qualities that exist among our present network of political and governmental leadership.

Throughout the world, eggs have long been symbols of fertility (naturally enough). They have a heavy, sinking quality that tends to resonate in the lower parts of the body. Chicken eggs have a twenty-one-day gestation period, and this can affect the female menstrual cycle either positively or adversely, depending on the condition of the person and how regularly eggs are consumed. I have known many women who were suffering from amenorrhea (lack of menstruation) and general nutritional deficiencies who have eaten eggs and were helped with both problems. On the other hand, I know many women who have eaten an abundance eggs and suffered from irregular menstruation and PMS— and the reduction of eggs in their diets helped tremendously with these problems.

All the eggs mentioned above produce a damp and hot condition in the human body.

Being a highly concentrated food, eggs are well complemented by spices and dispersing herbs. Though this is not a common way of eating eggs for most people in the modern world, it is important to learn and apply this simple act of balance. Pepper, hot sauce, green onions, chives, and other dispersing foods help to digest and release the enclosed potential of this highly nutritious protein food.

26
Mammals

Although poultry and eggs have become the most widely consumed animal foods in modern society, the term *meat* still most commonly connotes the flesh of mammals.

What's Your Beef?

Most beef cattle today are said to be crosses between the descendents of the mighty ox, or *aurochs,* whose origin can be traced back to India, and the Celtic Shorthorn. The domestication of cattle is thought to have begun with the taming of the wild ox about 10,000 years ago, possibly in Western Asia. How the genetic manipulation of the mighty aurochs into the modern cow occurred is still a mystery.

According to orthodox theory, domestication of the ornery aurochs, along with some unknown crossbreeding method practiced for thousands of years by Neolithic farmers, led to the extreme morphological changes found in modern docile cows. But this is a highly unlikely scenario, because entire sets of genes would have to be modified in order to change an animal's physical characteristics. The domestic traits of modern cows supposedly derived somehow from the ancient aurochs include reduced brain size, passive nature, early sexual maturity, and increased fertility. Such a shift in qualities is beyond current human capabilities and would certainly seem to be beyond the capabilities of our primitive

Neolithic ancestors. (Unless our Neolithic ancestors were not as primitive as we have been taught to believe.)

The aurochs was a strong and courageous creature known for its ability to stand up to almost any threat. Along with its long-held role as a food source, the aurochs also had secured a position in mythology and religion as a symbol of bravery and courage. Ancient Egyptians venerated the Apis bull through mummification. In Sumeria, the bull was a symbol of fertility and strength.

In some parts of the ancient world, cattle meat was once considered too noble a food to be entrusted to women, and therefore was usually roasted on an open spit by men. In Elizabethan England, excessive beef consumption was thought to cause stupidity and depression.

To the early settlers of America and to many other peoples in numerous parts of the world, the cow has served not only as a source of meat and milk but also as a dependable and patient draft animal that can endure many hours of backbreaking labor. As I mentioned earlier, anthropologist Marvin Harris makes a valid point when suggesting some food taboos are often more practical than mystical.

Before 1900, the average age of maturity for grazing cattle (that is, the age they would reach before being taken to market) was five or six years. In modern times, through industrial farming techniques, only breeding stock live longer than eighteen months. The modern factory-farmed cow bears little resemblance to its powerful and active ancestor; like other modernized livestock, this poor mammal suffers from overcrowding, drug abuse, and other forms of inhumane treatment.

Unlike with chickens, the overcrowding of cattle results not so much in aggression as in severe digestive disorders. Consequently, eating this kind of beef under stress is a guaranteed recipe for digestive problems. In fact, excessive beef eating alone can easily stress the digestive system, since digestive problems are some of the energetic qualities recorded in modern beef, owing to their confinement and lack of natural grass feed. Excessive consumption may even lead to insensitivity to anything or anyone exclusive of one's own immediate environment. The severe digestive disturbances common among cows can also become the human being's reality in the form of gastric problems (physically) and the inability to comprehensively digest and evaluate life (mentally and spiritually).

In a natural setting, cattle usually will select a comfortable distance from each other. Cows have a four-compartmented stomach. After it is chewed just barely enough to be swallowed, their food passes into the first of these compartments, the *rumen*. Through muscular action of the stomach, it is then returned to the mouth where it is thoroughly chewed and again returned to the stomach. It then passes through the other three compartments, to the small intestine and then to the large intestine. This extensive digestive process is what enables a ruminant to produce flesh from simple fare of grass and weeds.

Grass-fed cattle prefer to graze at twilight when the air is cool. Most feedlot cattle, by contrast, are fed in the morning, despite studies that have shown that afternoon grazing increases milk production by 10 percent and naturally increases the weight of cattle. Commercial cattle are given hormones for weight gain and fed an unnatural (for cattle) diet of grain, which in turn reduces the nutritional content of the meat. A high-grain diet can also affect the natural acidity of rumen (stomach) contents of cattle from a healthy pH of 7.1 (slightly acid) to an unhealthy 3.8 (extremely acidic). Again, cows are not meant to eat grain as their primary food. The healthy alternative is grass-fed beef.

Beef is a powerful food; unless the quality is good and it is prepared properly and eaten in moderation, it can induce fatigue and boredom and cause overheating. This is true for organically fed cows as well.

Cows cannot spit, but they can and do throw up, sometimes heaving violently. Their tongue is rough, and thus not very sensitive to taste; there is little need for it on a grass-based diet. It is not unusual for people who consume large quantities of beef to find simple food such as whole cereal grains and fresh vegetables tasteless when encountering them for the first time.

It's interesting to note that the food a cow eats is barely chewed until it first is sent to the stomach and then returned to the mouth— and only then is it thoroughly masticated. Like goats and sheep, also ruminants with four-compartment stomachs, cows easily thrive on a diet of wild grasses and other plants. Actually, they have one true stomach, along with three antechambers that house billions of bacteria and enzymes devoted completely to digestion and assimilation.

By contrast, humans are not ruminants—something worth considering when it comes to making the choice between vegetarian or non-vegetarian diet. With a digestive system more than 100 feet long, the cow can easily process the nutritional elements from tough plant cells and tissues through their elaborate digestive system. Humans are not so digestively endowed.

Cows do not chew well, and cows chew very well—a paradox, indeed. In humans, the practice of not chewing food well (that is, like the cow's "first round") sometimes results in digestive problems so severe that the person often has to use drugs to symptomatically relieve the problem or radically change his diet and finally learn to chew well. While the latter is the preferable choice, these days it is typically the path less traveled.

The cow's method of eating can manifest in humans in the form of *bulimia,* the eating disorder wherein the person afflicted routinely binge eats, followed by bouts of self-induced vomiting. (The word "bulimia" derives from *bull,* meaning "ox," and *limos,* meaning "hunger": together they mean "the hunger of an ox.")

Cows love attention, especially being talked to and scratched. They have a well-developed sense of hearing and do not like loud noise. They have trouble making decisions, can't take care of themselves, and tend to follow their keeper.

Cows have little facial expression, a kind of flat and blank look about them, and their verbal expression is limited to long moans. Cow people, like their counterparts, are often not the most communicative or open-minded characters.

When separated from cows and penned together, steers (bulls) will often ride each other. If there is more than one bull present when cows are in heat, the bulls inevitably will fight over the cows. Bulls also have an affinity for calves when the mother is not around. Incestuous acts as well as oversexed conditions have historically been associated with excessive beef consumption.

Cattle have a high metabolic rate and can sweat profusely. I surmise that the latter is due to their being confined with little room to roam; yet it still is a peculiar quality of this new breed of cow.

This humongous eating machine can certainly burn up the fuel. It takes an average of twenty pounds of grain to make one pound of meat, a fact often used to rationalize veganism. The problem with this position is that cows do not naturally eat grain; given their preference, they would rather graze in a field of grass. In fact, many traditional methods of raising cattle utilized rocky terrain for grazing, land that could not be used for growing crops—so the cost of feeding cattle in a traditional setting might add up to zero. Feeding cattle grain is simply a faster way to fatten cows for slaughter and is neither a traditional form of pastoralism nor a healthy way to raise cattle.

Veal, as we know it today, is an even more extremely unnatural way to raise cattle. A single calf can produce 100 pounds of veal in just three months. Veal comes from a baby cow, a calf that is allowed very little movement and is fed from birth to butchering on milk or an artificial substance called milk replacer. Such animals are usually anemic, very fragile, and extremely disease-prone. (Thinking about the energetics of that one makes you shudder, doesn't it?)

Feedlot cattle often experience what is called sudden-death phenomenon," a problem that usually occurs as a result of respiratory diseases, to which confined cattle are prone. A similar problem occurs among human infants and is called Sudden Infant Death Syndrome (SIDS), or simply "crib death." These infants of course are not eating cattle meat— but they *are* drinking homogenized and pasteurized cattle milk, which can adversely affect the respiratory system. (Unless they are being fed soy formula, which is even worse.)

Two other problems that commonly occur in cattle are cystic ovaries and mastitis, also common human problems.

Wild beef is more difficult to obtain than other wild animal food sources; however, there are sources of naturally raised, grass-fed beef. When choosing beef or any other ruminant, this is the only sensible way to go. The advent of "mad cow disease" only underscores the point.

Heavy beef eaters have other easily recognizable traits. They tend to be hot-natured (both physically and emotionally) and loud. They tend to have heavy and full faces and bodies with thick skin. Their skin often has a reddish color to it, and they are almost always hairy people.

While beef has been one of the most overconsumed meats, good quality beef can be a highly supportive food, especially for those with emaciated and very cold conditions. Grass-fed beef creates a hot and damp condition in the human body and contributes to endurance, strength, and stability.

Bison

Bison, also called buffalo, are an extremely hardy species and well suited to year-round range feeding. They easily cope with cold winter climates and the concomitant reductions in food supply by naturally slowing their metabolism. Even feedlot-raised bison have this natural ability.

Like beef but far stronger and more active, bison is now a popular alternative for those seeking a leaner meat than beef. Bison has a strong warming effect on the body and can be supportive for those suffering from chills, poor circulation, and lack of robust health in general.

Pigs: "To Market, To Market . . ."

According to some historians, pigs were the second animals domesticated, after dogs. Domestication of the wild boar may have occurred more than eight thousand years ago.

This four-legged mammal is the most prolific of domesticated animals, with the exception of the rabbit. The pig, of course, is famous for being sloppy, slovenly, uncouth, and living in squalor, hence its use as a derogatory epithet. However, the modern animal that inspires this dubious character profile bears little resemblance to its swift and powerful ancestor, the wild boar, who is lean, muscular, and capable of running twenty-five miles per hour for short dashes.

Boars are fearless creatures that thrive mostly at night and dwell in deep forests. The wild boar still roams the remote forests of southern and eastern Europe. (The term *boar* is applied to wild pigs, while the word *swine* is reserved for domesticated pigs.)

Boars are fierce and potentially dangerous animals that eat to live. Swine, however, are generally friendly, less nocturnal, more social, and live to eat. The wild boar is an omnivorous creature; it has been said that a wild boar's intestines are nine times the length of its body. Domesticated swine, on the other hand, have intestines fourteen times the length of their body and this purportedly improves their potential for digesting plant foods.

The pig is held by many cultures as the number one food source among animals, both for its nutritional qualities and for the simple reason that it is used in its entirety. In pig-eating cultures, no part of the pig is thrown away.

In non-pig-consuming cultures, on the other hand, the pig is abhorred as a filthy animal unfit for human consumption. Debates on the subject of religious condemnation of the pig by Jews and Muslims are continuous. Anthropologist Marvin Harris has offered what is so far the most sensible explanation for pork repulsion among those of the Middle East: it is fundamentally due less to religious beliefs and more to the fact that the arid environment of the regions where these religions were birthed is inhospitable to raising pigs.

Pigs naturally thrive in a lush forest environment where they can live healthy lives, root for food at their leisure, and rest in the cool shade of trees. This natural lifestyle does not adapt well to the arid climate of the Middle East. However, numerous Neolithic archaeological sites in this area reveal a history of thousands of years of pig domestication, long before any religious taboos set in!

Like any traditional animal food, pork can be an unhealthy food when raised improperly, but when raised naturally and prepared properly, it can be just as healthy and clean as any other animal food. This is evidenced in the populations of the world that do consume this animal.

Several years ago a good friend who was adamantly opposed to eating pork took a trip to Africa for a safari adventure. His guides on the trip were two powerfully built African natives who walked for the entire safari while my friend and others rode in a four-wheeled vehicle. My friend, a pretty big guy himself, couldn't help but admire the stamina and build of these two African men as they trekked for miles in the hot sun, never once complaining and all the while smiling and showing endless patience with their foreign tourists.

My friend has a long history of education in nutrition and health, so after many hours into the safari and unable to contain himself, he asked the two men what food they ate that gave them such strength and stamina. They both smiled at him and said, "Pig!"

My friend was stunned by this revelation at first. But the two men didn't hesitate in their answer, and clearly had no doubt whatsoever that it was primarily pig meat to which they owed their strength, endurance, and overall good health.

That day, my friend told me, he learned a big lesson about food. He learned not to believe everything he hears about a particular food, especially when so many other cultures may believe something radically different about that same food.

The Chinese and other Asian peoples have also kept domestic pigs for thousands of years; pork has served to nourish them for hundreds of generations and will likely continue to do so for hundreds more to come. To this day, wild boar are hunted and domestic swine are raised throughout Europe and many other parts of the world.

The pig is considered one of the most intelligent of all farm animals. This is partly due to the fact that pigs can easily be trained to do what man asks of them. It seems to me, though, that the willingness to do man's bidding is not necessarily a true sign of intelligence in animals, and I doubt very much that many wild animals, especially the wild boar, would ever prove this level of "intelligence."

The gestation period for pigs is three months, three weeks, and three days (114 days). Young pigs are unique among farm animals in that they are able to scuffle and run around an hour after birth. The wild sow gives birth to three or four young during her once-a-year breeding season in late December and early January. Domesticated swine have no season and can be bred any time throughout the year.

During copulation, the domesticated boar is rather quick to reach the point of ejaculation (after about one minute). But that doesn't mean the act is over, for the boar will continue to ejaculate for five minutes or more, releasing a cup or more of fluids. I can't say from experience, but I have heard from male pork fanciers that this particular energetic property is not far-fetched.

Another curious bit of porcine reproduction miscellany is that the sexual organ of the male pig is shaped like a corkscrew.

When not provided for, pigs are very capable of foraging for their own food. Their snouts, often called *rooters* because of their affinity for root plants, are used to dig and burrow into the ground. Unlike sheep, cows, and goats (all also ruminants), the pig has one stomach, and it is a highly efficient one capable of digesting just about anything that is edible—and pigs do just that. Like the lobster and other crustaceans of the ocean, or mushrooms and other fungi of the land, the pig easily qualifies as the leading candidate for the top scavenger among land animals—and this is not a derogatory statement.

The food-factory-farmed version of pigs is very competitive and will rarely eat alone. If a pig has eaten his fill but sees another get up to eat, the pig who has already eaten will get up to eat again out of fear of not getting enough.

Pigs are the fastest-growing farm animals, so it's not surprising that they would need large quantities of food. Unfortunately, though, these domesticated eating machines rarely have an outlet to dispel most of their accumulated food energy, so they simply get fat—unlike wild boars, which are lean and have little fat. The fat content of wild boar is approximately 4 percent, while that of the domestic, confined pig is approximately 35 percent.

Commercial pigs are prone to bacterial infections that cause abscesses. Some 30 to 50 percent of domesticated pigs raised in confinement are affected with *mycoplasmic pneumonia* (a cross between a virus and a mold) and, because of their susceptibility to stress, can die suddenly from *hyperthermia*. They are also very sun-sensitive and are extremely susceptible to sunburn and heat stroke. They have very few sweat glands and most of those are on their snouts. This animal food is hot! Energetically, these characteristics can manifest in humans as hot flashes, pneumonia, avoidance of sun and hot places with a preference for cold and air conditioning, irritability, quickness to anger, obesity, and rapid or labored breathing.

They are not attracted to the sight of blood, as chickens are; however, confined pigs are prone to excessive eating, nibbling, huddling, and tail biting, the latter often reaching a point where the pig doing the tail biting resorts to cannibalism and begins to eat the other pig. This excessive oral and anal behavior often contributes further to ear chewing and sudden outbreaks of violence and aggression.

Modern pigs suffer from social confusion, in that they often have great difficulty recognizing others in their group. This energetic characteristic often manifests in humans as a feeling of being out of place in social situations, or a constant need for acknowledgment, which, if it is not received, can lead to overindulgence and isolation.

Much of a domesticated pig's time is spent resting and sleeping. Because of this lack of activity, they suffer from inflamed joints and other joint abnormalities. The energetic equivalent of these traits appears in the human who consumes this quality of pig. In addition to their tendency toward developing gastric ulcers, pigs also suffer from an unusual wasting disease in which their muscles wither and lose their elasticity and strength.

One of the most dominant characteristics of confined pigs, especially those kept in darkness, is their tendency to sit on their haunches, depressed and with their heads drooping (as if in mourning) for long periods. Being a sensitive and intelligent animal, the pig abhors confinement and resorts to a stubborn and defeatist attitude in the face of the inability to do anything about its circumstance.

This is also not an unusual scenario for humans who find themselves in situations where they are uncomfortable or feel confined. The basic difference between a pig and a human in this scenario is that the human can usually make a choice to do something about it, whereas the pig cannot. It is not unusual for humans to *feel* they have no choice and as a result, often remain in a depressed situation where they can easily develop resentment, frustration, and increased depression.

Normal behavior in healthy, unconfined pigs has shown them to be especially hygienic. They will use one particular area for a latrine, another for sleeping and lying down, and another for birthing. In domesticated swine, of course, this relative fastidiousness disappears.

Heavy pork eaters usually have rounded facial and body features. Their bodies often lack clear definition from one body part to the next. Pork eaters are not always obese, yet they do tend to have an appearance of fullness. Their arms, from wrist to shoulder, often appear as one fully-extended appendage and their legs likewise. Their rounded faces usually include an extra fullness under the chin that tapers off down the neck, giving a lack of definition to the chin.

Traditional peoples who consume naturally raised pork do not have these traits; they rather have strong muscular bodies that are quite well defined.

While pork may be a religious taboo for some, for many more people in the world it has proved to be a highly useful and nutritious food. Quality pork can be supportive for conditions of dryness and underweight due to lack of assimilation. Its most pronounced effect can be noticed in the middle organs: the spleen, pancreas, stomach, liver, and gallbladder. It can also be helpful in stimulating metabolism and increasing strength and stamina.

Goats

According to the carbon dating of fossils, goats were domesticated around eight thousand years ago; some historians believe domestication of the goat occurred well before cattle.

Traditionally, goats have been raised for their milk and meat. Cheese, yogurt, and a number of other dairy products are made from goat's milk. The meat is called *chevon* and is a popular food among people of Spanish, Greek, Jewish, and other cultures worldwide. Kid (young goat) meat plays an important role in the meals of spring festivals of Easter and Passover. More than two hundred thousand goats are slaughtered annually in the United States alone. The most popular chevon for the Easter-Passover market are young milk-fed kids that weigh an average of twenty to thirty pounds.

The goat is related to the deer and like the deer is a browser. This simply means that the goat would rather reach up for its food than graze the ground with lowered head. Goats are partial to nibbling on hanging things and will taste just about anything at least once. While not all hanging items are edible to a goat, it doesn't really matter—these things are just too difficult to resist. If they don't actually eat them, they will nibble anyway, simply to entertain themselves.

Goats are ruminants. Like cows and sheep, they have four-compartment stomachs and prefer to feed on plant life that consists largely of carbohydrates, cellulose, and water. They prefer shrubs, weeds, saplings, leaves, bark, and grass.

Like their ancestors, goats prefer living on steep slopes. They appreciate their independence but can adapt to barn living with few problems. However, they do not like to be alone and prefer contact with their own species or with other animals.

Multiple births are not uncommon among goats. The female (doe) gives birth to one or more offspring, usually in springtime. She can become pregnant as early as the age of seven months. The average gestation period for a goat is 145 to 155 days. Does are dainty creatures, fastidious and intelligent—and very friendly. Contrary to what some people think, does are not mean and smelly creatures. The buck (male) is another story. He has scent glands, the strongest being just behind his horns, that give off a rather strong smell. Does don't seem to mind it, though, and they willingly accept the buck's other peculiar habits, one of which is their tendency to urinate all over their front legs and beards.

Goats are more economical to keep than cows. This small animal can produce more milk per pound of body weight on the same amount of feed as can a cow. A single cow will need to eat as much as six to eight times what goats would eat in order to produce the same amount of milk.

Goats are curious and adventurous creatures and will circumvent any boundary that isn't goat-proofed by jumping over it, crawling under it, or simply knocking it over in their quest to gain access to open space. Many goatkeepers consider goats to be the healthiest of domestic animals.

The energetic effects of regularly consuming goat meat or milk include a curious and adventurous personality combined with a stubborn abrasiveness. These qualities may manifest as a person being set in his ways, often rigorously imposing his opinions and beliefs on others. His eating patterns are usually haphazard at best and consist of strange and unusual combinations of foods. While this person usually has a few set meals, consisting of two to three items which he eats regularly, most of his eating is spontaneous and may include just about anything immediately available—usually one food at a time followed by another, then another, until he is satisfied.

These people like to talk incessantly on one subject. Their facial features are rough, with a tendency toward dry and matted hair. They generally appear unkempt, with a tight and gnarled body structure. While they are often obsessed with matters of physical hygiene (frequently to the point of being wasteful), their appearance does not usually make this obsession obvious to others.

These people are independent, yet they don't really like to be alone. In their relationships, they either keep their solitude for long periods or maintain a separateness with their partner through a lack of adequate communication.

Goat meat has a lean, stringy, and sinewy texture that creates a dry and warm condition in the human body. It can be a supportive food for those with loose muscles, low energy, and timid natures.

Sheep

There are many breeds of sheep, an animal valued for at least the past nine thousand years for its wool, meat, and milk. One of the more popular domestic type of sheep in the United States and Europe is the Delaine, which is a fine wool breed of Merino originally imported from Spain in 1801.

Wool is an amazing raw material with no equal among fibers natural or synthetic. It has the unique properties of bulk, elasticity, and absorption. It can absorb 30 percent of its own weight in water before it feels damp. A single sheep can supply from three to eighteen pounds of wool a year.

With the exception of traditional peoples raised around sheep, many people find lamb meat to have a strong or gamey taste. This is true among factory-raised sheep that often wallow in their own excrement; however, free-roaming sheep that get plenty of exercise do not have the same flavor.

Hardy, sure-footed animals, herded and chaperoned by a single sheepherder and often accompanied by a trustworthy dog, sheep did (and many in some areas of the world still do) roam the countryside and mountain ranges, freely grazing for their food. Most of the lamb produced in the United States and Canada are still raised on grass. However, like other livestock, many sheep suffer the perils of total confinement and abuse awarded them through man's insensitivity.

In fact, it is said that in order to wean a "200 percent" lamb crop (an ideal percentage), sheep must produce more triplet and quadruplet lambs at birth. Some of these baby lambs are grafted onto different mothers with more plentiful milk, or they are artificially raised on milk replacer. A 200 percent lamb crop is rarely achieved in America, and starvation is still the principal cause of baby lamb deaths. Ordinarily, if left to the wiles of nature, sheep will usually produce one lamb a year, with a gestation period that lasts an average of 145 to 148 days (twenty-one weeks).

Lambs have a keen sense of smell that allows them to readily distinguish their offspring from others. It has been said that their keen sense of smell is what determines how they react with people: by smell alone, they are able to distinguish between a gentle, harmless human being and one who might be potentially harmful to them.

Sheep are one of the least intelligent farm animals, and one of the most defenseless. They are very timid animals and will shy away from anything unless given a strong reason not to.

Sheep are known as followers: they are so dependent that rather than following one of their own kind, they will readily follow one of another species, e.g., the human shepherd.

There is an unusual herd of sheep in Scotland's Shetland Island beach; these animals are unusual among sheep in that they do not flock at all. Interestingly, these sheep eat sea algae. This reveals a fascinating conjunction of opposite characters: the normally conformist behavior of the advanced (and typically grass-fed) mammal, and the individualism of the "primitive" algae—which, though they aggregate in colonies that resemble fully formed plants, still maintain their actual form as independent, one-celled organisms.

Sheep do not like hot weather (not surprising when considering the animal walks around in a wool coat all year long) and prefer to retreat to a cool, shady place when the heat is on. It is not uncommon for them to eat nothing during the day when the weather is hot, choosing to graze at night when the weather is cooler. Sheep neither need nor drink as much water as most other livestock.

Some common health disorders experienced by commercially raised sheep include: stiff-legged lambs, usually the result of vitamin E deficiency; stillbirths, also linked to nutritional factors, as well as to over feeding; and worms, the most common of sheep's afflictions. When pigs and chickens are subject to worms, they usually do not cause great harm. But a worm-infested sheep can easily get run-down and die.

The energetic effects of eating an excessive amount of lamb include a timid and shy personality. These people often lack motivation and the initiative to start something new. They often complain and feel the need for much attention. They tend to be strong and stocky individuals, yet lean toward being inactive. Many will gain weight easily; however, when they gain weight, it is usually distributed evenly throughout the body. They are often easily confused by complex issues and usually require detailed explanations. Their sense of smell is usually very good and this makes them sensitive to body odors and environmental odors.

In relationships, they tend to take a passive role. They make dedicated partners that will do whatever it takes to make their relationship comfortable and relaxed. They tend to have soft and gentle yet full facial features.

Lamb is a dark meat and produces a hot and damp condition. Lamb is also considered the least allergenic meat. Lamb can be a beneficial food for people with weak constitutions, as well as for those who are underweight and have weak blood.

Rabbit

In America, the mere mention of Easter usually reverberates in praises by young children for the Easter Bunny and Easter eggs. For most adults, Easter has very different connotations. To them, it has religious overtones that chime with Sunday and church. The excitement, joy, and fantasy that children experience during Easter is actually closer to the original meaning of this holiday than the adult interpretation. Easter (named after the Babylonian god Ishtar) was on the lunar calendar long before the advent of Christianity and was originally a time of celebration that correlated to the springtime rebirth of vegetation.

The rabbit (it was actually a hare) became the symbol of fertility that referred to new life and the start of its periodicity. The rabbit was a logical choice for this symbol of fertility, considering its prodigious ability to multiply. The egg was another choice for a fertility symbol; when put together with the rabbit, it resulted in the Ishtar bunny that laid the Ishtar eggs. The combination of the bunny and the egg was a light-hearted combination, a harmless fantasy (since rabbits do not lay eggs).

Concerning the eating of rabbit, it might be best not to mention this to children, most of whom see the rabbit as a soft and cuddly creature, and certainly not something to eat. However, food they can be, and food they *have* been for thousands of years in many parts of the world. Hare bones have been found in prehistoric kitchen middens in New England, Africa, and Russia. Numerous Indian tribes ate rabbit long before the Europeans got to America. Although there are more than sixty-six breeds of rabbit in America, it was one of the last domesticated farm animals.

Rabbit was more popular as a food in early America than it is today. Thomas Jefferson had a fancy for rabbit meat and often had a good stock on hand. Today, in most parts of the United States, rabbits have yet to be accepted on a large scale as meat producers. This is not so in Europe, though, where rabbit is frequently eaten in stews, roasted, grilled, and in many other preparations.

Many rabbit-meat fanciers consider the meat superior to chicken, and as the world food problem gets worse they believe rabbit will emerge as the animal food of the future. Rabbit is a close-textured white meat and has a more delicate flavor than chicken. The protein content exceeds that of beef, pork, lamb, and chicken. The French, who are big rabbit consumers, favor wild rabbit over domesticated breeds for its superior flavor.

A female rabbit is called a doe and a male a buck. One buck can service up to ten does, and a ten-pound doe can produce up to 120 pounds of meat in her litters in one year. This means she can produce from three to five litters per year, numbering between six and twelve young per litter. The average gestation period for rabbits is thirty-one days.

When a doe accepts service by a buck, the buck will usually fall over to one side or over backward when finished. But it doesn't take more than a minute or so before he is ready to repeat the process again—that is, if the doe is willing. Perhaps this is where the saying "screwing like bunnies" comes from. A hardy and virile buck, however, does not fall over when finished; rather, once he has ejaculated he will stand up straight on his back feet and let out a piercing screech. (I have not observed that this trait carries over to rabbit-eaters; let us hope not.)

Wild rabbits come into heat only in the spring and fall, whereas domesticated rabbits have a four-day nonfertile period in each sixteen-day cycle. In commercial rabbitry, inbreeding is common. Sex becomes a free-for-all, father and daughters, mother and sons; the one exception to this orgy is brother and sister—this just doesn't work, and when it happens, the offspring are often born dead or very weak.

Although rabbits are highly sexual animals, overfeeding can easily lead to infertility.

Rabbits require lots of water and prefer to do most of their drinking at night. They do not require much care, and, if fed properly and allowed to live in clean surroundings, they are among the most disease-resistant of livestock. They can tolerate a great deal of cold, yet cannot tolerate windy or drafty conditions or strong sunlight.

Their heartbeat averages about two hundred beats per minute and they have very fast metabolisms. They can move in short spurts by using their two front feet together followed by their two back feet. But most of the time, they sit quietly in a crouched position. If startled, they are capable of a quick retreat at a dazzling speed. Rabbits like to dig burrows, but farmed rabbits do not have the opportunity to do so.

Rabbits are probably the most emotionally sensitive of all livestock and are thus one of the most easily stressed. Any deviation from the normal sequence of events in their environment, such as a thunderstorm, unusual sounds, or strange people, will tend to make them stressed. They may not reveal their stress in the same way as turkeys or chickens; instead, they tend to internalize it and this often manifests as infertility in does and sterility in bucks.

They are extremely adept at recognizing human fears and hostility. Just look into a rabbit's eyes when humans are around. What looks like fear isn't really. . . . It's more like they are aware of the human's deepest secrets. Perhaps they are.

Rabbits are sociable and affectionate animals. They like to touch each other's noses, eat together, burrow, and play together. They like things clean and sanitary. When deprived of these simple pleasures, they can easily develop health problems.

Coccidiosis is one of the major problems of caged rabbits. It is a parasite that damages the liver and is considered responsible for the deaths of many young rabbits. Fur chewing is another common problem, with the rabbit chewing either its own fur or the fur of another rabbit. This is usually due to boredom from being cooped up with nothing to do.

They also have a tendency to get fat, and when they do, they often become sterile. Other common rabbit diseases include rickets (fragile and crooked bones), enteritis (bacterial infection), pneumonia, viral infection, heat stroke, and eye infections.

Rabbit eaters are usually very affectionate, sexual, and emotionally sensitive people. They like lots of attention and they like to give attention to others. They like to express themselves more in an emotional way as opposed to verbally, preferring to be soft-spoken and quiet. Their faces appear soft and gentle and they will often nod their heads in approval or agreement during conversations.

Since rabbit is mostly white meat, it produces short spurts of energy with long intermittent periods of quiet. The meat has a warm and dry effect and can be helpful for people with low sexual energy and overly damp conditions.

Game

Game is a term given to mammals and birds that are hunted in their wild state for food, or it can be used to define farmed yet not fully domesticated wild animals and birds. If farmed, wild animals can still maintain much of their original character, as evidenced in naturally raised pheasant, guinea fowl, and deer.

Wild game is usually seasonal food, whereas farmed game may be (depending on the location) available year round. Though often milder in flavor, farmed game is not energetically as powerful as wild game and has slightly different effects.

Many people find game to have a strong flavor compared to domestic animal foods. If you find game particularly strong or unsuitable to your palate, you might want to reevaluate your perspective on meat: in its truly natural state, it is *supposed* to taste this way. The domestic creatures (this does not include free-running farmed game) you have eaten in the past are not only energetically inferior, they are also nutritionally inferior in their balance between proteins and fats, which influences the flavor of the meat.

While game may require more care in its preparation, it is among the healthiest of meats. Meat in general can be a powerful, heat-inducing food as well as a centering food, and the energetic difference between factory-raised animal meat and wild game is a difference between centered delusion and centered realism.

Aside from the emotional and physical responsibility it takes to eat any kind of meat, wild game, if it knows it is being pursued and hunted, will raise the adrenaline in its blood. This can deplete the store of glycogen in muscle cells, especially if the animal experiences stress for any length of time before being killed, and this can affect the meat by making it more acidic, which in turn alters the taste as well as texture, making it tougher and less palatable.

The essence of wild game is that it includes a variety of undomesticated animals that have not been genetically tampered with by man. Will eating wild game make one wild? Not necessarily, because each type of game has its own unique qualities and energetics. *Wild*, in the

sense of "aggressive and dangerous," does not particularly fit the qualities of deer, even though they may live "in the wild" with wild predatory animals. "Gentle and free" are words more fitting to deer.

One winter, my compost pile became a regular hangout for some
local deer. They became so accustomed to compost being a replenished
food supply, and to seeing me, that they would sometimes eat from my
hand. Free and independent, yes, but certainly not domestic.

Deer

Deer belong to a family of mammals call *cervidae* which include
moose, elk, and many other species of deer. Here we have an animal
that has survived virtually unchanged since prehistoric times, with
the exception of a few physical adjustments in size. This fact alone is
a strong statement for the energetics of any food source. With the deer
it is particularly interesting, since its only real defense against predators, aside from its keen sense of smell and hearing, is its agility and
speed. Any species that can exist and survive practically unchanged
while being the constant focus of numerous imposing predators
(including humans) for as long as deer have is truly a marvel of genetic
perfection.

Humans have consumed venison (deer meat) since prehistoric times;
indeed, venison has often sustained large groups of people as a principal
food. Once considered a robust and hearty food for feasts eaten during the Middle Ages and the Renaissance, for most people venison is
now a seasonal food, available mainly during hunting season. That is,
except for the hunter who is fortunate enough to kill one during the
season: for him, venison may be available all year round, with the help
of his freezer. Some states have laws that prohibit retailing venison in
supermarkets during off-season; others prohibit the retailing of venison
at any time, with the exception of menu fare at some restaurants. Other
parts of the world do not have the same restrictions when it comes to
hunting and consuming deer.

The doe (female deer) is wild, fleet-footed, and acutely aware, yet delicate, feminine, and beautiful. The buck (male deer), with antlers erect and
head held high, broadcasts a stoic, reserved masculinity, a distant mate,

cautious and proud, and prepared to defend the family if necessary. Deer are quiet and playful creatures, able to stop and hold a motionless pose at the slightest sound. At the same time, they are extremely agile: they can jump nearly fifteen feet into the air and run up to twenty-five miles per hour for several miles. In Medieval times, in addition to being an important food animal, deer were thought to be magical; to this day they play an important role in many shamanic ceremonies.

Deer have keen eyesight. In fact, the anatomy of the deer eye and the general organization of the neural circuits, the basic brain wiring, is virtually indistinguishable from that of humans.

A unique quality of the deer family is their lack of gallbladders.

The deer is a lean yet muscular animal that some experts say holds the mammalian record for defecation: apparently a single deer averages about thirteen piles per day. They have an incredible ability to rid themselves of excess waste, which is why venison is lean meat. Venison is powerful meat long known for its strength-inducing qualities and aphrodisiac potential. It is a meat so completely useable by the human body that little to none of the digested matter from it is excreted by the body. Ground and powdered deer horns are a common remedy in Chinese medicine for infertility and impotence. Deer are also polygamous by nature.

One particularly interesting family of cervidae (deer) are reindeer, called *caribou* in their wild state. (Some domestic reindeer are called caribou but are in fact reindeer.) Caribou are wild and bigger than domestic reindeer. Domesticated in Scandinavia and Mongolia thousands of years ago, reindeer are friendly, docile, and social animals with communication skills that extend beyond their own species. In fact, reindeer are known to communicate with humans to the point where humans do not even need to figure whose deer belong in which herd. The deer know and will stay or find their way to their designated herds (each herd often numbering in the hundreds) when separated, even if there are several other herds present.

The Laplanders of northern Scandinavia have immersed themselves in the reindeer lifestyle so completely that during the animals' seasonal migrations, they will pack up all their belongings and follow the herds. The reindeer supply the Lapps with extremely rich and nourishing milk and meat, as well as bone for tools and knives, and hide for gloves, bedding, and clothing. They pull sleds during migration and whenever else needed.

Other areas of reindeer herding include numerous parts of northern Eurasia. Many Arctic peoples, including the Sami in Scandinavia and the Nenets and other groups in Russia, also have a long history of reindeer herding.

Domesticated reindeer have uniquely structured hair that traps air, providing them with excellent insulation. They are strong swimmers and their hair helps to keep them buoyant when crossing wide rushing rivers and frozen stretches of the Arctic Ocean.

Reindeer physiology is designed to specialize in the digestion of lichen, an important food source in winter. Lichen is produced by a symbiotic relationship between algae and fungi, two very ancient organisms that have been present on the earth for millions of years.

There is an intriguing mystery of reindeer and caribou: they are the only species of deer whose males and females both grow antlers.

The shorter and stouter reindeer weighs an average of three hundred pounds; the wild caribou comes in at fully twice that weight. While the reindeer are a domesticated version of the wild caribou, all attempts to domesticate wild caribou have ended in failure. Both can breed together, but caribou tend to dominate. This has led to the theory that all domestic reindeer came from a single herd of caribou some five thousand or more years ago. Fair enough, but how did this happen, and who was responsible for it? Who was able to domesticate the wild caribou to produce the reindeer, genetically altering it in the process so that it would consistently weigh half the weight of the caribou? And why can't anyone repeat the process today?

At a time when our primitive ancestors were supposedly just beginning to crawl out of their caves, who were the Neolithic geniuses who were able to accomplish such an extraordinary feat of domestication?

Deer and its related species are powerful energizing foods especially supportive to those who lack a sense of adventure and motivation. These foods can also be very helpful for those suffering from depression, lack of clarity, and poor memory.

Elk

Elk is another common food in various parts of the world. Elk are strong and majestic animals; their meat is energetically more powerful than venison. Both tend to have a hot and dry effect.

In many countries—especially Scandinavian countries, where both deer and elk are common foods—they are often prepared with rich, creamy sauces that include mushrooms to balance the dry qualities. Other traditional preparations include marinating the meat in oil, vinegar, wine, and herbs, or smoking and drying the meat.

Boar and Bear

Another furred game animal is the wild boar. An impressive animal, indeed, and quite unlike deer, wild boar *are* wild—and dangerous. Energetically, wild boar meat has a hot and dry effect and is extremely energizing and stimulating.

The more extreme in behavior the animal, the more responsibility it requires to assimilate it. Wild boar would be most beneficial if you are going to be very physically active and outside in a natural environment, as traditional game eaters were. (Or you could curl up with your partner and a nice bottle of wine, then expend some of that wild energy together. No, better yet, follow the first suggestion, and then include the second. Now, that's being responsible.)

Some people eat bear, too. Here is one game animal that doesn't lack in fat. Personally, I have never tried this meat, and if trying it means I would have to shoot it first, then don't hold your breath. I stand five-foot-five and weigh 130 pounds. I can run pretty fast, but from what I understand about bears, not fast enough.

Good food for cold northern climates, and with its natural tendency to hibernate, bear may very well be the most heat-producing food there is.

Wild Rabbit

Wild rabbit is smaller and more active than domestic hutch varieties, giving it darker and stronger-tasting meat. Hare is larger than rabbit, and also has dark and gamey meat.

27
Creatures of the Deep

Like the land, the sea contains within its vastness both an animal realm and a plant realm. With edible creatures both large and small, along with numerous varieties of algae, the sea's gardens have long been an important and essential source for food. The ocean's bountiful harvest of highly nutritious sustenance has nourished coastal peoples and animals throughout the world, since recorded history and long before that.

Though the land provides the majority of our nourishment (as well as being our resident address), the seas cover approximately 72 percent of the earth's surface. These vast bodies of water share many of the same chemical and biological properties as the liquid portion of our blood. The salty, alkaline environment of the ocean lives within each of us through our own bloodstreams. The oceans of the earth represent the planet's blood and circulatory system, and the numerous varieties of food contained within these waters have a profound influence on the human internal ocean (our blood) and its relationship to health and well-being.

Oceans contain many life forms: microorganisms, bacteria, fish, shellfish, mollusks, and algae, all of which correspond to the structure and function of our white cells, red cells, bacteria, T cells, and other biological components that help to maintain a balance in our blood, our very own internal ocean. The pollution of the earth's water and rapid deterioration of one of our most important food sources is but a reflection of modern man's own internal toxification.

Our planet's circulatory system consists of two basic types of water—salt water and fresh water; both correspond to the circulation of body fluids, salt water energetically corresponding to the bloodstream and fresh water to lymph. The coastal environments—estuaries, marshlands, and other wetlands—are where the two types of water meet and exchange, and these are the sites of some of the greatest environmental devastation. Thus, this fluid metaphor does not bode well for our own immune systems. Here the recovery of a population-wide sense of *quality* is imparted with some urgency, and this puts the whole matter of energetics into a particularly relevant context.

The oceans supply a large portion of the world's food supply; sea algae (usually called "seaweeds"), fishes, and other life forms that exist in the salty environment of the oceans have a more pronounced effect on our bloodstream than those from fresh water. However, plant and animal life from freshwater lakes, rivers, and streams, have a greater influence on our lymphatic systems.

For the most part, fish, crustaceans, and mollusks cannot live and breathe on land, while human beings live on land and cannot live and breathe in water. Therefore, foods that live and thrive in a water environment energetically affect the human respiratory system as well. How they effect the respiratory system is largely dependent on each person's own respiratory strengths or weaknesses. For example, sea and freshwater algae produce and contain an extraordinarily high concentration of chlorophyll, which has the potential to enhance respiratory functions and regulate water balance in the human body through the function of the kidneys.

Let's take a look at some of the many forms of animal life that exist in water, along with some of their energetic properties.

The Bony Fishes

There are currently about thirty thousand known species of fish. They come in many shapes and sizes, some with scales and some without. Those with scales are scaleless when hatched but develop scales later, generally by the first year of growth.

Though fish have a rather poor sense of vision, they more than make up for this in other ways. (Perhaps it is their poor sense of sight that gives us the impression when we look into their eyes and find a vacant stare accompanied by what seems an almost paranoid appearance.) For example, current research has shown that fish are not driven purely by instinct, but are in fact cunning, manipulative, and very cultured. Their social intelligence is developed to the point where they easily recognize individual shoal mates. They even exhibit levels of social prestige, and scientists have been able to track specific ongoing relationships among individual fish.

In order to survive, fish depend mostly on their excellent senses of hearing and taste, along with their bodily sensitivity to vibrations and changes in environmental temperature and pressure.

Fish have four pairs of gills used for breathing oxygen, which they extract from water as it passes over their gills. Some fish (trout and salmon, for example) need more oxygen than others. More oxygen exists in colder waters than in warmer waters, so fish that require more oxygen for survival tend to dwell in colder waters, while those needing less oxygen tend to inhabit warmer tropical waters. Some fish are *anadromous,* meaning that they can live part-time in fresh water and part-time in salt water.

Coldwater fish, notably extra-fatty types, contain fatty acids called omega-3s, which have been shown to affect the disease process at the cellular level by blocking dangerous metabolic overreactions and thus supporting the immune system. These omega-3 fatty acids are important to human health because, as an animal source, they are already converted to DHA, which helps to make *prostaglandins.* Herring, sardines, mackerel and *wild* salmon are particularly high in omega-3 fatty acids.

Female and male fish discharge their eggs and sperm into the water, where the eggs then become fertilized and the young hatch and develop freely.

Fish are the most ancient group of vertebrates. All of the bony fishes have fins and a spine—with the exception of sharks and rays. Instead of spines, these two primitive fish have skeletons of cartilage (hardened with lime) surrounded by smooth, rubbery skin.

Some energetics of bony fish can be determined by their natural surroundings. Freshwater fish can be differentiated by where they live: lakes, ponds, streams, rivers, bogs, or marshes.

Saltwater fish can be differentiated by how and where they live as well. Some are inshore species while others are offshore species. Some are bottom dwellers while others are open ocean swimmers and still others are reef inhabitants.

Contrary to popular belief, not all fish are cold-blooded. However, neither cold-blooded nor warm-blooded fish can sustain a constant body temperature. Unlike mammals and birds, both of which have constant body temperatures, a fish's body temperature changes with its surrounding environment. Even though fish blood is thicker than human blood, it has low pressure because a fish heart has only two chambers (as opposed to four in a human) with which to pump its blood. This also accounts for the fact that fish blood flows slowly through its body and is lower in oxygen than human blood. A fish brain is not as highly developed as that of higher animals, since it lacks a cerebral cortex, the part of the brain that stores impressions and memory.

Unlike mammals, birds, and humans, all of which cease to grow after fully matured, fish continue to grow as long as they live, provided food is available for them.

Generally, fish eat less during cold months and more in warm months. When feeding less, their metabolisms slow down considerably.

Fish Families

There are two categories: the *pelagic,* or bony, fish and the bottom fish. The pelagic fish tend to be surface-dwellers and feed above the ocean floor. They are usually faster and more aggressive than bottom-dwellers, which feed more on vegetation and small animals on the floor of the ocean and are generally slower and less aggressive than the pelagic.

Some fish travel in large, well-organized schools, while others remain independent of groups. Most of the smaller fish are school fish (smelts, anchovies, sardines, herring, minnows, etc.); however, many larger fish also travel in schools. Among those that travel in schools, it is common for them to form a large mass that takes on the shape of an individual fish while cruising through the depths.

Each type of fish has its own peculiar characteristics, from the bass family—whose male guards the eggs until they are hatched—to flat fish such as the halibut and flounder—who camouflage themselves by changing color to match their background on the ocean bottom and whose eyes peer passively out of the same side of their heads. Other energetic effects of bony fishes can be determined by first distinguishing within which half of each of these four pairs of characteristics they fall:

- pelagic (surface) vs. bottom fish
- travels in a school vs. is independent
- freshwater vs. saltwater
- white-fleshed vs. dark-fleshed

The fat content of fish varies from lean to moderate and high. This does not necessarily determine whether one fish has more health benefits than another; it is simply another characteristic of their energetic properties.

The more fatty fish tend to become dry and tough when overcooked, whereas the leaner fish do not. Fatty fish tend to be more firm-fleshed, and lean fish more flaky in texture. Technically, a fatty fish is one that contains more than 1 percent fat; the fat often contains healthy doses of omega-3 fatty acids and other nutritional components.

Commercial fish farming is becoming more popular throughout the world. As with any animal food, fish that are free-running are generally superior in flavor and energy to those that are farmed in confinement. Unfortunately, due to a lack of concern for quality, the majority of fish farming has proven disastrous to both human and environmental health. However, a few conscious companies are working hard to change this situation.

Carp

Carp (called *koi* in Japan) have a long history with humans. They have been kept as pets in numerous places in Asia and will respond to the sound of a bell at feeding time. (Some carp owners say carp will even let their masters pet them.)

Carp can grow very large and live for a long time. Being scavenger fish (like catfish), they tend to keep their environment clean of debris and have long been an important fish of monastery ponds in China and Japan. Unlike most other fish, carp can prosper in mud and pollution; they do not fare as well in free waters, where they have to compete with other species of fish.

Trout

Trout are very sensitive to polluted water and will avoid it whenever they can. Like salmon, they need fast-running streams with highly oxygenated waters. They are similar in effect as salmon, but being freshwater fish, their energy tends to have more impact on the lymph system.

Pike

Pike are the largest of Britain's freshwater fish. The pike is a noble fish, though it is fiendish-looking, with razor sharp teeth, and vicious, too—so much so that pike are often known by the nickname, "river wolf." They have even been known to gobble up ducklings and other small animals.

Pike like to camouflage themselves among water plants, quietly waiting to ambush any fish that might happen by. When this happens, the pike will literally torpedo itself directly at its prey like a hurled spear—hence its name. Pike are undoubtedly the fastest freshwater fish, and they rarely miss their mark.

Salmon

Salmon and trout both belong to the *salmonidae* family. Salmon is a fish of mythological proportions and venerated by people all over the world for its unique health benefits. The ancient Ainu of Japan believed that salmon were a gift from the gods and recognized their strength and perseverance as qualities one would gain when consuming this special gift.

One of the most determined and persistent fish when it comes to spawning of their young, salmon are legendary for their breeding odyssey. They breed and hatch their eggs in fresh water; when mature, they return to live in salt water. Then, after four or five years in the open sea, salmon begin their long journey home, swimming against the seaward currents, to the rivulet or pond where they were born. Swimming through rapids and fierce mountain streams, and over razor-sharp rocks, if they are not first killed or eaten by predators, both male and female salmon finally reach their goal.

Battered and fasting from the hazardous trek, the female then digs a hole in the bottom of the stream, deposits her eggs, which the male then fertilizes. A few days later, the pair die together like an aquatic Romeo and Juliet—only in this case, not from unrequited love, but from a pairing that has been fully consummated. Salmon—honorable yet obsessive, determined to the death, together to the end. This is the nature of the Pacific salmon. The Atlantic salmon, though, often survives this ordeal and returns to saltwater, eventually to spawn again in fresh water.

In contrast to the noble wild salmon there exists another, more commonly consumed fish that in many ways does not even deserve to be called "salmon," since it has none of the redeeming qualities of wild salmon.

Commercial farm-raised salmon is what graces most people's plates these days, and it is loaded with PCBs, artificial colorings, and chemicals, many of which have been linked to cancer, reproductive problems, and vision damage in humans. These sad excuses for fish are treated with large amounts of pesticides and antibiotics to control the rampant parasite infestations caused by confinement and overcrowding.

Contrary to popular belief, these fish are not high in omega-3 but *are* high in omega-6 fatty acids—the ones you do *not* want more of! This is due in part to feed consisting of fish meal mixed with soy and other ingredients, most of which salmon would not normally eat. Wild salmon eat *krill* (a tiny crustacean) and this is what gives its flesh a natural deep red color. The red color found in farmed salmon is due to chemical coloring agents. Feeding a diet of fish meal pellets tends to turn the flesh gray, so colorings are added. In fact, a distributor of wild salmon once showed me what looked like a fan that he unfolded, revealing at least fifteen different colors ranging from white to red. There were several shades of pinks, pale orange, and so forth. He then went on to explain how the fan was used by distributors of farmed salmon for retail markets. One simply places an order for the color they would like the fish to be and the order is filled.

This type of salmon suffers from sea lice; the massive amounts of antibiotics given to them for this problem often end up polluting the environment and killing other aquatic life. Growth hormones are also added to their feed, causing them to grow at twice the rate of normal salmon. One study revealed that some farmed salmon contained six times the amount of dioxins as were allowed by the World Health Organization. Another study revealed that four to eight servings per month of wild salmon was safe, but *one* serving per month of farmed salmon increased the risk of cancer. Farmed salmon are so far removed from their original species line that they have lost the predatory instincts required to feed themselves, and therefore could not survive in the wild.

Salmon are difficult to farm because they are an active fish and need room to move. Conscious attempts to farm salmon on organic feed are an improvement, but most of the feed is still not something salmon eat in their natural habitat. As with any fish, but especially salmon, if you are going to eat it, eat it wild.

Eel

Eel share some of the characteristics of salmon, except that eel spawn in salt water and later return to live in fresh water. Both the American and European eel spawn in the same area of the Atlantic Ocean, at the northern edge of the Sargasso Sea.

At birth, baby American eels begin swimming toward North America, a trip that lasts about a year and spans approximately 1,000 miles. Baby European eels begin their 3,000-mile-or-more swim toward Europe, taking about three years. The peculiar thing about all this is that though one group of eels are about one year old and the other group about three years old, when they reach their destinations, both end up being the same size and looking very much alike.

As with salmon, both the adult male and female eel dies after spawning. Each female eel can lay up to ten million eggs, an ability that has undoubtedly contributed to their historical attribute as an aphrodisiac. They are very territorial and will dig tunnels several feet deep in the mud and then claim all of the adjacent area to themselves.

Garden eels live in colonies of 200 to 300. These snakelike creatures are extremely cautious and will withdraw into the safety of their homes at the slightest indication of movement around them.

Eels are scavengers and eat practically anything. American eels are nocturnal and tend to spend their days buried in mud, waiting to scavenge at night.

Unlike salmon, eels are fairly easy to farm. Current archaeological evidence has revealed that the ancient Gunditjmara people of Victoria, Australia were farming eels eight thousand years ago.

Dolphin

The dolphin, or *dorado,* is one of the fastest and most beautiful fish in the ocean. It is said to make dashes of up to fifty miles per hour. The edible variety of dolphin is not a mammal and is in no way like the popular porpoise often seen at Sea World; it more closely resembles a tuna.

Tilapia

Originally native to Africa and the Middle East, tilapia is now the second most widely farmed fish (after carp). Its mild-tasting flesh tends to take on the flavor of whatever the fish is fed, including soy and other ingredients they would normally not eat.

Mackerel

Mackerel are one of the most fatty fish, with a fat content ranging anywhere from 6 to 13 percent. Because of this, mackerel spoil easily when removed from their environment and must be eaten fresh, marinated, or pickled. They are voracious predators, traveling in large schools in the open ocean and spending most of their lives in deep water. Mackerel have poor eyesight and rely heavily on their keen sense of smell.

Tuna

Like the dolphin, the tuna is a very fast fish, a perpetual traveler that moves constantly, sometimes reaching speeds of forty-five miles per hour. It is also able to shift from high to low gear in a split-second. It just does not, cannot stop.

The tuna is a fascinating creature in that it *has* to move in order to breathe. High-speed swimming also is the tuna's way of keeping cool: if it should stop, it becomes overheated and dies. Think about these traits after your next tuna fish sandwich! Notice how your breathing becomes more shallow and you have intense cravings for something stimulating after eating tuna. This could be coffee, tea, chocolate, or anything that could stimulate. Why would this energetic effect occur with such a high-energy food like tuna? Simple: tuna need to move in order to breathe, and this quality will manifest in the person who eats the tuna as an increased need for oxygen. The human body recognizes this need for oxygen and triggers the craving for substances that will stimulate respiratory function.

A more natural way to benefit from the energetics of tuna is to do what they do when they need to breath: *get active*. Take a walk or do some brief exercise shortly after consuming tuna and notice how good it feels to breathe again.

When immobilized by a net, this extremely vital fish becomes passive and gives in to defeat. The bluefin tuna has dark red meat that closely resembles that of land mammals.

Bass

The bass has a voracious appetite and is often called the "wolf of the sea." A large number of unrelated fish are called bass. There are black, white, striped, and common sea bass. Interestingly, the Chilean sea bass reproduces every ten years in its natural environment. This is one reason it is on the endangered species list.

Bluefish

Bluefish are one of the most aggressive and bloodthirsty fish in the ocean. They are vicious and will kill for no apparent reason, long after their hunger is satiated. Deep-sea fisherman claim bluefish put up a tremendous fight when caught; they (the fish, not the fisherman) have actually been known to bite off fingers after they are pulled into the boat.

The only member of its family, bluefish travel in large schools that move swiftly through the ocean. Bluefish rarely attack their prey alone; rather, large groups rush into shoals of small fish, chopping them to pieces. The school will then circle around their prey and attack again. This goes on until the prey no longer reassembles.

I have twice had the opportunity to experience the power of bluefish when on deep-sea fishing excursions. On one occasion, the first fish I caught that day was a large, three-foot bass. How big? No, really . . . it *was,* and it was no easy task bringing it in. Needless to say, I was very proud of myself after bringing in that bass.

However, my second fish put up a fight that put that bass to shame. I thought for sure I had outdone myself and had an even larger bass on the line. It turned out to be a one-foot-long bluefish that just wouldn't quit. But I almost did—and if it hadn't been for the captain of the boat calling me every curse word in the book, I might have.

I took great pleasure in eating that bluefish when I got home—and it still got the better of me *after* I ate it, through its own unique energetics.

Energetics of the Bony Fishes

Some of the energetic properties derived from eating fish include: nervous, short-term energy; a tendency toward paranoia; sudden, sporadic physical movements; extreme adjustments in body temperature from hot to cold; increased metabolism; tightening in the chest and a need for more oxygen; lack of emotional warmth; quick, short spurts of verbal expression; skin irritations; and sharp mental acuity.

The physical and psychological effects of eating fish can be determined by each fish's particular energetic character.

Sushi (raw fish), a popular Japanese method of preparing fish and one of the few fish preparations where one may well consume a wide variety of different fish in the same meal, can include a wide spectrum of energetic effects. One energetic effect you will surely experience, should you eat a variety of fresh sushi, is what I call night flopping. This phenomenon occurs after one has retired to bed and has reached a deep sleep. The usual normal sleep patterns, where one gently rolls over from back to side or stomach, shift into a completely different pattern after an evening meal of fresh sushi (it has to be fresh to really get the effects). The gentle shifting of body position becomes almost acrobatic as one flips and flops to the desired position during sleep. This experience can sometimes be so pronounced as to wake the sleeper periodically throughout the night.

Sound outrageous? Check it out for yourself. My sense as to why this occurs is that it is because fish experience this flipping and flopping when removed from their environment and exposed to air. This energetic effect is further supported by the way the fish is handled by the sushi chef. With remarkable speed and agility, he will slap the fish into position and proceed to slice and dice. The fresher the fish, the more pronounced the experience of night flopping will be. Also, the different energetics of each fish combine into a potpourri of erratic effects. This unique way of consuming fish gives one the raw power of the fish one would not get through eating cooked fish.

Fish and seafoods tend to have long-term effects of cooling, due to their life in water; however, because of their high protein and short muscle fibers, they often produce an initial burst of warmth in the body. These thermogenic effects tend to be short-lived.

For example, darker-meat fish (tuna, bluefish, mackerel, and salmon) produce almost immediate warming effects, as well as an increase in energy, due to increased hemoglobin in their blood. Lighter-meat fish (cod, sole, halibut, etc.) are less aggressive fish with less oxygen-carrying hemoglobin and have a somewhat delayed energetic effect.

The exception to this would be if an individual were protein-deficient at the time of eating the fish. If this were the situation, both types of fish would likely produce more immediate effects.

Think about the times you have been swimming and tried to move through the water. Even if you are a good swimmer, it takes more effort for a human to move through water than it does to move on land. Fish have the energy to move through the water very quickly. Does this mean that if you eat fish you will move through the water more quickly? Possibly, but more importantly, fish will tend to give you its unique kind of energy—energy that will move you through your environment in a way that is different from chicken, beef, or other animal foods.

Fish can be supportive for health maintenance from both a nutritional and an energetic perspective. As with any foods, the effects of seafood are largely determined by the quantity *and* quality eaten. The larger the quantity consumed, the more intense the effect. The cleaner and less toxic these foods are, the more easily the human organism assimilates and processes the effects. The more toxic and chemicalized these foods are, the more complex and confusing the effects become.

At the time of this writing, people are still using these foods on a regular basis. However, many of our lakes and streams and large areas of the ocean have become so toxic that foods taken from them are becoming dangerously less suitable for human consumption. This is indeed a sad situation: one of the world's most important food supplies faces extinction due to man's ignorance and carelessness.

It also is worth mentioning that some authorities believe the irradiation of these (along with many other foods) does not adversely affect foods or those who eat them. I trust you haven't swallowed this one hook, line, and sinker!

Crustaceans (Marine Arthropods)

This group of sea animals includes the "lowly" lobster (so-called because of its scavenger qualities), crab, shrimp, and crawfish (also scavengers). These primitive *marine arthropods* ("water insects") are the first creatures, according to evolution theory, to include legs. They are all related in that each have five pairs of triple-jointed legs attached to the thorax, along with additional appendages; and all have a hard exoskeleton made up of *chitin,* composed of a combination of protein and calcium.

The exoskeleton of these creatures does not grow along with the rest of the animal, but it is molted and discarded as the crustacean grows, causing it to literally break out of its shell. The creature then eats its old exoskeleton in order to absorb the calcium in it, which it uses to grow another skeleton. The movements of lobster, shrimp, and crawfish consist of either crawling along the ocean floor or swimming backward with sharp jerks of their tails.

Shellfish once had a bad reputation due to their containing sterols, which were mistaken for cholesterol. Little of the sterols in shellfish are actually cholesterol, and even the ones that are have proved more beneficial than harmful.

Seafood in general has long been thought to be "brain food," and shellfish in particular does stimulate mental energy by elevating moods and mental performance. They are almost pure protein and this type of protein can deliver large supplies of the amino acid *tyrosine,* which breaks up to form *dopamine* and *norepinephrine,* which have in turn been shown to energize brain chemistry.

Lobsters

Lobsters tend to live near the shore in the summer and in deeper water during the winter. These unusual creatures are strongly attracted to decaying flesh and will feed on just about anything, including each other. They are ill-tempered, solitary, and aggressive creatures that live tucked away in crevices and rock ledges.

The aggressive quality of the armored lobster is most noticeable in its relationship with the loose and flaccid octopus—in fact, the two have a natural animosity toward each other. This is perhaps due to their both making their homes in the same places.

If confined to a trap or during molting, the cannibalistic lobster becomes subject to harassment and dismemberment and will often become food for its own kind. According to some biologists, the lobster feels little if any pain because it lacks a developed nervous system; however, it does have a highly developed sense of smell.

Crabs

Crabs move in a sideways manner along the ocean floor and sandy beaches. They can also crawl or use their last pair of flattened hind legs for swimming. There are 4,400 known species of crab, all of them edible.

This alert and aggressive beast is both a hunter and a scavenger, yet compared to other crustaceans, crabs are more adaptable to land. Swimming crabs lay their eggs in the summer, where they remain externally attached to the female for about two weeks until hatched as larvae. Once hatched, the surviving young molts, sheds its shell off and on for about a year, until fully matured.

Shrimp

Shrimp have many of the same characteristics as lobsters, with the exception of the two large claws that lobsters use for hunting and tearing apart their food. A single large muscle in the shrimp's tail allows it to thrust itself backward with quick strokes through the water.

Both the shrimp and the lobster contain their livers in their heads. The liver of these creatures is called *tomalley* and is considered a delicacy by many people.

Crawfish

The crawfish is a freshwater cousin to the lobster; in fact, crawfish are tiny freshwater lobsters. Like other crustaceans, the crawfish spends most of its time in water. However, during the cold winter months, it will venture out onto the shore and dig a hole in which to burrow, and there it will remain through the winter.

This unusual creature is blind, and neither nocturnal nor diurnal. Crawfish are *aperiodic,* which basically means they could care less what time it is.

The Energetics of Crustaceans

Some of the energetic qualities shared by all of these creatures and transferred to the person who eats an excessive amount of them can be seen through the following examples.

Their ability to create a hard, protective outer shell encasing a sweet, chewy, muscular flesh makes these creatures hard on the outside, soft and sinewy on the inside. This can manifest as an outward character that is stern, stubborn, aggressive, and a bit self-righteous; yet under this protective armor lies an inward character that is actually a bit shy and insecure, but easily malleable and capable of change, as long as one can penetrate the protective wall formed through past experiences.

The next time you have the opportunity, look into the eyes of a crustacean. Their eyes reveal a cold, heartless, penetrating stare. This intense squint and, in the case of the crab, downright menacing appearance, leads one to think that if these creatures could speak, they might say, "Come on, I dare you! If you can get through to me, you got me. I'm soft and sweet on the inside, but it's going to be messy getting there—and even if you do, you will still have to deal with the aftereffects of my character once I'm inside you."

These slow-moving creatures have no need to run and hide, for somehow they know they will get the last laugh when, a few days after eating them, your muscles tighten into knots (particularly around the neck and back) and your attitude becomes, well, a little crabby. The next time you eat shrimp or lobster, try to be aware of your sleeping patterns that evening. Chances are better than even you'll find yourself curled up in a fetal position periodically throughout the night. An interesting effect indeed.

Emotional insensitivity and decreased circulation are also energetic properties of crustaceans. Reversed motivation, with experiences of repeating and reliving the past, are common energetics that can lead to feelings of frustration and irritability. One may experience living life with keen mental alertness, yet perpetually *waiting* for something to happen because one feels too repressed to act spontaneously. The excessive consumption of crustaceans can also contribute to or exacerbate chronic skin conditions.

Crustaceans are certainly a unique food. They can be beneficial for conditions of kidney deficiency, low sexual energy, and flaccid muscles—especially the long muscles bordering the spine and those of the thighs and calves. Being scavengers who enthusiastically eat anything they might chance upon gives these creatures the energetic power to tighten the stomach and pancreas. This can manifest as overindulgence and erratic eating patterns.

Preparing crustaceans with olive oil or butter, cream or coconut milk, garlic and herbs, and spices helps to balance their effects as well as to neutralize any toxic effects they might have.

The crustaceans tend to delay their energetic effects from the time consumed to as far as two or three days later. I have counseled many clients who complained of waking up with pulled or strained neck or back muscles. When questioning these people about their consumption of lobster, shrimp, or crab, the usual response was that they had eaten these seafoods "a few days ago"—but what did that have to do with their cramps or pains?

Try to imagine me attempting to give an explanation to an individual about crustaceans being cold-blooded, slow-moving, consisting of pieces of muscle surrounded by a hard outer shell, and so on, and that these sensations and feelings are likely to occur if you should have such an intimate relationship with these creatures. . . . I usually get one of two responses to my explanation:

1. "Well, if you say so . . ."
2. This one is usually a mental response, but is so loud it might as well be verbal, and that is: "This guy is really out there!"

The first response opens the door for more stimulating interaction and the opportunity for both of us to further educate ourselves in the arena of food energetics. The second response usually results in a temporary shutdown of the right brain on my part until the opportunity to point out interesting correspondences should arise again.

The Mollusks

The mollusk family is one of the oldest and largest groups of water animals (more than one hundred thousand known species). They include clams, scallops, mussels, oysters, squid, octopus, and snails. There are three groups of mollusks commonly used for food: bivalves, cephalopods, and gastropods.

The mollusk group tends to have the longest delay in terms of producing their effects. These slow-moving, burrowing, clinging creatures can reveal their energetic properties sometimes up to a week after being eaten; however, some effects may be noticed shortly after eating them.

Bivalves

The bivalves include all the mollusks that consist of two shells containing a soft fleshy interior. The two halves of their shells are joined at a hinge and held together by one or two strong muscles. Some swim, some live in mud or sand, and some attach to rocks and pilings.

Most bivalves move by means of one muscular extension or foot, which acts as an anchor and is also used for crawling and burrowing. They eat by filtering water and food particles through their systems.

Scallops

Scallops are unique among bivalves in that their inner flesh consists of a single solid muscle, powerful enough, through its expanding and constricting motion, to give it the ability to hop or rapidly propel itself through the water. The scallop can literally take your finger off with one snap-shut of its shell.

The scallop is one of the few bivalves that do not burrow or attach to anything; rather, they live freely on the bottom of the ocean. They have forty to fifty eyes on the edge of their mantle, yet cannot visually distinguish forms, only light and movement. The majority of scallops prefer shallow waters.

Scallops are jumpy little creatures that alternate between quick, short bursts of propulsion, especially when predators are around, with long periods of being sedentary. While scallops can contribute to strong muscles, they also contribute to small muscular knots, particularly in the shoulders. They also contribute to extremes of energy output where one alternates between short bursts of energy and long periods of quietude.

Oysters

Unlike other mollusks, oysters have no foot or siphon, and they feed by opening and closing their shell to let water in and out. Oysters prefer shallow, warmer waters and will attach themselves to rocks, shells, and roots. When an oyster attaches itself to something, it is attached for life. When young, oysters are free swimming, but when they get older they attach themselves permanently.

Oysters' legendary trait as an aphrodisiac is revealed in their uncanny capacity to reproduce in stunning quantities—five hundred million eggs in one year. They also were once thought to resemble testicles and thus to have the power to increase seminal fluids in men and vaginal fluids in women.

Oysters are irregular in shape and are the most highly valued and expensive shellfish on the market. If you want your lover to become attached, encourage him or her to eat oysters; they contribute to attachment as well as to sexual vitality. However, they cannot guarantee that your lover will be monogamous! Their mucilaginous texture and high iron and zinc content help to tone the reproductive organs and stimulate sexual secretions.

Mussels

Mussels have been considered inedible in some parts of the world because they sometimes attach themselves to toxic supports and can easily accumulate toxic waste materials. Another surface-dwelling (non-burrowing) mollusk, mussels live attached to rocks and pilings.

In China, mussels, especially dried mussels, have long been used as a remedy for impotence and menstrual irregularity caused by cold conditions in the body. Like other bivalves that filter and perform similar functions as human livers, mussels energetically affect the liver as well as the reproductive organs.

Clams

Clams come in many different shapes and sizes, with life spans ranging from one to ten years. Growth ridges on their shells can determine their age. Their heartbeats range from one to forty beats per minute, quite slow as compared with the more lively mollusks such as the squid, whose heartbeat ranges from forty to eighty beats per minute.

Most clams have the habit of burrowing themselves in the mud close to shore. They move by dragging themselves with their singular foot along the ocean floor.

Quahogs are a group of five grades of clam that include, from highest to lowest: littlenecks, topnecks, cherrystones, medium clams, and chowder clams.

Like mussels, clams siphon their food through their bodies; the soft-shelled clam can filter up to a quart of water an hour through its body. The inner structure and function of clams, the siphoning process, closely resembles that of the human liver, thus clams resonate with and energetically affect the liver. Excess clam eating can also contribute to isolation and introversion, a dull, flat personality with a lack of motivation and the tendency to "clam up" and stop communicating.

Additional energetics of the bivalve group of mollusks include: burrowing, clinging, dragging (except for scallops, which hop), fertility, increased sexual vitality, and an overall calming effect (again, except for scallops). Because their lives progress slowly, one might experience the aftereffects from eating these creatures not immediately but gradually, even several days later.

Cephalopods

A group of nonbivalve mollusks called *cephalopods* includes the squid and octopus. Here the single foot of the bivalve is modified and differentiated into tentacles and a body with no outer shell. Unlike most other mollusks, cephalopods are predators and active swimmers.

Squid

The squid is the most active swimmer of the invertebrates. Their incredible agility and speed give them the ability to literally fly through the water—and, occasionally, through the air. When choosing their mates, squid will engage in a ritual where the male and female both rush at each other aggressively, coming as close as possible without making contact. This mating dance continues until the male chooses his mate. Once the mate is chosen, the male squid aggressively defends the female from all predators.

The graceful elegance of the squid in its natural environment is a sight to behold, yet when taken out of the water it becomes a flaccid, soggy blob.

Normally shy creatures, squid retire to the dark depths of the ocean by day and return to feed at the surface at night. Their ten arms are covered with suckers, which they use to grab swimming fish. They wrap their two longest tentacles around small fish, hold them steady with the other eight, and then proceed to eat with their sharp, pointed beaks.

Squid usually travel in schools. By contracting their bodies, they create a stream of water that propels them gracefully through the ocean. In addition to rapid propulsion, squid have a famous self-protecting mechanism: they emit an inky fluid that assists them in escaping and hiding from their predators.

I once had a client with prostate cancer who had decided to change his diet, based on suggestions from his doctor. He was told (and I agreed with the advice) to drastically reduce his animal food and junk food consumption and to include more whole grains and fresh vegetables. He was of Italian descent, had a strong constitution, and except for an excessive amounts of eggs, sausage, meat, and cheese, the remainder of his diet was quite balanced.

We discussed how he could make a dietary transition that could be both satisfying and supportive to his health. We agreed that he needed a break from processed animal foods, and decided to fill that void with small amounts of naturally raised animal products and seafood, especially fish.

Though he knew this was the proper thing to do, he had a look of deep concern on his face. When I asked him what was wrong, he replied, "Do I have to eat fish? I don't care for fish, but I love calamari [that is, squid]. Can I have calamari?" I assured him it was fine to have his calamari, but he should also have a wide variety of other foods.

I did not hear from him for about two months, but I heard about him from some of his friends. They said he looked great and was very busy with his business. Two weeks later he called me and said, "I feel great, lots of energy, my doctor is very impressed with what I've done, I've lost weight—but I feel like a rubber band. I mean, when I walk up the stairs, my legs feel like they are going to give out from under me and my arms feel real loose."

I asked him if he was perhaps overexerting himself and a bit tired, but he said he wasn't. I then asked him what he was eating. He was eating a wide variety of healthy foods prepared exquisitely by his supportive and committed wife. Everything looked great with his diet and with his progress in recovering from his illness. . . . But this rubber-band thing just did not make sense.

That is, until I spoke to his wife. She was a very optimistic, high-spirited lady, and when she took the telephone the first thing she told me was how she had learned at least fifty ways to prepare calamari. I said, "Really—does he like all of the other food he is eating?" "Loves it," she said, "but he can't wait for his calamari at dinnertime!"

The man did not like any other fish or seafood, and his doctor had taken him off all other animal products (due to his cholesterol levels) except for skinless chicken breast, which he didn't like either. So he was eating large portions of squid for dinner every evening. I explained the energetics of squid, with its loose and flaccid nature, and strongly encouraged him to add other animal products to his diet—any type, as long as it varied. This made sense to him. Within two weeks after reducing the squid and adding more variety to his diet, he had regained strength in his arms and legs.

When one food is used excessively, it becomes a dominant factor in one's life and has the power to energetically influence the effects of all other foods eaten. Even though this case is an extreme example, it is not uncommon for people to eat mono types of diets or repetitive diets—and I have yet to witness positive results from doing so.

Octopus

The octopus prefers shallow waters and may often be found hiding under rocks at low tide. More lethargic than the squid, the octopus prefers to crawl along the ocean floor with its eight arms, though it is capable of propelling itself through the water much like the squid.

This strange creature has no shell and can easily contort its body to squeeze through tiny holes and cracks. They live in retreats or lairs, coming out only to find food or to ward off predators. They feed mostly on crabs and other slow-moving creatures, which they grab with their tentacles and then inject with a paralyzing poison contained in their jaws.

Octopus lay their eggs in jellied clusters, about four thousand to a cluster; out of two hundred thousand eggs, only one or two will survive to reach maturity. The eggs hatch into miniature versions of the adults. After mating, the female rejects the male and establishes her home alone. At breeding time she stops eating and dies of starvation shortly after her eggs are hatched.

The octopus has an extremely well-developed sense of touch. Research and experiments have shown it to be one of the most intelligent of the invertebrates, especially in its ability to learn and memorize through touch and visual stimuli. Although research and experiments have been performed on the octopus, the work has been limited because of the animal's short life span (two to three years.)

Squid and octopus are carnivorous creatures and both can rapidly change color, especially when they get excited or when feeding. Their colors range from shades of browns and yellows to rose, depending on their temperament. These qualities energetically manifest in people as sudden or abrupt changes in mood and personality. They both contribute to muscular flexibility. Although both are predators, this is not obvious by appearance, with their flexible and graceful bodies. While squid travel in schools, the octopus is more of a loner.

Altogether, these qualities can energetically manifest as a shying from intimacy unless there is opportunity for domination—hiding the truth when it comes to emotional expression and the need to be surrounded or protected by strength and security.

Gastropods

Gastropods, often called *univalves* because of their single shell, include a large number of freshwater and saltwater snails as well as land snails. This group of mollusks mostly lives on rocks, sand, or mud. They have fairly well-developed sense organs, particularly their eyes, and easily detect light of varying intensities.

Snails

A snail's spiral shell is an ideal structure into which to retreat for safety and protection. Most snail shells have their opening on the right side and spiral clockwise. Some snails actually use their spiral-shaped shells to drill holes into clams and oysters. When reaching the inside, they then suck out the flesh. The two feelers on their heads allow snails to slowly and cautiously feel their way through life.

Escargot (snails) is a popular food in many European countries and has long been purported to increase sexual vitality.

Snails have an easygoing nature, not unlike a land slug, and are very sensitive creatures. They have a sensuous quality about them and energetically can stimulate the senses, especially the sense of touch, encouraging one to take it slow and easy. Is it any coincidence that snails often accompany a romantic candlelight dinner in places where they are considered a delicacy?

Conch

The conch is a large spiral-shelled creature found on the sandy bottoms of tropical waters. This unusual creature limits its food to algae and lives in a materialized version of the cosmic, logarithmic spiral, wherein lie the answers to so many questions posed by humanity through the ages.

Conch move by pushing themselves forward through a series of small leaps. They are also called abalone and are considered the filet mignon of the sea.

Snails and conch have a warm and damp effect on the body.

Sea Urchin

Sea urchins have a bony shell, made of calcium carbonate, which is covered with poisonous needle-like spines. They move slowly about the seabed by means of their spines, which they also use to defend themselves.

Scientists once thought the lifespan of sea urchins averaged around ten to fifteen years, but current research has revealed that they can live up to 200 years. They live on seaweed and contain five tonguelike sex glands on the inside of their hard shell. These pale orange-colored sex glands have long been a gourmet delicacy of the Japanese and other coastal peoples and have recently been referred to as "Viagra from the sea," due to their powerful aphrodisiac qualities.

Fish Eggs

Caviar and *roe* are two common names for fish eggs. Fish eggs can be an expensive food, Beluga being the most expensive and one of the largest types of fish eggs, Oestrova coming in second, and Sevruga third, as well as the smallest and most plentiful. These salty, bursting bubbles were once served free in coastal saloons as an accompaniment to beer.

While other fish eggs are commonly eaten, those of the sturgeon, whitefish, salmon, and lumpfish are the most common. Beluga, from the mighty sturgeon, are the fish eggs with the most prominent reputation.

The sturgeon is a fish that has changed little since prehistoric times. This is one ugly fish! Weighing in at up to hundreds of pounds, this wild and powerful fish was often bled alive in order to sap its strength. Sturgeon, a fish able to live for up to an incredible 150 years, used to be plentiful but is now dwindling because of its inability to adapt to polluted waters and industrialization.

The oceans are full of vital salts, gasses, and minerals fundamental to all forms of growth. In this fertile amnion float billions of eggs from many different species of fish, creatures that have to be immensely fertile in order for their species to continue to survive. Cod can lay from two to nine million eggs at once, hake one million, and mackerel up to one hundred thousand. These fish, like most others, are unable to protect their eggs, so most are ravaged by predators.

Eggs of any animal contain the as-yet-undeveloped potential of the whole animal; fish eggs also have their own unique energetic properties. They float suspended in the salty, mineral-rich, alkaline environment of the earth's bloodstream, just as human cells float in the bloodstream of the human body. Fish eggs thus have a profound effect on our cellular balance.

Osmosis is the process whereby sodium and potassium interact from inside and outside the body cell walls. Basically, sodium works from outside the cell and potassium works from the inside, yet a constant interchange occurs between the two within the cells and body fluids, as it must in order to maintain a healthy condition of blood and cells. Fish eggs can energetically stimulate osmotic interchange between the body cells and body fluids. The natural oil (high in essential fatty acids) contained in them also assists in the flexibility of surrounding membranes of our cells.

As with other very powerful foods, more is not necessarily better. They are very salty and can easily constrict and dehydrate body tissue, which in turn can produce temporary effects of warm and dry that later turn to cool and dry.

Fish eggs have long been considered powerful aphrodisiacs. Not surprising when considering their energetics!

28
Dairy Foods

Animal milk is the basic substance from which all dairy products are derived. Just how long humans have used animal milk as a food is still undetermined; new archaeological discoveries keep pushing the dates further back into antiquity. While six thousand years prior to the present (about 4000 BC) has been maintained by some historians as the point where cattle herding began, the practice likely goes much further back into prehistory.

How dairy has been used historically is of considerable interest here, in that most ancient cultures were not heavy milk drinkers per se. Rather, they tended to process dairy from various animals into cultured dairy products that could be kept without the use of refrigeration. These products included butter, cheeses, and a variety of fermented milk products. The ancient Sumerians, circa 3000 BC, were known to have made numerous types of cheeses along with other cultured dairy products. The ancient Egyptians and the Vedic culture of ancient India were also among those making healthy products from milk thousands of years ago.

Europeans introduced cow milk to the United States around 1625; shortly thereafter, the first U.S. dairy herd was established. Milk's appeal was strong, largely due to its vigorous promotion by an enthusiastic group of business people. By the 1830s, public demand had ushered in milking machines and automatic churners. Since that time, almost everything possible that *could* be done to milk to alter it from its natural raw state *has* been done, including irradiation.

With the advent of pasteurization, homogenization, and coast-to-coast refrigerated storage and transportation facilities, milk's availability increased dramatically. By the aftermath of WWII, it had become virtually synonymous with the emerging image of the clean-cut, nutritionally superior American way of life. What could be more American than Mom and apple pie? Only one thing: Mother Elsie and her frothy white stuff that washes that pie down—or tops it off, à la mode.

Milk became the "pure and perfect" food, so titled because of its high calcium, protein, and profit content. However, it has lately begun to be exposed as something not so perfect as we were led to believe. Many nutritionists (along with most of the world's lactose intolerant populations) have started to reconsider its importance and even its safety as a daily beverage.

Unfortunately, though, the excessive use of milk and milk products far removed from their natural states through the technology of modern processing has deeply and adversely affected a few generations of children and adults. Modern milk and diary products are perfect examples of how increased quantity of a product has had deleterious effects on its quality.

Surrogate Mothers

Milk is the first food of newborn humans, and is the one and only natural food that introduces us to the new world outside the womb. It secures and bonds us to our mothers, it prepares us for our life in the world of matter, it instills in us the feeling of oneness with the human species and connection to our world in every dimension, from chemical and sensorial to emotional and social.

Milk is of course also the first food of all other newborn mammals. When used by those of their own species, it doubtlessly bestows upon them similar virtues as a human mom's milk does on us.

The different milks of other animals, though far superior to soy formulas, when used as a substitute to nurse human infants create their own unique but related tangled webs of confusion.

Milk and other dairy products are singularly feminine in connotation. They are rich and creamy and derived from the female animal. The femininity of dairy products is undoubtedly one of its most appealing factors to humans.

Many of the misconceptions surrounding milk are based on the premise that milk contains all of the vital building materials of the animal, vegetable, and mineral kingdoms, and that it therefore must be the perfect food. There is much truth to that assertion: a healthy, well-nourished mother who nurses her newborn child may well be able to provide her child with ideal and essential nourishment. But it is absurd to think that the milk of a cow or any other animal could do the same for a human child (let alone a human adult!).

This does not mean that milk and products derived from it cannot be nourishing foods for many people. Quite the contrary: many people throughout the world thrive, and have for millennia, on natural raw milk and milk products. At the same time, many more people thrive on little to no animal milk products.

Animal milk contains precisely what is needed to support the physiology and character of the infant offspring of the animal that produces it. It is created by the mother animal solely to shape and form her offspring's character into the image of herself. This is precisely why traditional peoples since ancient times processed milk in natural ways to form butter, yogurt, cheese, and other dairy products: to alter the original form and make it suitable for human compatibility, as well as to help preserve what is normally a highly perishable food.

Milk is primal food and energetically corresponds to the character and personality of the species from which it originates. The fact that cow's milk is superficially somewhat similar to human mother's milk, and that this "pretty close to" equates to "just as good as" is one seriously incongruous leap of a conclusion. This is because that superficial and partial similarity exists solely in the world of *quantity*—not that of *quality*. (And in truth, even in terms of quantities, the nutritional profile of bovine and human milk is significantly different.)

One could argue (and many do) that humans have used the milk of animals as food for thousands of years; and besides, humans can eat anything. These are valid points. I'm not claiming that bovine milk and its derivatives are the sole source of plague and pestilence, or that they are of the devil. (That may sound extreme, but there are people who do take this sort of attitude about their pet "worst" food, be it milk, sugar, meat, alcohol, salt, fat, cooked foods, raw foods . . . the world of food fads has no shortage of villains.) No, far from it: nonhuman dairy food certainly has its place, as does any real food on this earth.

The point is that milk has historically been used mostly *in altered forms* and *moderate amounts*. The range-fed ruminants of antiquity could never have naturally produced milk in the kinds of quantities that would allow large groups of people to have their two to four glasses a day. Growth hormones and other artificial factors that unnaturally increase milk production in modern cows simply did not exist in ancient times. Cheese, butter, yogurt, and other cultured or artfully transformed dairy products were, for reasons of conservation and practicality, the primary forms that milk took in the dairy products of those traditional civilizations who utilized them at all. (Of course, there are always a few exceptions, the Masai tribe of Africa being one example; but they only consume a few foods anyway, more specifically, animal milk and blood.)

However, it is the *excessive* use of (or even the *pathological dependence on*) cow milk products and the processing of them from their raw state, along with the quality of what is being passed off as a nutritious food, that is so injurious.

Cross-Feeding

A major distinction between human blood and human milk lies in the fact that blood is an internal process, whereas milk is an external process. You'll recall that I spoke about things "seeking their own level" (in part 1); blood's level is *on the inside.*

You may notice, when you cut yourself and begin to bleed, that the medium of blood is not comfortable outside of the body; if subjected to this environment, it will react by coagulating. Blood flow is a continuously internal process, a process that is organized in such a way as to remain internal.

A mother's blood provides her child's internal nourishment at the stage of fetal development. Mother's milk emerges after birth as the next form of nourishment for her child. To a great degree, this second phase of nourishment constitutes the foundation of a child's character. It is organized and processed *internally* by the mother expressly for the purpose of *externalizing* as postpartum nourishment.

In other words, unlike blood, milk once formed *must leave* the body. Upon reaching the surface of the body, it separates, in contrast to blood's coagulating response to the outside world.

Because milk is connected in this way to its source (mother), it has the ability to bond or attach its consumer to this source. A perfect setup, indeed, for a little baby just entering a confusing world with little of its physical or mental capacity ready to plug in and use. This bonding of child with mother through her milk is one of the most important and assuring experiences a child can have.

The milk of each species is specifically designed to nourish and protect the immunity of the offspring of that species. Raw milk and raw dairy products are foods that are best introduced to a child after the foundation is set through its own mother's milk and the child is ready to incorporate other foods. The exception to this, of course, is if a mother simply cannot produce enough milk, or if her milk is nutritionally inadequate due to malnutrition or other unforeseen circumstances. (For example, there is evidence showing the transfer of HIV, herpes, and hepatitis to infants through mothers' milk.) Unfortunately, this is a growing concern in modern society and will continue to be so, as long as we remain disconnected from the natural world.

A Closer Look at Milk

Nutritional research is increasingly exposing the sacrilege of infiltrating human nourishment with processed cow's milk and other dairy products by linking them with such conditions as iron-deficient anemia in children, cramps, diarrhea, allergies, fatty deposits, and accumulations. Add to this the fact that a large majority of the world's population is flat-out lactose intolerant.

Cow's milk is composed of three basic ingredients: sugar, fat, and protein. The sugar is called lactose, a *disaccharide* and milk's sole sugar. A disaccharide contains two single sugars, in this case, glucose and galactose. Lactose is contained only in human and other mammal's milk; from the energetic standpoint, the lactose in each species is qualitatively very different.

Technically, human milk contains about seventy-five grams of lactose per quart, while cow's milk contains about forty-five grams. Because cow's milk comes close to human milk in its lactose content, it has been rationalized as being a viable substitute. But this similarity is a minor correspondence that misses several major points. For example, a calf is equipped with the appropriate enzymes and four-compartmented stomach to handle this type of sugar; a human infant has a stomach quite different from a calf's, and an entirely different enzyme profile.

Lactase is an enzyme that breaks down lactose. In human beings, lactase is found in the upper part of the small intestine (the *jejunum*) and appears during the last trimester in infants, reaching a peak in production shortly after birth. In the majority of the world's population, a decline in the ability to digest lactose occurs with aging after birth.

Lactase remains in the intestine up until about one year of age. It then begins to dwindle, yet can last up to four years of age, after which it no longer exists. If the amount of lactose ingested exceeds the amount of lactase present in the body, the lactose becomes indigestible and accumulates in the large intestine, where it ferments and reacts with the many types of existing bacteria. It is then converted to carbon dioxide and lactic acid, which causes water to build up as a result of osmosis. Undigested lactose remains in the intestines, where it continuously feeds bacteria, increases carbon dioxide gas, and builds water pressure in body tissue.

This intestinal drama has body-wide implications because the lungs and large intestine work together as a unit. The lungs receive oxygen and eliminate carbon dioxide; the large intestine receives and ferments bulk food matter, and once this is processed, eliminates what remains as waste. Simply put, the lungs process gasses and the intestines process solids.

Should the amount of carbon dioxide increase in the intestines beyond a threshold, it can produce acidic blood, resulting in fatigue and lack of mental clarity. This process can produce even more drastic results in young children, including colic, hyperrespiration, and excess mucus, and other problems.

These are just a few of the curses reaped by humanity from the extensive use of pasteurized and homogenized dairy products. More will be no doubt revealed through experience and research. Meanwhile, it is up to you to decide for yourself just how important and perfect milk and its products are for you.

While we repeatedly stress the importance of quality throughout this book, it cannot be stressed enough when considering the consumption of dairy products. This means that the smart choice of raw dairy products from grass-fed cows, sheep, or goats can have positive health benefits for many people when compared to their doctored counterparts that are pasteurized, homogenized, and riddled with antibiotics and hormones.

The protein found in milk products is called *sodium caseinate* or *casein*. Studies have shown that in sensitive individuals, lymphocytes—cells of our immune system that protect internal tissue—are activated to proliferate in the presence of milk proteins. Human milk contains 60 percent whey and only 40 percent casein, whereas in cow's milk the proportion is 18 percent whey and 82 percent casein. The percentage of casein, in other words, is *doubled* in cow's milk.

Casein is a sticky substance that when undigested will collect and accumulate in various parts of the body, particularly in soft tissue. This can result in restriction of healthy circulation, fat deposits, and a decreased ability to assimilate other foods.

Cow's milk has been described as "unstructured tissue," because after leaving the cow's body, it retains many of its original characteristics as living cow tissue. In other words, unless it is processed in a traditional, natural manner, the person eating it has to restructure it in order for the milk to take on a more human form. This is extremely difficult to do unless the milk is raw (or it is processed through fermentation or aged, as traditional diary products were and in some places still are).

This "unstructured tissue," after being ingested by an alien organism incapable of processing it adequately, will seek to influence the structure of its host body tissue. This can occur either by transforming the human tissue in which it bonds (and casein is well known for its ability to bond: it is used in the manufacture of glue and plastics) or by accumulating around this tissue to produce fatty cysts, tumors, and numerous other accumulations.

Milk contains large quantities of bacteria that contribute to its rapid spoilage. Pasteurization (the heating of milk) does keep this down to a minimum, but does not by any means eliminate it. And pasteurization contributes to problems of its own.

For example, in the process of heat-treating milk in order to kill bacteria, pasteurization unfortunately can cause the loss of up to 66 percent of vitamins A, D, and E. To make matters worse, pasteurization also destroys beneficial enzymes, antibodies, and hormones, and alters calcium into an insoluble form that cannot be absorbed. What's more, milk proteins are denatured through this process, thus promoting pathogens that can contribute to allergies.

Then there is the process of ultrapasteurization, wherein milk is heat treated at higher temperatures for longer periods, making the milk virtually sterile. And just when you thought nothing else could be done to alter milk from its natural state, they homogenize it.

When raw milk is left to set, cream rises to the top. Homogenization further treats milk by breaking up the butterfat globules in the cream and evenly distributing them so they can no longer rise. This causes oxidation and increases the rate of spoilage. It also changes the original fat globules: the original fat membranes are destroyed and new ones are formed with higher portions of casein. The enzyme lipase, essential for breaking down fat, is also destroyed.

And these are just some of the damaging effects caused by pasteurization and homogenization. For example, it is well established that magnesium is a supportive and essential complement to calcium. Commercial milk contains an added synthetic form of vitamin D called *calciferol*—which has been shown to bind with and remove magnesium from the body! Raw milk from pastured cows contains vital nutrients including vitamins A, B_6, D, and calcium, CLA (conjugated linoleic acid), probiotics, and enzymes. All are important in maintaining the integrity and nutritional profile of milk—and they simply cannot withstand the torturous effects of modern processing.

The point is this: many of the benefits people think they are getting by drinking processed milk are just not there in milk rendered into this unnatural state.

Commercial milk is slightly acidic, with a pH of about 6.5. When milk is ingested into the human body it is warmed to the temperature of the individual's metabolism. In this warming oven, the acid medium of milk creates the perfect breeding ground for further bacterial growth—which can adversely affect the immune system and create or encourage the growth of *Candida albicans* (a common opportunistic yeast). Pasteurized milk has the tendency to coagulate into tight globules when exposed to the stomach's strong acids, thus making it even more difficult to digest.

Moderate amounts of high-quality, raw dairy products are, for many people, healthy foods and should always be consumed with complementary foods from traditional sources.

The Calcium Question

Calcium caseinate is another substance found in cow milk. Milk is rich in calcium (as you have heard time and time again!) yet that calcium is bonded to casein, and this calls into serious question its usability and absorbability by humans.

Just because calcium exists in milk does not mean you can absorb it (though the TV commercials don't mention this). Pasteurization changes calcium into an insoluble form that decreases its ability to be absorbed.

The majority of the world's population does not depend on dairy food for their calcium needs, and many that do ingest less than half the quantity of calcium recommended by the dairy industry and their supporters. Both groups of people (dairy and nondairy consumers) still have strong bones and teeth. In fact, among some groups of people who consume *less* calcium than Americans, there exists *greater* bone density and *less* osteoporosis!

Interestingly, the calcium in an infant's body raised on cow's milk may be as much as twice that of one raised on human milk; as a result, the cow-milk-raised child can easily become metabolically dependent on high calcium intake throughout his or her growing years.

So when you consume lots of processed milk and milk products, you get more calcium, right? Wrong: along with a stockpile of unusable calcium, you create a *greater need* for calcium!

Cream and Skim

Traditional cream was obtained by allowing raw milk to stand until the fat globules would rise to the top of the container. The rich fat layer that accumulated at the top was removed and stored as cream. Eventually centrifuges were developed to speed the process. Whether by centrifuge or natural process, cream *rises*—and if eaten in large quantities, it can contribute energetically to stagnation of blood and lymph, particularly in the upper body and brain. It produces a cold and damp effect in the body.

Skim milk is a by-product of whole milk. The fat has been removed (along with its vitamin A and D) in the hopes of appealing to the weight-conscious people of the world. This does nothing to improve milk, however, for it still contains lactose and casein, and without the fat-soluble vitamins A and D to aid in its digestion, skim milk becomes truly unsuitable for human consumption.

Vitamins A and D are also needed for the assimilation of calcium and protein in the water faction of milk. The removal of the butterfat content of milk removes short-chain and medium-chain fatty acids, the very ingredients that protect against disease and support the immune system. Also removed through this process is the very important conjugated linoleic acid, which has strong anticancer properties. This process (removal of butterfat) is one of the most ridiculous things done to milk. It is not healthy for anyone—and it helps no one lose weight.

Regular use of skim milk can contribute to loss of minerals in the body. Additionally, it creates a cold and damp condition with pallor of the skin, and it can create small, hardened deposits throughout the body.

For all of you weight-watchers who drink skim milk, please take note: hog farmers use skim milk—*not* whole milk—to fatten their hogs! And if that isn't enough to discourage you, take note: calves fed skim milk develop sterility and failure to thrive. Leave it alone—and if you consume milk, make it only whole raw milk.

Cultured Dairy Products

Cheese, yogurt, buttermilk, and other cultured dairy products are practically free of lactose, because the fermenting bacteria use the lactose as fuel. With yogurt, the lactose has been broken down into glucose and galactose through fermentation; yogurt is a predigested food with partially broken-down sugar, fat, and protein.

Yogurt

Yogurt is created by adding a mixed culture of *Lactobacillus bulgaricus* and *Streptococcus thermophilus* to milk in order to increase its beneficial bacterial content. Through fermentation, the mixture becomes a type of health-promoting product that has been used for thousands of years by certain populations. The problem with most modern natural yogurts (the unnatural ones are worthless) is the additional processes of pasteurization and homogenization, processes that really defeat the purpose of yogurt, although some health benefits may still be gained by adding probiotics to the mix.

There are many healthy qualities in original yogurts as used traditionally in cultures throughout the world. These yogurts were and still are made from the raw milk of yaks, llamas, and other creatures that roam freely and live an extraordinarily active lifestyle, running and playing about the land and rocks (as do the people who consume the products). It was never made from the milk of a confined, factory-farmed cow that does literally nothing except eat, brood, and wait to be milked.

Energetically, yogurt has a cold and damp effect on the body. People prone to yeast infections and damp conditions should minimize the consumption of this food. Note, however, that quality yogurts do indeed exist, and they can often be supportive in moderate quantities for individuals who have a long history of having adapted to dairy foods.

Cheese

Potsherds found in archaeological digs in Switzerland reveal evidence of cheese-making in that part of the world as early as 6000 BC. As a naturally preserved source of protein and fat, various cheeses have nourished much of Europe, the Middle East, and other parts of the world for many thousands of years.

As in other cultured dairy products, the lactose in ripened cheese is converted to simple sugar. Enzymes are used to coagulate the casein (rennet, the inside of a calf's fourth stomach, is often added to accomplish this), the whey is pressed out, and bacteria work on the fat, protein, and lactose until they are broken down into simple molecules. The result is cheese, compressed curds containing a concentrated form of protein and fat.

Bacteria and mold are instrumental in the making of cheese, and this alone reveals much about the energetic properties of this particular food. Being acidic, cheese contributes its acidic bacteria to the bacterial pool of the intestines; when produced raw from pastured (not pasteurized!) cows, it can be supportive to digestion and assimilation as a good and reliable source of nutrition. However, when processed with modern methods and if eaten in large quantities, cheese can contribute to candidiasis, allergies, infections, and many other problems.

Any type of natural cheese, when consumed with a variety of plant foods as traditionally done, offers numerous health benefits.

The energetics of fresh or soft cheese includes a warm and damp condition in the body. In excess, soft cheeses can contribute to pallor, damp skin, water retention, and occlusions.

Aged cheese or hard cheese hardens and tightens, produces a warm and dry condition, and when eaten in excess can create an aged, dry, and wrinkled appearance to the skin.

Butter

A food once used extensively and exclusively by those who herded animals for a living is now an international sensation. The Japanese, who have now grown accustomed to butter and the other ways of the West, used to think their European friends who ate butter exuded a body odor that smelled particularly rank.

This is not a particularly astute observation for the rare individual who does not eat butter. However, for those who do, it seems perfectly natural to smell this way. While this is an interesting observation, it is not entirely accurate. People whose diet lacks vegetables and consists mostly of animal products and refined carbohydrates can and often do exude strong body odors—but this is not the case with people whose diet consists of moderate amounts of animal products with a high content of natural plant foods.

To make butter, cream is removed from whole milk and then churned until butter granules form, expand, and merge together. The end result of this process is a somewhat solid mass called butter and a liquid called buttermilk.

Butter is composed of about 80 percent fat, 18 percent water, and 2 percent milk solids. Butter contains a good amount of short-chain fatty acids, which are easier to digest and healthier than the long-chain fatty acids found in polyunsaturated plant oils.

People who follow low-fat and vegan-type diets often have cravings for butter, especially if their diets contain little or no fat and limited protein. This is not unusual when one considers the roles played by fats, proteins, and minerals in the process of metabolism. They need each other!

Unlike most plant oils, butter is good for frying because the saturated fatty acids it contains are somewhat stable to heat, light, and oxygen.

Excessive butter consumption, a common phenomenon, can result in difficulty in "letting go," whether it has to do with resentments, negative memories, or just about any other emotional experience. The person who loves butter and consumes it excessively will do almost anything to rationalize the case for butter and proclaim it better than any other fat. Some butter extremists eat up to a pound of butter a day.

To the butter lover, butter makes just about anything taste good. Butter is: holding on, yellow, mother, comfort, home, what is missing from toast, "I don't want to think for myself," "I prefer to dwell on the past," and "Life without butter is not worth living."

Excessive indulgence in butter produces a warm and damp effect in the body as well as a lack of healthy blood flow to the brain. It can also contribute to physiological and psychological heaviness.

On the other hand, when consumed in moderation, butter offers a host of health benefits. It is easy to digest, warming to the body, helps to maintain cellular integrity, and contributes to smooth and healthy skin. Raw butter from grass-fed cows is the ultimate butter; once you have tried it, you will be hard-pressed to go back to the usual pasteurized product.

Clarified butter, or *ghee,* is butter that has been heated, had the whey proteins skimmed off, and casein and salts removed. The result? Pure fat, and a healthy one at that. In India, ghee is a most precious substance because it comes from the ever-so-important and sacred cow, a creature long subjected to man's symbolism and mythology. Sometimes called golden fire, traditional ghee was made from the milk fat of buffalo. Like butter, ghee is even more effective at maintaining a consistent burning of one's metabolism. This can be helpful for those suffering from low blood sugar and extreme mood swings.

Ice Cream

Ice cream . . . yessss—NO! Frozen milk, cream, sugar, embalming fluid, and other what-have-you. And then there's the "natural" version: frozen milk, cream, sugar replacement, no embalming fluid, and what-have-you. Either way, what little passion may possibly exist in milk is totally eliminated in ice cream. Use it to rid yourself of passion, compassion, and warmth. It works! You and I both know it does.

Rich, creamy, and sweet, yes, but a substitute for sex and love, no. Ice cream offers a cold and unrewarding affair, indeed, one that is guaranteed to leave you lonely and frustrated.

Miscellaneous Milk

"What about goat's milk and cheese?" Goats are more playful than cows and they do have a sense of humor. Goat's milk has roughly the same protein and water content as cow's milk but *more* fat (4.3 percent, as compared to cow's milk's 3.9 percent) and *less* lactose (4.3 percent versus cow's milk's 4.9 percent).

It is more easily digested than cow's milk, because the fat globules are smaller and the fat is finer and more easily assimilated. It is also rich in antibodies and tends to have a lower bacteria count than cow's milk. Pasteurization of goat's milk is unnecessary because of the absence of tuberculosis; however, it is usually done anyway.

Reindeer have the richest milk: 22.5 percent butterfat, only 2.5 percent sugar, and 10.3 percent protein—almost three times the amount of protein of cow's milk. The problem is that the deer give only about one cup a day at the height of their season.

Dairy products seem to be such innocent foods. They are animal products, yet blood does not have to be spilled in order to obtain them. They are freely given, not won through slaughter or coercion. They are "perfect"; they are nature's own matronly, Mom-and-apple-pie recipe for building strong bodies and photogenic smiles twelve ways.

Not quite. Still, they have for thousands of years secured their place among some of the most important foods of the world and may be quite helpful and even necessary for many people in moderate quantities.

However, like all foods, dairy products must be eaten in a way that is supportive for human health, not as a mono food or as a meal replacement. Look to time-tested traditional preparations for balanced uses and consume only the highest quality available.

29
The Animated Life of Plants

Plants have the most important job on the planet: They supply the earth with oxygen. They do this by purifying the air of carbon dioxide, which they absorb and process through *photosynthesis,* a chemical reaction that results in the release of oxygen.

This process is reversed in animals: animals take in oxygen and discharge carbon dioxide.

Plants are also indispensable in that through this same photosynthesis, they have the capacity to transform light energy from the sun into chemical energy needed by other life forms. Not only can plants transform this vital energy, but they can also store it for later use. This stored chemical light energy, when eaten by animals and humans in the form of plants, is used as fuel.

In addition to being a primary food source, plants also are the true origin of proteins, carbohydrates, and other complex molecules, all vital components necessary to human and animal life. Without plants, the planet would be a lifeless spinning orb, sterile and barren.

Our planet has two main groups of land plants: the flowering plants, which include all plants with roots, stems, leaves, flowers, and fruits; and the nonflowering plants, which include ferns, mosses, algae, and fungi. Flowering plants are thought to have appeared 130 to 150 million years ago and have since multiplied to become about two hundred thousand known species. Most of our plant foods come from families of flowering plants.

The word *vegetable* has its origin in the Latin verb *vegere,* meaning "to animate or enliven." The most highly developed group of flowering plants is seed plants. This group contains more varieties than all the other plant groups put together; what's more, seed plants comprise most of the vegetables and crop plants eaten by humans.

Many vegetables can be eaten in their entirety, while others are eaten only in part, or during a particular stage of their development.

The Stages of a Plant's Life

Life cycles of flowering plants vary. Plants that live and die within one season are called *annuals*; those that live for two years are called *biennials*; and plants that live longer than two years are called *perennials*. These life cycles, or developmental phases from seed to flower, closely resemble our own unfolding life experiences of growth and development, and plants at their various phases of development energetically correspond to and influence the same phase in human unfolding.

The first phase of plant development occurs during seed planting. This is when germination and respiration take place in the seed, before it sprouts. Germination begins when a seed absorbs large quantities of water, usually in the spring, when environmental conditions are appropriate. Shortly after germination, the root burrows downward, while the upper end of the plant, the shoot, begins to form additional light green chlorophyll-containing cells.

The second phase of growth includes cell division, cell enlargement, and the initial stages of cell differentiation. This preflowering phase also includes the development of stems, leaves, and absorbing roots. While cell division is but a small part of the total process that growing plants experience, it is through this process that plants create new plant tissue. These early stages are similar to the gestation period we go through after conception. The consumption of seeds (grains, beans, etc.) therefore energetically brings to light our most ancient memories and the seeds of past experiences.

Unlike animals, whose growth depends largely on cell division, approximately 90 percent of a plant's growth takes place through the elongation of already established cells. Plants do this by absorbing large amounts of water, which causes their cells to stretch, mostly lengthwise. An interesting fact about this process is that the elongation of cells is not reversible. Plant cells grow and stretch to the limits of their capacity, then they harden—making growth more or less permanent.

The third phase of development is the reproductive phase and includes the development of flower buds, flowers, fruits, seeds, and further enlargement and maturation of the stems and roots. Other important processes occurring at this phase include the making of new cells, tissue maturation, fiber thickening, and the formation of hormones. The consumption of these parts (buds, flowers, fruits, etc.) of plants directly correspond to our hormonal development as well as sexual and creative potential. The unfolding of the plant into maturity carries the energy of the unfolding of life's potential.

The fourth and final phase is that of maturity, the termination of a plant's process so that it may relive again through its offspring seed.

These processional stages of plants closely resemble the human developmental process of childhood, adolescence, adulthood, and maturity; consuming plants at these varying stages nourishes us on levels far beyond mere biological nutrition.

Seeds

All possibilities exist in the seed. The hidden potential of life is held in check until perfect environmental conditions unlock and reveal the mystery of a plant's life. The sole purpose of a seed is to reproduce its kind in the final stage of its growth. To begin its life in the darkness of the earth, to unfold into light, to adapt—and to refold by reproducing its likeness—such is the journey and mission of seed.

A plant in seed form is called an *embryo;* once germinated, it consists of two parts. The upper part is called the *plumule,* which will become the stem; the lower part is called the *radicle,* which will become the root. After germination, the plumule strives to reach the surface and light, while the radicle probes deep down in the earth to anchor the plant. Attached to the plumule and radicle are the remnants of the seed, one or two *cotyledons,* which provide the young plant (seedling) with food until the roots and leaves have grown enough to be independent.

Four basic conditions are necessary for a seed to germinate: moisture, warmth, air, and darkness. Seeds need a warm, dark, and moist environment to release their energetics. Some seeds will not germinate even if the conditions are ideal, unless they first have been through a prolonged period of cold. Others need plenty of warmth and rainfall to start the process.

Many seeds are used for food before they become full-grown plants. These include seeds derived from fully mature plants, such as sesame, pumpkin, and sunflower seeds, nuts, legumes, and cereals (grains).

Seeds get around. Nature supplies the means for broadcasting seeds through the following methods:

- Wind dispersal: Lightweight seeds like dandelion are blown about, sometimes far from their original birthplace.
- Animal dispersal: Some seeds cling to the fur of animals or are swallowed by animals and birds, who then excrete the seeds during their travels.
- Explosive dispersal: Some pod plants dry in the summer sun and literally explode, scattering their seeds.
- Water dispersal: Some seeds travel by falling into water and can be carried for many miles by streams and rivulets before settling.

Seeds represent the beginning and the end of the life of a flowering plant, and they energetically correspond to the human nervous system and brain.

Roots

More than being simply the part of a plant embedded in soil, the vegetal root corresponds to the ancient art of sacred geometry. Just as a whole plant depends on its root for stability, nourishment, and proliferation, so too does the square or cube depend on its mathematical root to progress geometrically and logarithmically.

Plant roots are selfless foods. Their efforts at transforming mineral into vegetable are for the sole benefit of the plant as a whole. The root has the power to stabilize a plant, anchoring it and providing it with nourishment. It is in your small intestine, your root, where vegetable roots impart their energetics.

The first part of a plant to break through a sprouting seed is the root, in its pursuit of its main functions of anchorage, absorption, and storage. Of all the functioning parts of plants, the root is the only part that does its job in complete privacy. Hidden beneath the ground in the dark recesses of its place of birth, the root dutifully taps its surroundings for the essential minerals and resources it needs to insure the future life of the plant.

Roots, like human intestines, function and thrive according to their external supply of nourishment. Through absorption and assimilation, roots supply plants with vital nutrients. If adequate nourishment is not available, as is the case in much of today's malnourished land, the whole plant will suffer. However, if the soil is rich and vital, the plant will thrive. This is no different from your ability to digest and assimilate your food and environment through your small intestine, depending on the quality of the nutrients in that food.

Roots energetically supply an increased potential of absorption and assimilation to the human digestive tract. This is one of the most important energetic qualities of the relationship between roots and people. Another energetic quality of roots is their ability to stabilize the whole plant, giving it stamina and endurance.

The private nature of the root, demonstrated by its work underground in darkness, is energetically manifested in us as stamina, confidence, grounding (physically and mentally), persistence, and strength. On a spiritual level, roots help to define the inner meaning of our biological existence and secure the foundation for spiritual progression into the unfolding flower of awareness.

Different kinds of roots include long, round, diversely branched, and fibrous. Some plants have a large central root, called a taproot. These roots store food for plants to use in winter. They include such varieties as dandelion roots, carrots, and parsnips, along with many other edible varieties.

Unlike leafy greens, roots are fixed-goal-oriented: their goal is to dig deep and get to the point. Leaves, on the other hand, are more diversified in their goals. They sway with the breeze, expand into light, and openly expose themselves to their environment. The fixed-goal quality of roots records in us the qualities of attachment and holding on to life.

Roots demand the very quality of attention from us that they have so aptly given to their role in nature. Place a bunch of leafy green vegetables on a cutting board accompanied by a few carrots, turnips, or other roots. The leafy vegetables, exposing themselves with light and luster, give the impression of freedom. The roots, those roots, no lightness here, no, these are serious—bring you right back to reality, don't they? It's as if they are telling you to pay attention. They conjure up images of organization, attention, focus, order, and, again, getting to the point.

The shape and structure of the root as well as the flavor can determine the energetic effects of root vegetables.

Tubers

Botanically, tubers are roots swollen with the plant's winter food supply. Potatoes (see nightshades), Jerusalem artichoke (often called *sunchoke,* this is the tuber of the sunflower plant), and sweet potatoes and yams are a few well-known tubers that have served as staple foods for thousands of years.

Sweet potatoes are native to tropical America, particularly central coastal Peru; archaeological evidence places them back in prehistory to 8000 BC. Often confused with yams, sweet potatoes are perennial herbaceous climbers and a member of the species *convolulaceae,* the only member of its family raised for food. Like that of maize, also native to Central America, the ancestor of the sweet potato is lost in the mists of time.

Although they are native to both Africa and southeast Asia, we still have yet to find a definitive origin for yams. Yams are also herbaceous climbers, but from an unrelated family, *dioscoreaceae.* While yams are nutritionally inferior to sweet potatoes, both are starchy, rich, sweet-tasting vegetables that have been consumed as staple foods by traditional peoples for thousands of years.

Both sweet potatoes and yams tend to have a warm and damp effect in the lower body.

Long Roots

Carrots, burdock root, salsify, and parsnips are just some of the root vegetables in this category. Long root vegetables are particularly effective, energetically, on the large and small intestines, bladder, and the central parts of the reproductive organs (uterus, cervix, and prostate). These roots tend to concentrate or gather energy in these organs, especially when the roots are cooked.

Still, each root vegetable is unique. For example, a carrot is firm and stiff due to water pressure that builds up in its tissue. Burdock root contains less water and is drier than carrot, yet the burdock is more flexible than the carrot. While the carrot may well encourage strength and stability in the human body, it also creates a harder, less flexible condition in the lower body. Burdock root, on the other hand, can create similar conditions in the lower body, yet it provides more flexibility than carrots.

Long roots, particularly when cooked, tend to create warm and dry or warm and damp conditions in the lower body. Their energetic properties are to penetrate downward and inward. Daikon (long white radish) is one exception: it creates a cold and damp condition in the lower body, especially when eaten raw.

Round Roots

Turnips, radishes, onions (onions are actually bulbs, but do grow underground), beets, celeriac, and rutabagas are just a few examples of round root vegetables. The edible roots of this group usually contain more water than long roots and, like all roots, have flavors of spicy, sweet, or bitter. Round roots usually reach maturity earlier than long roots.

Because these round vegetables grow under the ground and share the same basic properties of absorption and assimilation as long roots, they too have an energetic effect on the lower organs of the body. Their swollen and rounded character give them the ability to mildly relax the lower body organs, especially when these vegetables are cooked. However, the spicy or more pungent varieties (onions, turnips, etc.), when eaten raw, have the ability to rapidly release tension and excess heat in the lower organs.

Round roots tend to create warm and damp or cool and damp conditions in the lower body. Their energetic properties are to sink downward and outward.

Irregular Roots

This group includes multistructured and odd-shaped roots such as dandelion, horseradish, and gingerroot. Most varieties of this category tend to have strong spicy or strong bitter flavors. The spicy varieties have a strong dispersing effect on the body, and the bitter varieties a drying, purging, and strengthening effect.

These varieties, along with echinacea, ginseng, and others, have long histories as medicinal plants. The energetic properties of irregular roots can be either dispersing downward and outward, or gathering downward and inward.

The symbiotic relationship between the human intestines and root vegetables can be understood through the following example. A person suffering from constipation resulting from a dry condition has available onions, burdock, and turnips.

- If he eats the onion raw, it will disperse stagnation and produce an aftereffect of cooling in the intestines.
- If he cooks the onion, it will have a sweet taste and a soothing, warming, and relaxing effect on the intestines.
- If he uses the cooked burdock root, it will strengthen, constrict, and dry the intestines.
- If he uses the turnip raw, he will get a less dispersing and cooling effect than the raw onion.

- If he cooks the turnip, the taste will be bitter and he will get a warm, slightly drying, and relaxing effect.

Get the idea? Of course you do. Eating the burdock doesn't make much sense in this situation—but if this same fellow were suffering from diarrhea, it would make the most sense.

Stems and Shoots

The stem part of a plant is the structure that connects the roots to the leaves. Aside from making this structural connection, the stem serves two other purposes: it holds the plant erect and in some plants, like melon and squash, the stem acts as a trailer and creeps along the ground.

A second important function of the stem is the role it plays in transporting water and minerals throughout the plant. The stem is the central part of a plant's circulatory system.

Stems consist of a tubular structure with many little tubes that extend through leaves. They are composed primarily of a hard, fibrous tissue called cellulose. Some plants have edible stems, while others have stems that are simply too tough to eat. The energetic qualities of edible plant stems are most influential on the circulatory system.

There are many varieties of stems and one can easily see the difference between short erect stems, such as those of the broccoli, where large amounts of moisture and mineral salts are pumped abundantly through the stem to the leaves and buds; and the long crawling vine stem of the buttercup squash, where nourishment is siphoned in slow but consistent streams. Then there is the unusual storage stem of the potato (potato is actually a portion of a stem called a tuber), where the plant's nourishment is stored in a somewhat stagnated mode, in terms of its circulation.

Some plants are grown specifically for their young stems and leaf stalks; these include celery, bok choy, rhubarb, asparagus, okra, endive, fennel, bamboo shoot, and artichokes.

The energetic properties of stems include upward and slightly inward or upward and outward. They also tend to have cooling effects on the body, particularly on the circulatory system.

Leaves

Leaves are an electrifying, logarithmic progression of a flowering plant's life cycle. They convert the energy of light into chemical energy. Reddish and bluish rays of sunlight are absorbed by pigments of leaves and converted into electrical energy.

Yes, *electrical* energy: all energy is electrical in varying degrees. Absorbed light electrifies the object that absorbs it and gives it life. The leaf, like all organisms, is given light, which it absorbs only to regenerate the absorbed light in the form of life. This fundamental law of give and regenerate abounds in all of nature, and leaves are perhaps its prime example. Leafy vegetables, along with all other green vegetation, do this through a process called photosynthesis.

The word *photosynthesis* stems from the Greek *photos,* meaning "light," and *synthesis,* which means "putting together." Plants put together light with carbon dioxide to make sugar and starch. Photosynthesis is the most important function of plants that produce chlorophyll (not all plants produce chlorophyll), the substance that makes leaves green.

This process occurs during daylight hours. Leaves manufacture food for the whole plant, and any surplus sugar that is produced through photosynthesis is changed into starch, which is then stored, usually in the leaves. During the night, the stored starch is changed back to sugar and carried by the veins of the leaf into other parts of the plant. At this point, any extra food that is not used immediately for growth and other basic functions is stored in the stem, roots, seeds, and fruit for later use. This built-in survival mechanism of the plant kingdom is prevalent throughout nature and has been one of the most difficult lessons for modern man to learn and apply to his life on this planet. Plants are consistently recycling.

The need for light is reflected in plants by the way they lean in the direction the sun is positioned. In the morning hours, when the sun is rising in the east, plants lean toward the east, and throughout the day plants follow the sun to its resting place in the west.

The green leaves of plants are biochemical factories: the photosynthetic process is essentially an energy-fixing reaction. The contrasting process to photosynthesis in plants is *respiration*. Respiration is essentially an energy-*releasing* reaction. The reserve of light energy built up by plants is stored and fixed through photosynthesis and released through respiration.

The green color of leaves comes from chlorophyll, a chemical that, with the assistance of light, changes carbon dioxide and water into sugars. The carbon dioxide processed by leaves comes from the air and enters through small holes in the leaves called *stomata*. Leaves can also lose moisture from these holes. Leaves do not work at night or in very dry weather; at these times, the leaf closes down and stores water for the plant.

Closely observe a leaf and you can see tiny veins or branches extending out from the main stem. These tiny veins are the leaf's transport system for the circulation of water and minerals. In between these veins lie smaller units of plant tissue, which are made up of even smaller units called *cells*. The tissue and cells are what leaves use to capture light energy to store as sugar.

All leaf cells are similar, and within each cell exists tiny green bodies called *chloroplasts*. It is within the chloroplasts that the green pigment of the leaf is stored and the processing of sugars takes place. The chloroplasts are the work force of the leaf and are constantly in motion.

Inside these organisms exists a system of double membranes arranged in spiral layers forming structures that resemble stacks of coins. These structures are called *grana*. Chlorophyll is arranged in thin layers in the grana, making them very efficient for catching light. The molecules of chlorophyll, like all molecules, are made up of atoms. The five kinds of atoms found in chlorophyll are carbon, hydrogen, nitrogen, oxygen, and magnesium.

The leaf of a plant is the organism's respiratory system and corresponds to our lungs. Green leaves are in essence the lungs of the plant, as well as the lungs of the Earth. Energetically, leaves embody light and lightness. They stretch their limbs upward in a centrifugal direction, or outward horizontally. They reach for their light source, graciously absorbing the generous offering of warmth from the sun.

Leafy green vegetables physically affect the upper part of the body, especially the lungs, heart, and throat. They encourage cosmic rhythm, the breath of life, and oxygenate the human body, feeding the cells so as to produce hemoglobin. This, in turn, lights and enlightens the darkened areas of the body and soul.

Leafy vegetables tend to grow in a centrifugal direction and therefore energetically stimulate the mental processes of imagination, openness, creativity, and spiritual awareness. These foods energetically manifest qualities of freshness and life. Their role as a food is to produce a gentle cooling effect in the body, particularly in the upper body (heart, lungs, and throat). All leafy greens have a tendency to balance body density and heat, and this makes them beneficial for conditions of excess.

Leafy greens vary in effect according to their structure. We can classify leafy greens into four basic categories according to structure and effect.

Broad Structure

This group of green vegetables includes plants with the broadest leaves: collard greens, bok choy, chards, romaine and leaf lettuce, and any others that sport a rounded and wide leaf structure.

These varieties of leafy vegetables produce the most cooling effect in the body and are beneficial for people who experience tightening, constriction, or excess heat in the chest area. For individuals who are rather expanded in the chest area or are cold in this area, these particular greens may not be the best choice of green vegetables for these problems; however, they are harmless. These leafy greens tend to contain more moisture than others, have a sweet or slightly bitter flavor, and their energetic properties are upward and outward.

Serrated Structure

This group of green vegetables includes mustard greens, kale, rapini (broccoli rabe), escarole, turnip greens, radish greens, and any other ripple-edged greens.

This group comprises the largest selection of edible greens. As green leafy vegetables become tighter from the broad category, they also tend to become more bitter in taste. The more bitter the taste, the more drying the effect on the body. These greens are especially helpful in ridding the upper body of excess mucus and water, yet they may not be the best choice for individuals with a dry and constricted feeling in the chest area. The energetic effects of serrated greens are upward and inward.

Tightly Serrated

This group consists of the most bitter as well as the tightest leafy greens. They include dandelion greens, carrot tops, watercress, chicory, and any other narrowly structured leafy vegetable.

The effects produced by these vegetables are cool and dry. The use of fat or oil in preparing these greens will contribute to a more warming and less dry effect. The energetic properties of these greens are upward and sharply inward.

Straight and Smooth

These green vegetables include chives, scallions, and leeks. They tend to have a pungent or spicy flavor and can help disperse excess heat and stagnation in the upper body. The energetic properties of these greens are strong upward and dispersingly outward.

Buds

Plants produce two kinds of buds: leaf buds and flower buds. Leaf buds contain the future leaves of the plant, intricately and logarithmically folded together. They can also contain additional stems. Flower buds contain future flowers, but unlike leaf buds, flower buds don't grow new stems. Flower buds are surrounded by a set of leaves called *sepals*. This spiral whorl of leaves is collectively called a *calyx*.

Energetically, buds—both leaf and flower—represent a plant's ability to reflect on its past and prepare for its future. The plant at the prebud stage has released and unwound itself to the point where it then temporarily retracts and concentrates its energies in order to go through its final stages of reproduction.

The bud is an area of very active cell division. It represents a building of momentum, with the explosive capacity to create a complex structure different from any the plant has previously experienced. The bud is a fertilized womb and contains a tremendous amount of active yet contained energy.

Cultivated plants whose buds are used for food include the cabbages and their relatives, broccoli and cauliflower. These buds are milder in their energetic effects than those eaten and enjoyed among wild food enthusiasts. Three delicious and powerful wild plant buds eaten by traditional peoples are young dandelion buds, milkweed, and daylily buds.

Buds have the potential to energetically support fertility, both physically and mentally, in the form of ideas. They also resonate in and help to cleanse the lymphatic system. They have energetic properties of upward and gently outward.

Ground-Level Vegetables

This group of vegetables includes a wide variety of flowering plants that exceed the number of varieties found in the leafy and root groups. Some of these vegetables are round, some elongated, some stalked; all are found at the end of a stem and all lie on or close to the ground. Some of these vegetables are buds and others are the fruit of the plant.

Cabbages, hard squashes (butternut, buttercup, acorn, etc.), cauliflower, broccoli, cucumber, zucchini, and summer squash are just a few of the examples of the many varieties of ground-level vegetables.

Being in between leafy and root vegetables, ground-level vegetables energetically have an effect on the middle organs of the human body: stomach, pancreas, liver, gallbladder, and spleen. Those varieties with high water content (cucumber, summer squashes, and head lettuce) energetically cool, dampen, and relax these organs, whereas hard squashes and cabbage will tend to create a dry and warm relaxing effect. Like different leaves and roots, each ground vegetable has its own unique energetics.

These are the more social vegetables of the plant kingdom and they relate to the social and human relations side of us. Calming, soothing, comforting, and just plain getting along with each other are some of the energetic qualities available through these vegetables. The energetic properties of ground vegetables include: slightly upward and outward, slightly upward and slightly inward, or sinking downward and outward. Overall, their energy is of a steady circulating nature.

Flowers

Flowers further develop a plant's character by giving it color beyond the green stage. They also reveal the hidden beauty of a plant's reproductive process.

Flowers embody the beauty of transformation and they let us know that a plant, at this stage of development, is reaching the final stage of its transformation process. The process of plants up to the flowering stage can be compared to the human being who has created major breakthroughs in his or her fears and anxieties and has now become a more social and loving person due to this awakening, realizing a greater sense of self-worth.

While this may be a wonderful and colorful experience, there still exists the further stage of transformation where we must then think about what to do with this newfound realization.

The flower's next stage of transformation consists of reproducing its likeness in the form of fruit and seeds. With humans, it is no different; it is simply a matter of production, or more simply put, using our transformed self in some way as to contribute to other budding organisms in some creative way.

Essentially, edible flowers correspond and contribute to our right-brain function of creativity.

Flowers contain various parts, each with a specific function. The petals are the most recognizable part of a flower and serve to help protect its delicate core from varying weather conditions. A flower's bright colors also help to attract insects. In wind-pollinated flowers, the petals are usually small or nonexistent, whereas petals of insect-pollinated flowers are large and brightly colored.

Stamens

Some flowers contain a single *stamen,* while others may contain many. Each stamen contains both a *filament* and an *anther* which, when ripe, contains pollen. Each grain of pollen contains a male cell capable of fertilizing a female egg cell. These are the male reproductive organs of a flower.

Carpals

These are the female reproductive organs of a flower and, as with a stamen, some flowers may contain one or more *carpels.* The carpel contains a *pistil* and *ovaries,* both located at the central bottom part of the flower.

Flowers are often used as decorations for culinary preparations; however, there are a number of flowers used for food and a large variety of flowers are (and have been for centuries) used in the preparation of herbal remedies and concoctions.

Some edible flowers include red gladiolus, yellow calendula, yellow marigolds, lavender chicory, lavender borage, hollyhocks, yellow squash blossoms, orange nasturtiums, violas, white and red runner bean blossoms, apple and plum blossoms, and Johnny-jump-ups. When consuming edible flowers, we are consuming both the male and female reproductive organs of the plant and their energetics.

Flowers have long been equated with love for another person. Energetically, they represent open sexuality. And they do evoke a special type of sexual energy. The next time you create a particular food preparation that you are proud of, garnish it with a few flowers—they needn't be edible flowers—then stand back and observe what the addition of the flowers to the preparation has done to the food. Yes, it makes the food sexy. That is the nature of flowers, exposed male and female reproductive organs together with bright colors. Only plants can get away with this kind of exhibitionism in public.

The energetic properties of flowers are strongly upward and strongly outward. They also contribute to bright and colorful personalities.

Full Circle: Fruits and Seeds

After its brief streak of copulation and sexual exposure, the colorful flower now prepares itself for the final stage of responsibility, the fruits of its labor. When a flower is pollinated, whether by insect or wind, seeds begin to form in the flower's ovary. The ovary begins to grow, the petals fall to the ground, and the fruit remains. Every plant has its own unique type of fruit, and each and every fruit contains a seed or seeds, either inside or outside of the fruit, each seed being capable of growing into a new plant.

Fruits are the final stage of reproduction for a plant, the final product, the children, and these children contain the seeds for the next generation. They now need only to ripen to maturity so they can pass on their knowledge (genetics) to their offspring.

Well-Known Vegetable Families

Another way of looking at different groups of plants is according to the particular families to which they belong. There are numerous species and subspecies of vegetables, and members of each species vary in terms of energetics and placement within the categories of root, leaf, stem, and flower categories.

Cruciferae

The cruciferae family of vegetables, so named because all have flowers with four petals that resemble a crucifix, includes the subspecies *brassicas*. Brassicas include:

- kale (leafy category): a strong and durable plant as well as one of the earliest forms of cabbage cultivated
- cabbage (budding heads of the ground category): a versatile vegetable responsible for the development of broccoli, cauliflower, kohlrabi, and brussels sprouts, due to the natural development of parts of the cabbage by early plant cultivators
- bok choy (leafy and stem category)

- Chinese cabbage (ground category)
- cauliflower (bud and ground category)
- broccoli (bud and ground category)
- kohlrabi (stem and ground category)—not a root but a swelling of the stem
- brussels sprouts (bud and ground category)

Other cruciferae include mustard greens, collards, watercress (a plant widely known and used in ancient times; it grows best in cold running water and grows wild in every state in the union), and land cress—all leafy category—and turnip, rutabaga (an offshoot of the turnip), radish, and horseradish—all root category.

Cucurbita

Cucurbita is another species of vegetable that includes summer and winter squashes, all ground categories. Pumpkins and hard squashes were cultivated by Native Americans as part of the "three sisters," their triad of principal foods: beans, corn, and squash.

Hardy foods with strong personalities, pumpkin and winter squashes grow slowly, have tough skins, and store well.

Cruciferae and curcubita are just a few of the numerous plant families.

30
Some Unusual Characters

The vegetable realm includes a huge range of varieties, many more than could possibly be covered individually in this book. However, several specific families are especially interesting in that they not only have become very popular, commonly used foods, but they also exhibit most unusual traits.

Fungi

The fungi family includes a wide variety of mushrooms, all of which are relatives to molds and yeasts. They are saprophytic plants, which means that they are unable to photosynthesize sugars (unlike other vegetable plants) and therefore must survive on the decaying remains of other organisms. They do this by excreting digestive enzymes, which help to further break down decaying matter.

Some varieties of fungi have a symbiotic relationship with tree roots, the fungi borrowing sugars from the roots and in exchange giving the roots minerals (especially phosphorus).

Unlike the higher seeded food plants, fungi do not contain chlorophyll, nor do they have roots; rather, they have short hairlike filaments called *mycelia* (singular: mycelium), which make and disseminate spores for future fungi.

The composition of their cell walls also differs from that of the higher plants. Instead of having a cellulose structure, fungi cell walls are composed of chitin, the same chemical complex that makes up the outer skeletons of crustaceans and insects.

Fungi are one of the most primitive species of food. Remains of puffballs have been found in Stone Age settlements. These and many other exotic species of mushrooms have been eaten throughout the world, and still are today. Their meaty flesh is actually the fruit of the fungus; when cooked, it adds a distinct, rich flavor to almost any plant or animal food preparation. This is partly due to the fact that mushrooms are unusually high in glutamic acid, a substance reported to be beneficial to brain and nervous system functions.

Most mushrooms prefer a dark, cool, and damp growing environment. However, once picked, mushrooms do not like moisture; once they get wet, they tend to spoil much more rapidly than if kept cool and dry.

The common white mushrooms often found in grocery stores, though grown in great abundance, are one of the most highly chemicalized plant foods available. The fact that there are so many varieties of mushrooms, some poisonous enough to induce immediate death, along with the fact that mushrooms experience numerous color changes on their road to maturity, has contributed historically to much of the fear and denunciation attending these lowly scavengers.

When considering the use of mushrooms for food, it is important to choose those from a healthy environment—that is, wild or cultivated on healthy soil. Do not let the idea of fungi thriving on decaying matter dissuade you from enjoying what many believe to be one of the most delicious foods available. If you prefer to leave mushrooms out of your relationships with food because of previous experience or taste, okay—but do not be too quick to judge this unusual food.

Bacterial Breakdown

Bacteria, germs, and viruses exist everywhere, and the fact that we are taught by medical science to fear such things has not helped us any in opening up to the idea that some of these particular substances may actually be beneficial to our health. Miso, for example, is simply soybeans, grain, and salt mixed together, then left to ferment and produce bacteria by eating and digesting itself.

Mushrooms, from an energetic perspective, may assist in the absorption and elimination of some types of troublesome bacteria. After all this is what they do in nature: eat bacteria. Numerous studies in Japan have shown that some mushrooms (shiitake, reishi, enoki, straw, oyster, and tree ear) have the ability to interfere with the growth of cancer by supporting the immune system.

The traditional use of mushrooms to help balance meat preparations can be found throughout the world. Meats tend to putrefy once exposed to oxygen; since they thrive on bacteria, mushrooms may actually help reduce and control some forms of harmful bacteria.

This does not mean that eating meat is a bad thing, by the way. Quite the contrary: simply avoiding meat does not mean you will not create harmful bacteria and putrefaction in your digestive tract. Some vegetarian-oriented diets have a tendency to produce more acid fermentation and thus more bacteria from the overconsumption of simple carbohydrates than does heavy meat-eating.

What's more, overeating itself tends to produce unhealthy bacteria in the body, especially overeating carbohydrates, and cooked mushrooms help to reduce these unhealthy bacteria and other organisms that can disrupt a healthy homeostasis.

On the other hand, mushrooms prefer cool, dark environments, so they also have the potential to induce those kinds of feelings in the eater, especially if one tends to feel shy or inhibited in the first place. They also change color throughout their developmental stages, and this is energetically indicative of emotional volatility in human temperament. When cooked, mushrooms tend to have a cool, damp effect on the human body. Eaten raw, they will have a cold and damp effect.

The Nightshades

The most common nightshade plants used for food are the tomato, potato, eggplant, and bell pepper. These unusual plants, once considered poisonous by many, are relatively new to Europe and North

America. They originally came into prominence as ornamental plants. A sight to behold, these beautiful plants decorated many a landscape of European and American homes during the seventeenth and eighteenth centuries.

The term *nightshade* derives from *nihtscada,* meaning "the shade or shadow of night," an evocative name that refers to the narcotic qualities allegedly exhibited by any of the various flowering plants of the genus *solanum.*

Their above-average nitrogen content gives this family of plants a strong link to the animal world. Unlike other flowering plants, nightshades contain an imitation of the animal *gastrula,* the basic reproductive form from which an animal develops. The gastrula in nightshades is located just above the seed bud of the blossom.

Some of the toxic substances found abundantly in commonly eaten nightshades are *solanine, glycoalkaloids,* and *alkamines.* The green substance found on many potatoes indicates the presence of *solanine,* a poison that has been linked to rashes and other skin diseases. Glycoalkaloids have been shown to cause red blood cells to self-destruct in vitro, and alkamines, which are absorbed by the intestines, have been shown to contribute to nervous disorders in humans and animals.

Altogether, these substances found in nightshade plants have been linked with kidney stones, calcium depletion, nausea, abdominal pain and swelling, loss of red blood cells, ulcers, jaundice, rashes, muscle wasting, breathing difficulties, trembling, drowsiness, and paralysis. The most famous negative association of nightshades, though one that is still debated, is with rheumatoid arthritis.

Needless to say, this is a fairly exhaustive list of technically researched symptoms—symptoms that should stimulate some thought as to how much and how often you might want to intimately involve yourself with these foods!

In addition to being highly animated during the cool night hours, the nightshades are not very social plants: they thrive best when growing alone in their own soil, away from other vegetables. They do, however, grow well with their own kind. All of these traits suggest quite interesting behavioral energetics in the nightshade eater. Keep in mind that scientific research based on isolating one or two components from a food does not always mean the whole food is something to be avoided. One could find something toxic in any food if one were to look hard enough.

While harmless in moderate amounts, any of the common nightshades can, when eaten in excess, contribute to:

- physical and mental weakness (they are weak and fragile plants, without a central core)
- premature aging (if you should meet someone who appears more wrinkled and older than they really are, more than likely, they are eating these foods as a regular part of their diet)
- a dirty grayish complexion, often accompanied by sagging skin
- physical and emotional coldness
- poor circulation resulting from stiff and rigid joints and muscles
- a preference for engaging in late-night activities
- insomnia
- a strong desire for flesh and blood

The latter, on a mechanical level, means the person has a tendency to crave animal products, especially dairy products and red meats. Symbolically, it means the person feels the need for more attention, support, and strength from others; psychologically, these needs often manifest as emotional vampirism.

Potato

The potato originated in the high Andes Mountains of Peru. One hundred and fifty varieties were known by the time of the Spanish invasion. It can grow at elevations of thirteen thousand feet above sea level. A starch-producing plant (yet quite unlike cereal plants, which are seed carbohydrates), the potato is a weak plant with straggling, though somewhat erect, branching stems. The average height of the plant is one to three feet. It can, but rarely does, produce a fruit about three-quarters of an inch in diameter with a greenish color.

Potatoes can be grown almost anywhere, with the exception of low tropical regions. The undergrowth of the potato plant consists of fibrous roots with additional branching stems that become swollen at the tips to form *tubers*. In winter these tubers—the actual potatoes—survive and the leaves of the plant die. Young shoots then develop from the eyes of the potato, feeding off the mother potato until it withers and dies—truly a self-absorbing, self-satisfying plant with little concern for its mother, other than to suck the life from her until the young become mature enough to sacrifice their own lives to the next generation of young shoots.

This rounded, watery, gutless tuber (not a root) is the second largest cash crop in America, after wheat.

Poisonous alkaloids called *solanines* appear as a green color on potato skins, particularly when they are exposed to light. The solanine level of most potatoes is about 90 parts per million (ppm), which is about one quarter of the danger level determined by researchers.

The potato has a most unusual history. In 1530, the Spanish conquistadors found the Incas eating tiny potatoes the size of peanuts. They observed the Peruvians first soaking the little potatoes in water and then letting them freeze in the cold mountain air. They then dried them in the sun and proceeded to rub off the skin by walking on them in their bare feet until the tiny potatoes turned black and hard as stones. They were then soaked for three to four days before being cooked in soups or ground into flour to make bread.

These tiny little forerunners of the bloated modern potato were subjected to some serious processing before being considered fit for consumption! Traditional peoples throughout the world have long practiced various methods of detoxifying particular plants, in order to make them edible; potato may very well be one of the earliest examples.

Introduced to France in 1540, potatoes were at first considered an ornamental plant and not yet accepted as a food. Thirty years later, the French forbade the cultivation of potatoes, based on the belief that they caused leprosy. By 1771, most of Europe (with the exception of France) had finally accepted the potato as a food. However, there was still much concern and doubt throughout Europe about the possible dangers of this new food, particularly among the farmers and peasants. In 1663, the Royal Society of England urged the planting of potatoes to prevent famine—a request that was vehemently opposed by the peasants and farmers.

Many believe the Irish were the first to consume potatoes in any substantial quantities. This is probably due to the history-making "potato famine" in Ireland that wreaked havoc among both young and old. This tragedy was largely due to the Irish attempting to replace much of their original cereal agriculture with potato farming. Potatoes did not become the basis of the Irish peoples' diet until late in the eighteenth century.

However, the Germans were the first big potato eaters. In 1720, Frederick William I imposed on the Prussian peasants (under the threat of draconian punishment) the mandatory planting of potatoes. The peasants, still convinced that potatoes caused leprosy and other skin diseases, refused and pulled the potatoes from the ground. They were then told they had to grow them—or have their ears and noses cut off. Given this set of alternatives, they grew potatoes.

Up until 1770, the Presbyterian clergy of Scotland maintained their stand that potatoes were not good because they were not mentioned in the Bible.

In Elizabethan England, the potato, having not yet reached its bloated condition so common today, was known as being small as a human finger. In Shakespeare's *Troilus and Cressida* (act 5, scene 2) this reference occurs: "How the devil luxury, with his fat rump and potato finger, tickle these together."

Once accepted, the potato grew in both size and popularity; however, in America potatoes were still not widely eaten until the start of the nineteenth century.

Energetically, potatoes can contribute to mental and physical weakness. The physical effects of excess potato-eating can result in pallor, withering and wrinkling of the skin, skin moles, and rashes. They are very difficult to digest, contrary to popular belief, and contribute to flatulence, intestinal swelling, and the reduction of minerals in the body.

During the 1600s and 1700s, potatoes were thought to weaken the human reproductive cells and thus cause hydrocephalus and general stupidity among those adults and children who ate them. An interesting piece of art by Vincent Van Gogh called *The Potato Eaters* clearly depicts the debilitating qualities then attributed to potatoes.

Because of the potato's self-satisfying nature and laziness, it can contribute to mental symptoms of fatigue and drowsiness, scattered thinking, inability to pay attention, mental dullness, simplemindedness, blind allegiance, and blind faith, as well as unthinking devotion to dogma and an overall dull spirit with a lack of creative thinking. It is interesting how red meat, having essentially the opposite qualities, is the most common match for potatoes in developed countries. When one eats compliant potatoes, it is wise to eat them with dominant strong, stabilizing foods (such as meat) to counter some of the weakening effects inherent in the potatoes.

Potatoes are weak plants, susceptible to disease and rapid decay; if eaten in excess, they can foist these qualities on the human immune system. Unlike cereal grain carbohydrates, which have a nourishing and vitalizing effect on the brain, the potato, with its large, expanded, and watery starch molecules, tends to have a weakening effect on the midbrain. This, in turn, stimulates the forebrain to substitute for the usual functions of the midbrain—hence, the manifestations of blind idealism and a lack of common sense.

While potatoes may be lacking in the areas of strength and endurance, they do have positive qualities. They are a supportive food for conditions of tension accompanied by excess heat and dryness. They are effective at absorbing salt and can be very helpful for reducing the sodium in tissues of people who have consumed far too much salt. Referring back to the character types of dominant and compliant, potatoes are one of the most compliant foods.

Tomatoes

Like potatoes, tomatoes have their origin in South America, most likely Peru. The Peruvians gathered the wild fruit in season; at the time of the Spanish conquest of Peru, this fruit was yellow in color and the size of a cherry.

Except for Peru and possibly some other places in South America, the tomato was regarded strictly as an ornamental plant and was introduced as such to Italy, France, England, and Portugal shortly after the close of the sixteenth century by visiting Spaniards. The Italians appear to have been the first to use the tomato as food, and even for them, it took about two hundred years of growing it as a curiosity and ornamental plant before they did. By 1827, the use of tomatoes as a food had increased throughout Europe, yet both England and France were still hesitant and had not yet fully accepted the fruit.

The Italians called the yellow tomato "golden apples," a title later mistranslated by the French to "love apples," accompanied by the myth that tomatoes had aphrodisiac qualities. Perhaps this is what finally influenced the French to accept the tomato.

In America, the first tomatoes were grown as ornamental plants around 1832. Americans had heard the French were eating them and by 1844, they had begun to increase in popularity. Still, the tomato did not find its place in America's kitchens until World War I. It wasn't until 1929 that the Bureau of Home Economics launched its promotional campaign that claimed the ideal diet for Americans should include fifty-five pounds of tomatoes per person per year.

The tomato is actually a fruit; however, in 1893 the Supreme Court, by decree, ruled that because it was used as a vegetable, it should be considered one for trade purposes. It is ironic that nearly one hundred years later, the Reagan administration raised a howl in the press by its claim that tomato catsup and French fries (themselves not yet renamed in a puerile fit of political-rectitude as "freedom fries") qualified in school lunches as "vegetables."

The tomato plant is a weak-stemmed herbaceous plant that, under natural conditions, forms a spreading, straggling bush about two to four feet high. The leaves are extremely toxic and have been known to cause arthritis and even kill grazing livestock. In addition to containing poisonous alkaloids, the leaves and other green parts of the plant have golden yellow glands that give off a most unusual odor and toxic substance when touched.

The tomato's growing pattern is one in which the plant shuts itself off from its environment. This has often reminded me of the pattern of individuals suffering from a degenerative illness who also can develop a tendency to isolate themselves from their natural environment. This may not be as subjective an observation as it seems: blood crystallization studies done in Germany have shown that cancerous blood and the juice of fresh tomato reveal a striking structural similarity.

This unusual plant, like its relatives in the nightshade family, does have positive qualities: it can help to reduce excess fat accumulations in the body, and can have a cooling effect on an overheated metabolism. Another beneficial property is that they can calm and clear excess heat from the liver.

It is not unusual for a woman in the early stages of pregnancy to crave tomatoes: the fruit has the uncanny ability to deplete the body of minerals, and eating tomatoes during the early stages of pregnancy can stimulate the release of calcium into the bloodstream, making it readily available to the growing fetus. The mother, however, does not benefit—unless she has an abundance of calcium reserve.

Tomatoes keep best in a cool, dark place and this preference can manifest energetically in the human who consumes large quantities as a cold, dark, and reclusive character. It is a soft and fragile fruit that bears little resemblance to other more commonly known fruits that spend their daylight hours thriving on sunlight. Like other nightshades, it has been strongly linked to arthritis and skin diseases, especially the seeds, with their mucilaginous coating.

In addition to making one feel cold and dry, tomatoes also contribute to stiffness in the joints and muscles. Its juicy, acidic flesh and seeds have an almost immediate effect of thinning the blood. Unlike potatoes, which give the skin the appearance of a loose, withered look, white with pallor, the tomato gives the skin a dark, dirty, sallow, and tight appearance.

Aubergine (Eggplant)

The eggplant is native to Arabia and more specifically to India. The plant derives its name from one of the original species of eggplant, which was small, white, and shaped like a hen's egg. It was introduced to England as an ornamental plant in 1587, but not then used as a food. During the late 1700s, the French claimed it provoked fever and epilepsy.

The United States got its first introduction to the eggplant as an ornamental plant in 1806; it was not recognized here as food for well over a century, until late in the 1800s, when the famous restaurant Delmonico's made it a regular part of the menu.

Once called the "mad apple" because it was rumored to cause insanity if eaten daily for a month, the eggplant has yet to play a major role in American cuisine. Its greatest devotees are southern Italians and Arabs, especially Syrians and Turks.

Eggplant has been linked with cancer in that its slightly mutagenic qualities have caused genetic damage to cells in vitro. Nigerians once regarded it as a contraceptive or natural abortive. Its mucilaginous texture can be helpful for constipation, and it can assist in the reduction of abdominal swelling. It can also help to balance fatty foods, especially cheeses and cream. It has a cold and damp nature, and like potatoes and tomatoes, energetically affects the blood and bones.

Peppers

The most common peppers are the bell varieties. These are available in numerous colors and sizes and should not be confused with the table spices—black and white pepper, which are not nightshades. The two families of peppers are the *piper* from the family *piperaceae* which includes the seed varieties of black and white pepper (both non-nightshade), and the *capsicum* of the family *solanaceae*, which includes bell peppers and hot peppers (both nightshades). The latter are native to the tropics and the highlands of Latin America.

Like the rest of the nightshades, with the exception of their country of origin, peppers originally were regarded as ornamental plants and only later accepted as food plants. Again, with the pepper we find a weak and delicate plant that was once considered difficult to grow until hybridization made it more convenient.

Some of the more traditional techniques for preparing peppers involve subjecting the plant to a whole gauntlet of steps, not unlike the original Andean method of making potatoes run the gauntlet. The Italian method of preparing roasted peppers is a good example: the peppers are salted, literally burned to a black crisp, and the skins and seeds are then removed before eating.

Peppers are hollow and crisp with the usual acrid taste found in other nightshades. Energetically, they contribute to feelings of cold and emptiness. One may not experience the energetics of peppers in the way one would normally experience potatoes or tomatoes, yet all four of the commonly used nightshades have similar overall qualities, differing mostly in textural details. Some peppers are spicy, giving them a unique quality among nightshades.

The potato, when cooked, is soft and mushy and has a loosening effect on the intestines and nervous system. The pepper, when cooked, also has a weakening and loosening effect on the intestines, yet is not as soft and smooth as the potato, unless it is peeled. It tends to have a more abrasive effect on the intestines. Peppers can also be supportive in stimulating appetite, circulation and digestion, and to promote urination.

Essentially then, the nightshades represent a phenomenon that exists somewhere between the plant and animal kingdoms, and the relationship you choose to have with them as foods requires a little thought—and a lot of common sense.

31
The Staff of Life
Cereal Grains

Grasses are a family of plants that include all of the cereal grains (*cereal* deriving from Ceres, the Roman goddess of agriculture) and represent the most important food source of the human species.

Einkorn, emmer, and barley are thought to be the first domesticated cereal grains, with origins in the Fertile Crescent (modern Iraq, Syria, and Lebanon). The domestication of wild related grasses by our Neolithic ancestors was originally thought to have occurred around ten thousand years ago, but new findings have pushed this date back by an additional ten thousand years. I am certain that archaeological discoveries in the near future will push this most recent date even further back into prehistory. Grain grinding stones have been discovered on the Solomon Islands in the South Pacific dating back twenty-six thousand years.

Although academics have proposed theories on cereal domestication, just how our ancestors were able to domesticate wild grasses by altering their genetic profiles to become the foundation food of civilization is still an unsolved mystery. Whoever they were, somewhere in our distant past, these unknown ancestors created an unparalleled food source that continues to nourish and, to a large extent, *define* the majority of the world's populations to this day.

Most grasses are perennial and have flowers without petals. Grains constitute the fruit as well as the seed of grasses, and all of them have the ability to recycle themselves by utilizing the raw materials of their basic construction. Botanically, almost all the grasses commonly used for food are cereal grains. There are others, however, such as buckwheat, amaranth, teff, and quinoa, that while not considered grasses from a technical point of view still have the same basic structure as other grasses.

Cereals contain the most highly developed seeds of food plants. Their embryological roots, stems, and leaves reveal the same pattern of nodes that exist in the fully mature adult plant—an embryological process that closely resembles the developmental processes of the human fetus.

The edible part of a cereal grain is the *kernel*—technically, a complete fruit with a thin and dry ovary-derived layer. Some cereals grains (for example, rice, oats, and barley) bear tough outer husks that protect the kernel, while others (wheat, corn, and rye) are often called naked grains because they do not have to be hulled before milling.

Cereals have the capacity to reproduce in abundance from a single seed and when eaten by human beings can be supportive energetically to reproductive strength—not only sexually but psychologically as well. They are highly productive plants with a unique built-in mechanism for reproduction. Energetically and nutritionally satisfying, each whole cereal grain represents both the beginning and the end of a grass plant's life cycle, containing all the possibilities and potential of the whole plant. Grain is the primary fuel for the brain and nervous system and contains the genetic memory of how humanity rose from the dark recesses of primitivism to become the civilized species we once were during that lost piece of history called "the golden age" by our ancestors worldwide.

Grains are the most versatile foods on the planet. Porridge, bread, and noodles are just a few forms grain can take to flexibly combine with almost any vegetable, legume, or animal to produce healthy and satisfying nutritional preparations.

Grains are self-preserving foods that store well and have long been used in times of famine and other situations where humans have had to survive. In the 1800s explorers found sealed underground grain silos in Hungary, Spain, India, Africa, Turkey, Central and South America, Germany, France, and Egypt—some thousands of years old and some with grain still intact and in good condition. Well-preserved grain has also been found in tombs thousands of years old.

By way of stark contrast, the United States Department of Agriculture, with its state-of-the-art technology, currently has the capacity to store grain for only about four years without mold and insect infestation. Could this be simply the result of a dramatic decline of grain quality over millennia? Or did our ancestors know something we have yet to learn about natural storage and preservation?

More than any other food, cereals have the greatest capacity for increasing human potential on all levels of life. Their ability to reproduce en masse along with their adaptability and versatility bestow on cereals and on cereals alone, the highest position in the world of food. Additionally, these tiny seeds contain within them one of the most promising solutions to world hunger.

A sacred and principal food among all the high civilizations of antiquity, these pivotally important seeds have experienced many changes and abuse from man's technological developments. Certainly, factory-farmed cows and chickens are abused and neglected, and many people (especially vegetarians) express their compassion and sympathy concerning the massive slaughter of these creatures.

But what about *grains?* Is the refinement, chemicalization, and sterility of these most nutritious foods not as important an issue as the abuse of livestock? Is it because we cannot look into their eyes, as we can with livestock, and see the anguish and suffering that might be expressed there? And if we could, would we see clearly enough to notice it?

Like all living organisms, grains are sensitive to their surroundings and interactions with humans. Numerous studies revealing immune properties of plants are now shedding light on this subject. Within the food chain, the animal kingdom represents the final stage before humanity. Likewise, the plant kingdom precedes and represents the primary food source for animals. It's time we start to establish Grain Rights (and even more importantly, Soil Rights), or there won't be any animals (with or without rights) to worry about.

One way of understanding the crucial importance of grains is to recognize that they play the role of *source* within the food hierarchy. The majority of domesticated animals eaten for food in the United States is unhealthy and riddled with both degenerative and infectious disease. Is this the direct result of abuse to animals? Is man's inhumanity to animals the *cause* of these problems—or are the heinous actions that so greatly contribute to the pain and suffering of animals but a symptom of a greater *cause*?

Continuous disease and animal abuse will not result in the elimination of the animal kingdom; but the neglect and abuse of their food source—the plant kingdom, water, and soil—ultimately *will* determine the fate not only of the animal kingdom but of the human species as well.

Clean up the environment, and the plants will thrive. When the plants thrive, the animals will naturally follow suit. The human species can continue to survive only if the plant and animal worlds thrive.

Energetically, grains may very well hold the biological key for establishing the desperately needed balance in human/Gaia relations. It is therefore urgently important that they be restored to their rightful position as our principal food—and in the process, returned to the qualitative and highly nourishing state in which they once were.

Within the human species lie the seeds of future generations, generations who will largely determine the fate of the earth. Within the plant kingdom lie the cereals, seeds of nourishment, the past, present, and future blood that has for thousands of years determined, is now determining, and will continue to determine the fate of the human species.

Energetically, whole cereal grains finely tune the human nervous system in such a way as to affect every part of the body, to the extent of unifying it with the soul as one whole functioning organism. This was the legacy given us by our ancestors.

Whole cereal grains are unique among carbohydrate sources—but not the hybrid form of wheat or other cereals designed through modern genetic alteration in such a way as to not be able to reproduce. These latter are rather the source of the health *problems* experienced by so many people today in the form of gluten intolerance, digestive disorders, and more. No, I am speaking of the original heirloom varieties of grains that have carried their seed from twenty thousand or more years ago to modern times.

These sacred seeds were the mainstay of highly evolved peoples and the foundation of great civilizations that once spanned the globe. If you think about the importance of cereals to our ancestors and ponder why it was that they considered them sacred, you must also give some thought as to who these ancestors were—and not necessarily through the filter of conventionally accepted evolution theory that upholds the idea that "monkey men" were our ancestors.

Consider the evidence left by people who have proved their advanced knowledge of the solar system, mathematics, engineering, agriculture, and many other sciences. These people used this knowledge to create civilizations that conformed to nature, unlike our civilization today that attempts to force nature to conform to it. Everything upon which we base our understanding of early history consists of the natural remains—stones, pottery, metals, and bones—derived from these ancient culture-bearers. The ancient Egyptians, Sumerians, Indus Valley peoples, Mayans, and Olmecs are just a few of the great civilizations of the past whose knowledge was handed down to them from previous generations of great men and women of remote prehistory.

The more such evidence surfaces, the more obvious it becomes that not all or our prehistoric ancestors were simple primitives. Some of them developed great civilizations that included a wide variety of foods with cereal grains as the most important food of all. In fact, one of the primary reasons grain was considered sacred is because it was handed down from generation to generation, and our current understanding of how long this has been going on is still in its infancy.

In his classic book, *Atlantis: The Antediluvian World,* Ignatius Donnelly discusses the development of plant species and quotes Darwin, enlightening us to the very likely possibility for the origins of cereal grains.

It is Atlantis we must look to for the origin of nearly all our valuable plants, as Darwin says: "It has often been remarked that we do not owe a single useful plant to Australia or the Cape of Good Hope (South Africa)—countries abounding to an unparalleled degree with endemic species—or to New Zealand, or to (South) America south of the Plata River; and according to some authors, not to America north of Mexico." In other words, the domesticated plants are only to be found within the limits of what I shall show hereafter as the empire of Atlantis and its colonies; for only here was to be found an ancient, long-continuing civilization, capable of developing from a wild state those plants that were valuable to man, including all the cereals on which today civilized man depends for subsistence.

The mystery of how cereal grains and numerous other plants were cultivated from wild species by hunter-gatherers without sophisticated scientific knowledge more than ten thousand years ago still perplexes modern agronomists. In fact, many of the questions that arise from this mystery have not been answered satisfactorily even in modern times, and most professionals in the field of horticulture prefer to avoid the issue altogether by simply falling back on the generally accepted—though unproven—theory of hunter-gatherer intervention.

Rice

Along with being one of the most versatile grains, rice is the staple food of one half of the world's population. There are many varieties of rice, but only two basic ways of growing it: on dry land and in flooded paddies.

Dry land rice acts and grows pretty much the same way other cereal grains do.

Paddy rice, the most commonly grown rice in Asian countries (about 90 percent of rice grown today is paddy rice), requires vast quantities of water, along with a tireless, labor-intensive workforce. Paddy rice is most definitely a "high-maintenance" grain, but its long history as the principal food of Asia has proven it to be worth all the effort and energy put into it.

Paddy rice not only requires large quantities of water, it also utilizes large tracts of land with the sometimes unfortunate consequence of making much of the land barren in the process. This in turn can contribute to scarcity of fuel and foliage. Even though vast amounts of water are used, rice, unlike other grains, will not drown in water. However, it does require much oxygen to grow, and it gets all that oxygen by sucking air through spores in the leaves above the surface. This is one of the reasons the ancient Chinese, in their sophisticated medical treatises, associated rice with the lungs.

Rice consumption varies widely among Asian peoples. For example, the Chinese eat twice as much rice as the people of Japan (and that is not per country but per capita). An interesting bit of history pertaining to rice-eating and its influence on health can be found in the disease beriberi.

In some poverty-stricken areas of Asia, rice can often be the only food available. During the late 1940s, the deficiency disease beriberi came to the attention of the United States government. Believing that rice was the cause of the problem, the government planned a solution: enrich the rice. This was effectively accomplished with rice in America—however, most of Asia found that the increased cost of enriching the rice, along with the yellow color that appeared when the enriched rice was cooked, did not appeal to them, so they did not want the enriched rice.

In the 1950s and afterward, beriberi did indeed recede in Asia—but needless to say, it did not do so as a result of enriching rice (which the populations there refused to eat), but rather as a result of nutritional diversity in general. Yet even today, the assumption persists among many that white rice causes beriberi, when in fact, it is a lack of nutritional diversity that is the actual cause. As evidence, white rice has been consumed for many thousands of years in Asia, with only isolated incidents of beriberi among traditional Asian cultures and not among those with varied diets.

Rice, like other traditional grains, has long played an important role in the structure of Asian communities, the family, relationships in general, and even spiritual beliefs.

In Japan and other islands of the Indochina seas, rice is held to be synonymous with the perfect woman: pure and white, soft and tender, beautiful yet timid—and most of all, dislikes being touched and handled by men. It was, and perhaps still is in some places, thought ideal for women to do all the weeding and cooking of rice. Japanese women believed that if they did the planting of the rice, it would enhance both their own fertility and the productivity of the rice.

Rice has an unusually compelling, almost addictive quality: the more you eat it, the more you *want* to eat it. Its somewhat bland flavor makes it the perfect staple for accompanying flavorful preparations of meats, vegetables, and fermented foods—healthy traditional fare that has been the norm among traditional rice-eating cultures for thousands of years. In the past few hundred years rice has crossed many borders to become a principal grain among foreign lands and cultures, and along with it have come many of its traditional Asian accompaniments.

An unusual and still relatively minor influence in Western culture is that of brown rice. Today, it is not unusual to find brown rice consumers who hold the belief that brown rice is the best, healthiest, and most nutritious grain to eat, even though evidence for the extensive use of brown rice by any traditional culture has yet to be found. Nevertheless, many Western natural food proponents conform to an exaggerated rice creed thought to be rooted in Eastern (particularly Asian and Indian) influence, and taught by new age spiritualists who believe in the manifest superiority of rice and race, probably as a result of their own cultural background. Many of these masters of manipulation lead their flocks on the path to nirvana through teachings based on cultural beliefs that are more often rooted in theoretical idealism than actual traditions.

The protein quality of rice is about 66 percent higher than wheat or corn and just below that of oats. Milling brown rice to white rice can result in a 50 percent loss of B vitamins and iron; however, the amino acids, especially lysine, are not affected. Why then has rice been traditionally hulled for thousands of years? Did ancient Thais, Chinese, Japanese, Indians, and others mistakenly consume white rice for thousands of years when they could have been eating brown rice? Could they have known about the harmful effects of *phytates* found in the hulls of rice—or was it as simple as balancing their diet with a diversity of supportive proteins, fats, and minerals from a variety of food sources as they have done to this day?

Not too long ago rice was thought to have originated in China about 1,500 years ago. Then discoveries from Thailand carbon-dated rice at 9,260 years ago, quite a stretch from the previous date. Newer findings reveal that China had developed advanced rice-growing technologies as early as 9,000 years ago. Currently, rice domestication has been dated at 11,500 years ago in China's Yangtze River valley. Japan too has its unique rice history. The prehistoric Jomon people, the first pottery makers, left rice in some of their ancient wares that have been dated at 12,000 years. Attempts to find the wild ancestor of modern rice have been inconclusive and have left many researchers with the uncomfortable realization that most of the "could be" ancestors are but free-running varieties from domestics.

As one of the least allergenic of grains, rice is truly a remarkable cereal grain. It has qualities of endurance and adaptability; pride and honor; and most of all, it is one of the few foods with enough power to control and mobilize the masses. There are many varieties of rice (*Oryza sativa*) including black, red, glutinous, long, medium, and short grain—but wild rice is not one of them. Wild "rice" is actually a type of aquatic oat and has no relationship to *Oryza sativa*.

Wheat

Some historians believe wheat and barley are the two oldest cultivated cereals. While still mostly shrouded in mystery, what we do know about the story of wheat and its diverse cultural influence is that it is a fascinating one indeed, and it reveals much about the importance of this versatile cereal. If it were possible to choose one cereal to rank at the top of the list in importance in Western culture (though this, as you must have gathered by now, is not possible!), it would have to be wheat.

The ancient Sumerians were making bread five thousand years ago as if they were given instructions on how to do it. I say this because there is no evidence that it was an accidental discovery, nor a gradual, step-by-step process of learning. The Sumerians are known to have made breads of barley, millet, and emmer wheat by using wild yeasts, sourdoughs, and sweeteners. These nourishing loaves were most likely enjoyed with their more than one hundred different soup and stew recipes, which contained a wide spectrum of herbs and spices (they used four at a time). The same meals may also have included one or more of their eighteen to twenty different kinds of cheeses.

At the same time that the ancient Sumerians were practicing this dazzling display of agricultural and culinary skills, their not-too-distant neighbors the Egyptians were also enjoying a wide variety of breads, including fruit cakes sweetened with honey.

One ancient archaeological site where evidence of wheat has been found is Çatal Huyuk in Turkey. Here we have the remains of an advanced culture dating back some six thousand to eight thousand years. Among the fourteen food plants identified was an evolved form of emmer wheat along with cultivated bread wheat (*Triticum alstivum*), the latter having no wild progenitor *anywhere*. In fact, none of the grains found at Çatal Huyuk have progenitors from that area, meaning that they had to have come from somewhere else. From somewhere else—six thousand to eight thousand years ago? This means that whoever brought them to Çatal Huyuk had already cultivated them—for who knows how long before that—at another location.

Along with the unique form of bread wheat found at Çatal Huyuk, equally perplexing is the technological mystery of how the inhabitants polished their ornaments of obsidian (hard volcanic glass) without scratching them, and how they were able to drill holes so small in obsidian that our smallest modern needle cannot fit through them. They also smelted copper, lead, and other metals.

Conventional theory holds that Paleolithic man was eating wheat in the ninth millennium BC in the Upper Tigris Valley, and although this was thought to be wild wheat, it was still powerful enough of an influence to inspire the creation of settlements that would eventually anchor people to the spot where it grew. Thus, it is said, hunter-gatherers abandoned their lifestyle and the cultivation of wheat became a priority that would later influence economy, trade, spiritual beliefs, and just about every other aspect of human life and living.

Aside from the fact that not all peoples abandoned the hunter-gatherer lifestyle, this theory has additional flaws that make it untenable.

These issues will be discussed further in part 5, "A Forbidden History of Food and Agriculture."

Of all the cereals, humans consume wheat and rice in the largest quantities. Wheat's prevalence and long history in Europe has had a phenomenal impact on the development of Western culture and agriculture. Unfortunately, however, modern hybridized denigrated forms of wheat have now become the norm as one of the most widely consumed grains in the world, and as a result of this decline in quality, it has become one of the most problematic grains in its influence on health.

Wheat is easily one of the most if not *the* most versatile of cereal grains; there are more than thirty thousand known varieties. The maximum life of wheat seed is about ten years. The storage proteins of wheat have rather unique chemical properties; when ground and mixed with water, the proteins bond and form a concentrated structure called *gluten,* a flexible substance that assists in the rising of bread and is used in numerous other products (including pasta) and numerous Asian specialty foods.

Winter wheat has an interesting built-in genetic memory called growth habit. Planted in early autumn and harvested in early summer, it has a dormancy period and is genetically programmed to sleep through the winter. This hardy wheat requires exposure to freezing cold weather in order to reproduce. On the other hand, spring wheat is planted in spring and harvested in early autumn, with no dormancy period.

These two types of wheat can produce numerous colors of wheat, leading to many different varieties, each with its own unique properties.

Wheat is a virtuous grain with self-fertilizing flowers that are bisexual and so tight that pollen cannot escape to produce natural hybrids.

"Whole Wheat"

The misleading term *whole wheat* is often associated with breads, pastas, and numerous other products made from whole wheat. While these products do start out with whole wheat, most are *not* in fact "whole" wheat, but whole wheat that has been cracked or ground into varying grades of flour.

An exception is sprouted wheat, sometimes used to make unleavened sprouted bread. Here the whole grain is sprouted, molded into shape, and then baked slowly at a low temperature into a loaf of bread.

Another method of preparing "whole" wheat is to dry roast it until it pops like popcorn, producing puffed wheat. Still another method is to soak wheat berries overnight, then cook them for a long time until somewhat soft. While this sequence of processing does soften and tenderize the wheat berries, it does little to render them digestible, even if chewed well.

It is no coincidence that, when considering the tough outer hull that surrounds the germ of wheat, this tough grain was historically ground and sifted, soaked, fermented, sprouted, and naturally processed in some form wherever it was consumed.

Bread

The two most common types of bread are yeasted or leavened bread, and unyeasted or unleavened bread, also known as sourdough bread. I must clarify here that the discussion that follows does not include those varieties of imitation breads containing preservatives and chemical additives. While such bastardized loaves have widely replaced the original staple foods in many parts of the world, there is nevertheless an abundance of the real item available. Fortunately, there *are* enough real grain breads available so that I can limit my discussion here to those, and not bother with the counterfeit items.

A recognizable difference between the yeasted and unyeasted breads is that yeasted breads tend to have a lighter and more airy texture, compared to the usually more dense and heavier unleavened breads, although some sourdough breads can have the same light qualities as those of yeasted breads.

Some whole foods enthusiasts consider unleavened bread as superior to leavened or yeasted bread, due to the belief that yeast proliferates in the intestines, thus producing an increase in harmful bacteria. While it is highly doubtful that this occurs, it is worth pointing out that many other foods contain yeast as well. Perhaps an even more important counterpoint is that unyeasted breads are perfectly capable of creating digestive problems, too, especially when eaten beyond the threshold of appropriateness, and especially when not thoroughly masticated.

Yeasts belong to a group of single-celled fungi that contain many different species. Some can be harmful when they proliferate (*Candida albicans,* for example); however, one species long put to good use in bread baking is called *Saccharomyces cerevisiae,* or *brewer's sugar fungus.* This and other forms of yeast were widely used for both brewing and baking culinary practices dating back at least six thousand years by the Egyptians and Sumerians.

For those who believe baking yeast is a harmful and proliferating monster that destroys or weakens the intestines, take note: yeast cells in a loaf of bread die when the temperature of the baking bread reaches 140 degrees Fahrenheit.

Yeast imparts its own unique flavor to bread and, through the metabolism of sugars, produces the by-products carbon dioxide and alcohol. Other leavening agents do the same, to a degree, including sourdough starter. *Saccharomyces exiguus,* sourdough yeast, differs from the usual baker's yeast in that it tends to thrive in acidic environments and leaves a more sour taste to the unbaked dough. It is still a form of yeast, however.

In ancient Rome yeast was made by sealing barley cakes in clay pots until they soured, or by combining wheat or millet with grape juice and allowing it to ferment, after which the cakes were dried in the sun.

Why all the elaborate processing? Because wheat (as well as rye, oats, barley, etc.) has a highly developed, independent, and tough character. It contains many elements and qualities that make terrific raw materials for creating new human material—but effecting this transformation is not simply, as they say, a piece of cake. Grinding it into flour, sifting to separate chaff (depending on the grain and the bread type), adding salt and water, soaking, rising, and baking, all contribute to transforming a cereal grains' structure and energy.

Common sense suggests that bread is most nutritious and beneficial to those individuals who actively engage themselves in life through physical activity and eat a wide variety of fresh foods.

White or Wheat?

It is almost startling to realize how routinely the dualistic concepts of good and bad or right and wrong are applied to food, and the eating of bread has had its share of dogmatic criticism. One way to stimulate a religious fervor among a group of health-food fanatics (or for that matter, among a group of newly enlightened fiber fanatics) is to step into their midst and declare, "Wheat bread is *not* better for you than white bread." Then step back again and watch what happens.

You might get a couple of interested or curious reactions; but most of the group will probably interpret your statement to mean, "White bread is better for you than wheat bread," or, "Wheat bread is not really very good for you," or from the real fanatic, "The whiter the bread the sooner the dead," or, "You're wrong, my doctor said . . ." What's the truth here?

In days of old, it was more difficult to remove the bran from wheat flour to make white flour, but it was done nevertheless. Some of the ancient Egyptian wheats were sifted of up to 80 percent of bran. Around 400 BC, Hippocrates, the "father of modern medicine" (why he is still associated with a modern medical model that has even less to do with genuine health than it does with his own philosophical understanding is beyond me) stated in his *Regime:*

> Wheat is stronger and more nourishing than barley, but both it and
> its gruel are less laxative. Bread made of it without separating the
> bran dries and passes; when cleared from the bran it nourishes more,
> but is less laxative.

Now, he wasn't talking about chemically bleached and bromated white flour, so that needn't even enter the picture here. These days, the hoopla surrounding whole wheat bread is concerned primarily with the presence of the vitamin-rich germ and fibrous bran of the whole wheat for laxative purposes. While wheat bread may be higher in vitamins and fiber, it is only slightly higher in protein than white bread. The bran is mostly indigestible, and the aleurone layer of the wheat contains phytates, which can affect calcium absorption. Therefore, much of the nutrition of whole wheat bread may be lost through the laxative effects of the bran, and thus may pass through the digestive system without being absorbed. Traditional agricultural peoples throughout the world consumed large quantities of vegetables, making the bran/laxative issue a nonissue.

White bread is not as high in nutrition nor as laxative as whole wheat bread, yet good-quality, organic, unbleached white flour used alone, or in combination with other preferably ancient grains (see ancient grains) flours for bread, can be nutritious and easier to absorb. For people who eat a heavy meat, egg, and dairy food–based diet with little plant foods, whole wheat bread will undoubtedly be the best choice, yet it still does not balance the excess extremes as evidenced among fiber-obsessed dieters.

For those who eat a diet high in fiber (from a wide variety of vegetables) along with moderate amounts of quality fats and proteins, good-quality homemade baked products made from sifted or partially sifted flour can be a welcome change and may actually be helpful, as well as more satisfying. That goes for other baked flour products as well: muffins, cakes, cookies, pie crusts, and so on.

It is simply not true that because white flour is white and wheat flour is brown, white flour is devoid of nutrition and not good for you. Neither may be good for you, or both may be: this is something each person must discover individually through experience.

Speaking of experience, most whole foods enthusiasts likely have had negative experiences with white flour, due to their backgrounds where white flour was present in a highly refined form and combined with refined sugar, hydrogenated fats, and various additives (not to mention all of the other junk foods). This, along with several scientific studies and the claims made by health food fanatics, has pretty much convinced people of the deleterious effects of sifted flour. The new whole foods religion teaches us: "Eat foods only in their whole form." And, like most other religions, idealistic yet unrealistic rules are often established to rationalize the belief system.

Throughout my years of counseling and teaching natural foods, I have met many people well entrenched in whole foods ideals whose greatest dietary concern was their craving and excessive consumption of flour products, primarily whole wheat flour products. Many of these people thought it bad to eat flour products because they weren't whole grains, and that broken or cracked grains, as opposed to whole grains, cause distorted thinking—"because they cause mucus . . . because they stagnate the brain . . . because they stagnate the intestines . . . because they are cancer-causing . . ." and still other more fear-inducing beliefs. Nevertheless, beliefs or no beliefs, they just could not stop eating flour products—and whole wheat flour products were the preferred form, because ground whole grain is a more politically correct choice than sifted whole grain flour.

My first impression concerning this common problem of cravings and indulgence in baked flour products was that people simply had to create order in the rest of their diet to make it more satisfying. Needless to say, this did not work. Assurance that their brain would not deteriorate and crumble into dust if they did not completely stop eating flour products helped a little.

Yet there was something else. That "something else" was that flour in its myriad of forms was and still is a strong constitutional element in many people's genetic backgrounds.

I doubt many of our ancestors had such difficulty overconsuming flour products. They certainly didn't have fearful beliefs surrounding this food, and most ate some type of flour product on a daily basis.

I would often ask people who consumed excessive amounts of flour products how they felt when they ate large quantities of whole wheat or coarse grain flour products, and the general consensus was usually that they felt full and yet, in a strange way, unsatisfied. They generally would feel that when they got started they wanted to continue to eat more, to the point of eating a whole loaf of bread slathered with nut butter, or six muffins, or a tray of homemade cookies.

(At this point I must interject that in addition to extremely unbalanced diets, there are some important psychological issues involved with eating this way—but let's leave that alone and continue with the issue of the physical feeling.)

I'd ask them how they felt when they ate white flour products.

And the general consensus was that they couldn't handle much, or only small quantities at once. The interesting point here is this: their white flour consumption invariably would be a compulsive detour from their usually healthy diet to poor-quality commercial products, otherwise known as junk food—not to white flour products made from wholesome ingredients.

It is my sense that these people, who were eating primarily grains, vegetables, and other high-fiber foods in their daily diets, had enough roughage in their diet already. When they ate large amounts of coarse whole grain flour products, it did little more than to add still further roughage, giving them the temporary feeling of being full and satisfied, but at the same time moving their other food (as well as the flour products themselves) through their digestive system all the faster. This can not only limit absorption, it can also create gas and other digestive distress.

Hippocrates was definitely on to something when he spoke of the difference between the two types of flour, something he obviously gained from years of experience. The Egyptians too were aware of this, as they were known to have sifted much of the chaff from their flour when making bread. It is doubtful that the ancient Egyptians did this for all their bread, but the point is that bread was not the whole meal. The Egyptian diet consisted of a wide variety of plant and animal foods that accompanied their staff of life.

To return to our overconsumers of flour products: When these people would eat commercial white flour products, they would eat a smaller quantity than when they ate high-fiber whole wheat flour products— yet they still craved them. When these same people started to make homemade flour products with organic unbleached low-fiber flour, sometimes combined with small amounts of flours from ancient grains (quinoa, amaranth, kamut, and teff), they not only found it easier to reduce their flour consumption altogether, but most of them also lost interest in commercial junk-food flour products as secret binge foods.

I include this lengthy history not only to make a point about flour, but also to illustrate a larger point. It often takes experience, experimentation, and willingness to follow seemingly "bad" or "unhealthy" desires to their logical conclusion, only to discover that the human body and appetite knows something that dogma has overlooked! The Orwellian doctrine of "Whole Wheat, Good—White Wheat, Bad" turned out to be only adding to some people's intestinal burden, not to its nutrition, and a common craving for sifted flour products was an expression of body wisdom, not the craven corruption of an impure appetite.

Bread of any type has a tremendous capacity to absorb fluids when introduced to the human digestive tract. (See the section on baking for an explanation.) Because bread is baked and therefore requires some additional digestion, it can tend to induce feelings of heaviness as well as increased thirst. A lighter yeasted bread may not make one feel as heavy as unleavened bread, but it also doesn't feel as substantial nor as satisfying as unleavened bread. (Unless one eats a large quantity of it in a single meal, which is not a smart thing to do.)

Whether it is white or whole grain, leavened or unleavened, bread is a wonderful and nourishing food, and negotiating a healthy relationship with it is based largely on your individual digestive capacity and your level of activity.

Truly the staff of life, bread tends to produce a warm and dry condition or a cool and dry condition in the body.

Pasta

Noodles, unlike breads, are not baked. Pastas (the Italian term for noodles) consist of ground flour with water and salt; often additional ingredients are added, such as egg, vegetable powders, and so forth. The ingredients are then mixed to form a dough, which is then shredded or otherwise cut into different shapes, then dried. The dried noodles are boiled until soft.

Pasta is a pleasant and highly enjoyable way to eat grain and is easy to digest as well. There are many different types of noodles and it is important to experiment with variety.

There are the brown, coarser types of wheat noodles and the whiter *semolina* types. The basic difference is in their heaviness or lightness. Some people are concerned about the white flour used in semolina noodles; however, they do have their redeeming qualities, one of these being that they're much easier to digest and more enjoyable (just ask any child) than many of the brown wheat varieties (which often taste like sawdust).

While Western cultures have a relatively short history of noodle consumption, the same is not true for China and other Asian cultures, who have eaten noodles in some form or other for millennia.

Noodles have energetic qualities that can help one relax and feel more flexible, both physically and mentally. Unlike bread, they are not eaten dry; therefore, they are not as absorbent as bread, and instead add moisture *to* the body. Noodles tend to produce a warm and damp condition when eaten hot, and a cool and damp condition when eaten in the form of noodle salads or other cool preparations.

Cracked Wheat Products

Cracked wheat, bulgur, and couscous are three different products made from cracking and sometimes precooking wheat.

Cracked wheat is simply whole wheat that has been cracked and sometimes roasted. It makes a hearty breakfast cereal, especially when cooked with enough water to form a thick porridge.

Bulgur and couscous are more processed than cracked wheat, both being forms of cracked wheat that have been precooked and dried. Because of this, neither couscous nor bulgur need to be "cooked" in the usual sense. One simply needs to add boiling water to these dry cereals, and within minutes you have a light, fluffy grain that can be eaten as a side dish or used in a variety of salad preparations.

When prepared so they are light and fluffy, bulgur and couscous produce a cool and dry condition. When cooked as a thick cereal, they both tend to produce a warm and damp condition.

Wheat Gluten (Seitan and Fu)

When wheat flour is kneaded into dough and the bran is rinsed from the dough, the resulting product is *wheat gluten*—a pliable and chewy substance that is sometimes dubbed "wheat meat" because of its resemblance to meat.

When gluten has been simmered in a soy sauce broth, it is called *seitan*—flavored wheat gluten. *Fu* is dried wheat gluten and is more porous and spongy than fresh wheat gluten. It is used in many of the same ways as seitan and must be reconstituted by soaking in water before using. Both are Asian specialty products and tend to produce a warm and damp condition.

These products are not that easy to digest, unless prepared with a variety of vegetables. Though they are considered high in protein, they are not adequate protein substitutes for animal protein.

Wheat Relations: Spelt

Spelt is another grain of mysterious origin. The earliest strains of spelt have been found around the European Alps; the most current historical date for the earliest spelt specimens is nine thousand years old.

An heirloom grain and possibly an ancestor of modern wheat, spelt has been found in some of the earliest European farming communities. Spelt is a hard-grained type of wheat with an unusual mixture of botanical genes. Research has shown that the genetic foundation of spelt reveals an odd mixture of genes from several plants. Unlike many grains that tend to be either a genetic development of one source or a genetic mutation of another, spelt appears to be a nine-thousand-year-old product of genetic manipulation. Now, who could have accomplished such an incredible feat back then?

Spelt has a hearty flavor and earthy taste. It tends to be a bit more sticky than most varieties of wheat.

Wheat Relations: Kamut

Like spelt, kamut is considered one of the "ancient grains." (I put this in quotes because, really, when you think about it, which of the grains are not ancient?) It is a nonhybridized relative of modern durum wheat, yet is nutritionally superior in protein and amino acids.

Kamut is thought to have originated in Mesopotamia at least six thousand years ago, but it is possible that it originated in Egypt as one of its earliest grains. It is not known for sure, but some specialists believe it may have survived among peasant farmers in Egypt. Perhaps the most original and unique tasting forms of wheat—if it is in fact a form of wheat—I dare say kamut is without a doubt the finest-tasting wheat relation there is.

Modern kamut has an interesting story behind its modern rediscovery.

In World War II, a pilot took a handful of kamut from a stone box he found in a tomb in Dashur, Egypt. (Who this person was is not mentioned in the original story.) He gave thirty-six grains to a friend, who sent them on to his father, a farmer in Montana, who grew a small crop from the grains and displayed it at fairs as a novelty, calling it, "King Tut's Wheat."

As the years wore on kamut was somehow forgotten, until 1977, when Bob and Mack Quinn located a small jar of the grain, and, based on what they had heard about it, gave it the title of *kamut,* which in Egyptian means "soul of the earth." They could not have chosen a better word to describe this grain. After the Quinns' discovery (or rediscovery) of kamut, they began to grow it and it is now available in many health food stores.

The modern product contains much of the original integrity of the ancient seed, because of its short history of being grown without pesticides. It is usually grown organically and produces a high yield. It is also hypoallergenic and considered safe for many suffering from wheat allergies. Although the true history of kamut is still a mystery, we can thank the Quinns for reawakening this golden wonder from its deep sleep and mysterious past.

Kamut is a highly nutritious, delicious, and satisfying grain with a warm and dry nature.

Quinoa

High in the snow-capped mountains of the Andes on the altiplano of Peru and Bolivia, there exists one of the world's most ancient native grains, a staple of the Aymara and Quecha Andeans. Here in the cloud-covered mountains one can find quinoa (botanical name: *Chenopodium quinoa*) growing more than two miles above sea level.

The word *quinoa* comes from the Quechua Indian language and means "mother." There are hundreds of species of *Chenopodium,* yet only a few are cultivated and the rest are weeds. At some point many thousands of years ago, ancestors of the ancient Inca people somehow transformed a wild weed chenopod into a superlatively nutritious grain chenopod that would be handed down to their descendants.

Strikingly, this same unique transformation of chenopod weeds to grain can also be found in several other parts of the American continents and the lofty Himalayan Mountains of Tibet.

Like other chenopodium grains, quinoa is extremely adept at adapting and even thriving under extreme environmental conditions, a strong energetic quality indeed. Because of its high protein (almost ideal amino acid content) and its exceptional nutritional profile (high lysine, iron, magnesium, and zinc), quinoa continues to sustain many of the less fortunate of those native peoples lacking animal protein in their diet.

The quinoa plant ranges from twelve inches high in Peru to twelve *feet* in the Himalayas and contains a rather unique immune-defense chemical. *Saponins* are a bitter-tasting coating that covers each grain and serves to protect the plant from insects and high-altitude sun. This chemical is easily removed by soaking for a few minutes, then rinsing with cool water. If the saponins are not rinsed, quinoa tends to have a bitter taste.

While living in Colorado in the early 1980s, I experienced eating quinoa for the first time. It had just arrived in the States and within a short time would become available to the public through the efforts of some ambitious people who knew its time had come—again. It was not long before it gained in popularity and quickly adopted its well-deserved alias, the "Super Grain" because of its exceptional nutritional profile.

When I took that first mouthful of quinoa, my first thought was, "Where have you been all my life?" It was love at first bite. I not only loved it but also, unlike many other things I ate, it loved me too. It was the beginning of a wonderful relationship that would prove to be more stable and long lasting than some of my other relationships. . . . But that is another story. Since that first mouthful of quinoa, I have been and will continue to be an avid proponent of this truly unique ancient grain.

The conquering of the Incas by the Spanish resulted in what they hoped and thought would be the demise of quinoa. Fortunately the grain survived the conquest, and today one can view acres of different varieties of quinoa at various elevations in Peru. It also can be found wild or rather free-running, sprouting from crevices of ancient stone temples and ruins scattered throughout the towering mountains, subtly reminding the tourist of the rich cultural history of this enigmatic land.

Quinoa can grow with little water in places other grains would not survive, and while it can be prepared in numerous ways, it cooks very quickly for a whole grain, in about twenty minutes. Its essential temperament is warm and dry; however, like other cereals, this can be adjusted by your choice of preparation and added ingredients.

One particular preparation from the Peruvian highlands is a hearty and delicious stew of quinoa, vegetables, chicken, and hot peppers. When trekking though the highlands of Peru one can find, usually in small villages, several variations of this stew. During my travels to that part of the world, every time I had the opportunity to eat this stew, it was consistently delicious, invigorating, and satisfying.

Amaranth

Another chenopodium, amaranth consists of a plant group of sixty species and is grown on five of the seven continents.

During the conquest of the Americas, everywhere the conquistadores found amaranth it was considered sacred and used ceremoniously to make sweet cakes, tortilla-type breads, and gruel. To the Aztecs, amaranth was truly a "food of the gods."

Cortéz did not like the ritual use of this plant and found the Aztec ceremonies with it to be sacrilegious; and so, toward the end of the conquest, he ordered a massive destruction of the plant, nearly eradicating it. Thankfully, he did not entirely succeed, and we thus have this extraordinary grain available to us today. (Incidentally, on the subject of those barbaric sacrifices that we have been told were daily rituals among these "primitive" indigenous peoples: in his later years, Cortéz came clean with a report that he never once in fact witnessed a human sacrifice.)

Amaranth was also a ritual plant of the Pueblo Indians; the Hopi Indians too used the plant at their Kachina (sky gods) dances, where they made red rolls (called pika bread) of the chewy grain and handed them to children as gifts from their beloved Kachina friends.

But I am getting ahead of myself here. The true history of amaranth goes much further back into the past and it too (like that of many other grains) is shrouded in mystery.

Among the many species of amaranth, most are plants that produce edible leaves but not grains. Among those plants that do produce grain, there is one that stands out above the rest. It is the pale- or blond-seed amaranth and it is a domestic. No wild species of amaranth produces pale seeds—and that is where the mystery begins.

Domestic pale seeds are better for popping, have better flavor and faster seed germination than other species. Pale amaranth seeds have been found in a cave at Coxcatlan in Vera Cruz, Mexico and dated at 6000 BC. Pale or blond amaranth seeds are thought to exist because of genetic mutations brought about through selection by some unknown domesticators at some point thousands of years ago. The reason for this conclusion is that there are no pale seeds found anywhere in any wild weed species.

Conventional theory holds that grain domestication is a process that begins by carefully selecting the largest and best mutated seeds from wild grasses and planting them. This process is then repeated at each harvest until one has a crop with the desired results: a domesticated grain with larger and easier-to-harvest seeds.

This theory begs some basic questions. How would the "domesticators" know what the desired result would be, since it would take many generations—perhaps a thousand years—before results could be realized and it would be only their distant descendants who would see the results? How is it possible that these larger mutant seeds, simply through selection, end up being far more productive than the wild parents? And how did the nutritional profile of the domestics dramatically increase from mutated wild seeds?

With respect to amaranth, here is yet another question: How did the unknown domesticators select their marginally larger amaranth seeds to start with—when it is barely possible for someone with 20/20 vision to see these seeds, let alone differentiate slight variations in their size? Amaranth seeds are so tiny that these assumed slightly larger mutated seeds would be extremely difficult to sort out without using a magnifying glass.

To compound the mystery of the "unknown genetic manipulators" is the fact that the very same blond species of amaranth found in Mexico has also been found many thousands of miles away, among remote isolated peoples in Tibet. In fact, amaranth has been a sacred food among these *and other* remote and isolated peoples in India and Africa since antiquity.

Now more questions arise. Who were these people who presumably domesticated this blond species of grain from a wild weed—and how did they do it, when we cannot seem to do it today? Was this extraordinary feat of domestication accomplished in one place and somehow transported by Neolithic people (who are thought to have been just emerging from the safety and seclusion of their caves at the time), or was the domestication from wild weed to grain accomplished independently in several different places, many thousands of miles apart?

What are the odds of *that* happening?

Whether in Mexico, China, Africa, India, or Peru, all traditional amaranth-using cultures have the same beliefs about amaranth, as well as the actual same species of blond amaranth. It is believed to be a sacred grain capable of feeding the soul as well as the body. Amaranth may very well have more metaphysical qualities than any other grain, both in traditional lore and in energetic reality. It is certainly a highly nourishing "superfood."

The word *amaranth* stems from a Greek term for "immortal" or "everlasting," and was so titled because of the durability of its seed. In India it has been known since ancient times and is called *ramdana,* grain of the god Rama. In other parts of India it is called the "immortal grain from heaven." In China it is called "millet from heaven."

Amaranth is a close botanical cousin of quinoa; like quinoa, it is loaded with superior nutrition. It contains a high iron content, and its protein is easily digested and nearly complete in its amino acids. Three and one-half ounces of amaranth provides more calcium than a glass of milk. It has no gluten and is high in lysine (often low in grains) and minerals.

It is a processor of solar energy and belongs to the unique group of plants call the C_4 group, which are photosynthetic superfoods in that they are extremely efficient at converting sunlight, carbon, soil, and water into plant tissue. This group also includes maize, sorghum, millet, and quinoa. The C_4 group of plants grows faster and use less water than plants of the C_3 group.

Wild species of amaranth offer tasty leaves similar to spinach and can yield thousands of seeds. On the other hand, domestic amaranth can yield hundreds of thousands of seeds. There are sixty species of grain amaranth. The tiny seeds are the size of poppy seeds and stem from shoulder-high plants with seed heads that can measure four and one half feet in length, each containing up to fifty thousand seeds. The large seed heads are strikingly beautiful and are red, gold, or purple in color. Amaranth is grown at altitudes exceeding thirteen thousand feet, but the plant is just as comfortable at sea level or, for that matter, almost anywhere; it produces high yields wherever it is grown.

One amaranth plant can plant one acre; one acre of seeds can plant twenty thousand acres. With this kind of productivity in such an extraordinarily nutritious food, one wonders why anyone needs to go hungry.

Consider for a moment the energetic effects of a food that is resistant to drought and pests, easily handles stress and adversity, is astonishingly prolific, and amazingly adaptable.

That is amaranth.

Teff

The world's tiniest grain is so small that five grains can fit on the head of a pin. Teff is said to be the smallest of the millets; there have been two thousand strains collected. Like amaranth and quinoa, teff has the highly adaptable characteristics of being drought-resistant, highly nutritious and a low-risk, highly productive crop.

The domestication of teff goes back at least five thousand years, but its true origins (are we surprised?) are unknown.

A staple food and a genuine lifesaver among African peoples, especially Ethiopians, teff has long been their life support system, ensuring their survival in times of drought and famine. For these people, teff is bestowed with the highest honor and respect as a gift from the gods, a sacred food.

The young seedlings are fragile and delicate, requiring much care and attention until fully grown. When they are young, there is considerable danger of suffocation by weeds, so Ethiopian farmers are most attentive to weed eradication. When fully mature and able to deal with weeds on their own, the seed heads form a heart-shaped display that has earned teff the nickname "lovegrass." To Ethiopians, the precious lovegrass is an expression of love returned from the loving care given to it in its youthful days as growing seedlings. Indeed, it is a perfect example of the intimate relationship of humans and food through food energetics.

Teff is one of the grains that is highest in minerals; its iron content, for example, is higher than that of most other grains. Its protein is almost complete; it is chock-full of vitamins and is gluten-free.

Teff is most commonly available in health food stores as a dark brown or a light blond grain. While numerous breads are made in Africa from teff, the most well-known and popular is *enjera,* a flat bread that looks like a large pancake with a spongy texture. Enjera is eaten as a staple food in Ethiopia and is absolutely delicious, especially when eaten with several side dishes, as is the norm among Ethiopians.

Like amaranth, teff has a warm and damp nature.

Barley

According to some historians, barley is one of the oldest cultivated grains and the ancestor of many others as well. Although it has a relatively short growing season, barley is extremely adaptable. It has a hardy nature that gives it the ability to grow in both hot and cold climates and withstand both drought and frost.

Barley was the principal grain of the Greeks and was a primary food of the gladiators. A highly nutritious grain, barley falls somewhere between rye and wheat in terms of nutritional essentials and is higher in protein than rice. Unfortunately, more than half the world's barley harvest goes to feed cattle; a good amount more goes to make beer.

When cooked, barley has a chewy, almost gummy texture that gives it interesting energetic qualities. When cooked in traditional stews with a meat bone and hardy root vegetables, it adds a thickness to the stew that can create a warm and damp condition. It cooks well as a hot porridge and also makes a delightful, cooling grain salad. In general, barley tends to create a damp condition; where it is grown and the particular type of barley determine its warming or cooling qualities.

Rye

Rye is one of the hardiest of all the grains. It has an incredible ability to tolerate cold weather. Rye was first considered by farmers to be a weed, an unwanted growth that invaded and contaminated wheat fields. Not only could it survive in infertile soil, it also could flourish at fourteen thousand feet above sea level and farther north (which it prefers anyway) than wheat.

Like so many grains, rye has an unknown history. In 1837, an attempt to cultivate wild rye into a new form of domestic grain was carried out at the Botanical Gardens in St. Petersburg, Russia. The experiment did not work, and although many attempts have been made to do the same since then, they continue to fail because the wild rye seed simply refuses to lend itself to domestication by giving up its fragility of stalk and tiny seed. Hmm . . . so how was this done thousands of years ago?

Like wheat, rye is one of the most important cereals for breadmaking, as it contains the gluten that makes bread rise. Rye flour contains a high amount of pentosans (long chains of five-carbon sugars) that give it a strong capacity to bind water, a property that makes it a bit harder to digest than most other flours. The ability of rye to retain water has led many to believe that rye was a good appetite suppressant and dietary aid for losing weight. Russian peoples eat large quantities of rye and are fit examples of its hardiness and stamina.

The greatest and perhaps the only real weakness of rye is its susceptibility to *ergot,* a parasitic fungus that rarely appears in any other cereal grain. Ergot can cause uncontrollable muscle contractions in people who eat it. (One theory about the Salem witch trials episode in colonial Massachusetts holds that the young girls were poisoned by an ergot-contaminated rye crop, leading to hallucinations and other symptoms.) Don't let this dissuade you from eating rye, though—ergot is easily diagnosed and recognized by farmers and thus is no longer the threat that it was many years ago.

Rye is particularly good for building bulk and stamina. It tends to create a warm and dry condition.

Oats

More rye is eaten today than in days past—but still more oats are produced, and most of the oat crop (all but about 5 percent) is used as feed for livestock. Oats prefer cool climates with lots of moisture. They are second to rice when it comes to water requirements, but oats do not need the attention that rice requires to grow.

Oats have long been an important cereal among the Scots, Germans, and other northern Europeans who eat oats cooked as a thick porridge high in protein and fat. Oats have the ability to extract nutrients from soil that will not support barley or wheat. The endosperm of oats contains a natural antioxidant that helps preserve them and make them an easy cereal to store, even when cracked.

Once criticized as food fit only for horses and people too poor to eat anything else, the lowly oat is today one of the most convenient and popular foods of the natural foods movement.

Oats also have the ability to absorb salt and therefore can be helpful for those with an accumulation of excess sodium in their bodies. They are also recognized as a valuable food for health maintenance. With credentials that include the ability to lower cholesterol, help stabilize blood sugar, and regulate the bowels, the once lowly oat's future looks promising, indeed.

Oats are available whole, cracked, steel-cut, rolled, and as flour.

In any and all of these forms, it can be cooked as a hearty thick cereal and garnished with seeds, nuts, dried fruits, cream, milk, or one's choice of natural sweeteners for a nutritionally satisfying and warming breakfast. Rolled oats and oat flour make great piecrusts and cookies. A favorite breakfast cereal of mine is two-thirds rolled oats and one-third amaranth, soaked overnight and cooked the next morning. Served with cream or coconut milk, this combination makes for a super-nutritious start.

Energetically, oats have a warm and damp effect on the body. They can be especially beneficial for people who are weak and have difficulty gaining weight, and for those who are high-strung and stressed. If eaten in excess, however, oats often give a pasty white pallor to the skin.

A friend of mine who owns a couple of horses once told me that her children could no longer ride the horses, because the horses had grown impatient and hyper. She asked me if there was anything in terms of food that could calm them down. Not knowing a hell of a lot about horses at the time, I couldn't think of anything that might help her.

When I next saw her, about four months later, the children were riding the horses. I asked her what had happened, and she told me she had changed the animals' diet. She had stopped giving them corn, and instead gave them oats.

When I first saw the horses (when they were still eating corn), I couldn't help but notice their lean, vital bodies and restless nature. They were beautiful. The second time I saw them, they looked like different animals—still beautiful, but with increased muscular definition, and much sturdier than before. In four months of eating oats instead of corn, the horses had completely changed both psychologically and physically.

This is a good example of food energetics in action. Animals often eat a mono diet, so changes in their diets often reveal dramatic and obvious differences. Humans, on the other hand eat (or should eat) a wider variety of foods; as a result, the energetic effects are less obvious and often go unnoticed.

Corn (Maize)

Ten thousand years ago, someone took a tiny finger-size wild weed and altered it to become the large forearm-size ear of corn we have today. Some botanists believe that *teosinte* is the forerunner of maize; however, a roughly equal number of botanists believe it is the other way around, and that teosinte is actually an offshoot of maize. In any case, there is no such thing as wild maize, only farm escapees.

In 1948 scientists found six-thousand-year-old popcorn in a New Mexico cave. This very same popcorn was soaked for two days and later popped, just as if it were fresh. This is a dramatic illustration of how tough and resilient the grain is. Maize clearly has power that does not fade over time.

Experts are still not sure if maize has its origins in Peru or elsewhere in the lowlands of Central America. The oldest known remains of the supposed "wild ancestor" of maize are pollen grains found on a drill core (for sampling soil layers) used to excavate a foundation for a new building in Mexico City. The pollen grains were dated at seventy thousand years old. That is not a misprint: *seventy thousand* years old. In fact, one of the principal reasons these prehistoric pollen grains are assumed to derive from a *wild* plant is that for many scientists, it is simply unacceptable to think that civilized humans could have been cultivating plants at such an early date.

Some of the most advanced civilizations in the world were built on a foundation of maize. The Olmec, Maya, and Inca were people whose agricultural practices and lifestyles surpassed many of our present, so-called civilized endeavors. Many of their accomplishments are still a mystery to modern man, and to this day are either rationalized away through scientific intellectualism or romanticized by new age mysticism.

One thing is for sure: the processing and production of maize requires sophisticated knowledge. It is low in lysine and tryptophan; therefore, eating maize without combining it with foods that contain these ingredients can lead to the nutritional-deficiency disease *pellagra*. Happily, these ingredients are found in squash and beans, both of which were domesticated about the same time as maize, and these three food plants have served as central ingredients of many traditional diets. To South and Central Americans, they formed the "Sacred Trinity," known as gifts from the gods.

One Native American legend about maize relates that one day, a long time ago, three sisters arrived from the Pleiades constellation, each bearing a different gift. One held out her hand and offered maize, another squash, and the third beans. They then told the people to plant them together and they would be happy and healthy. It is interesting that the Iroquois Indians grow corn, beans, and squash in single plots in a form of sophisticated polyculture. They say that each of these three siblings has different personalities that support the other two. The corn is austere, standing straight and tall, and protecting its beans and squash from weeds and insects. It also acts a scaffold to support the beans. The beans produce nitrogen, which is essential for plant growth. And the squash controls the growth of weeds and recycles crop residue, thereby promoting fertility. Not only are these three foods a harmonious trinity in their own environment, they are equally so as nourishment for the human body.

Maize is a plant of immense versatility. In addition to being North America's most popular native cereal, it was the most important food plant contributed by the so-called "New World" to the Old. (I say "so-called" because civilizations in the Americas, especially South and Central, are turning out to be just as old as those of the Middle East.) The United States produces more than half of all the harvested corn in the world; it is grown in every state in the union. Corn was the staple food of all Native American cultures (with the exception of nomadic tribes) and to this day remains the fundamental food plant of the United States. This is due in part to the fact that three-quarters of it goes to feeding livestock.

Corn produces a tremendous yield, yet it cannot reproduce itself without the aid of humans. Its loose flowers allow for free-flying spores and its promiscuous female organs openly receive wandering spores. With the largest seed head of all grains, each plant contains one or two ears with seeds set in rows, always in even numbers, and covered in husks that prevent it from reproducing itself. Corn must be shucked before the seeds can be planted, and as tedious as this might sound, it is not so bad when considering the resultant yield—it can exceed three hundred bushels per acre.

Apparently, there is only one species of corn, but there are many varieties and subspecies with colors of red, white, blue, and yellow. Some are sweeter than others, but all are versatile. Corn bread, muffins, porridge, and masa are just a few of the preparations one can make with corn.

Alkaline substances such as ashes or lime traditionally were used to process whole corn by the Aztecs and Maya; many North American Indian tribes used wood ashes, naturally occurring soda, or burned mussel and clamshells. Some of these methods, particularly lime and ashes, are still used today. This allows one to use whole dry corn without grinding it. Dry corn tends to create a dry and cool condition in the human body. Sweet corn, more a vegetable than a grain, tends to create a damp and cool condition.

Millet

Known mostly as a feed crop or birdseed in the United States, millet is a staple food of great importance elsewhere, particularly China, India, and Africa. It has a remarkably high protein content and contains more amino acids than wheat, barley, oats, rice, or rye. It is easily digested and has a high alkaline mineral content.

Millet is a hardy and flexible cereal. While it can easily fend for itself in a wild state, it also will respond graciously to limited care through cultivation. It has one of the lowest water requirements of any cereal, making it an important grain in arid lands. Millet does need water to grow, but it is not as demanding in its water needs as most other grains. If millet does not get enough water, it tends to go into a dormant stage and wait patiently until it does get the water it needs. When it does get water, the millet plant excitedly sucks up the water and grows at an extremely rapid rate.

There are many genera of millets and all can be divided into two categories: tropical and temperate. The tropical varieties tend to have a higher proportion of minerals.

Sorghum is another important cereal to Asia and Africa and is similar in many respects to millet.

Millet is considered by many to be the least palatable grain. I must say this is not a sentiment that I share. However, millet does tend to take on the flavors of added ingredients, particularly sautéed or stir-fried vegetables, herbs, and meats, or pretty much any traditional recipe. It is a very dry grain and fats help to enhance its palatability as well as its warmth, and at the same time reduces its drying effect.

It is a very light and airy grain, with a tendency to create a dry and warm effect in the body. In Chinese "five element" theory, millet is associated with the earth element, which corresponds physiologically to the spleen, pancreas, and stomach.

Buckwheat (Kasha)

Although consumers treat buckwheat as a cereal, it is not a true cereal grain. Rather, its kernels are actually dry fruits called *achnenes,* which are similar to the seeds of the strawberry. Buckwheat is of Asian origin and a relative of the sorrel family, which includes rhubarb. It is high in lysine, a nutritional component deficient in most grains. In addition, it has very few insect and disease problems.

Buckwheat thrives in cold, damp, and windy climates, and it is in these environments where we find the greatest consumers of this food. For the robust eaters of Finland, Northern China, and Austria, buckwheat is an important food, ideally suitable for consumption in cold climates as well as mountainous regions. A fast grower, buckwheat can produce two crops a season.

Buckwheat is especially beneficial for individuals with frail bodies and low self-esteem, as it has greater potential than any grain to bring warmth to the body. It also has an unusual ability to absorb liquid, making it a supportive grain for those lacking the ability to absorb nutrients from their food.

There are many other whole grains that are not mentioned here and I encourage you to explore and experience the energetic properties of all of them in order to fine-tune your brain and nervous system. Here are a few tips to consider when eating whole grains:

Soaking whole grains overnight or several hours before consuming increases the absorbability of their minerals, amino acids, and vitamins, and neutralizes phytates. Soaking grain also helps to neutralize enzyme inhibitors and increases important enzymes normally locked in the grain. Gluten is also partially broken down by soaking.

Finally, be sure to consume grains with reasonable amounts of fats, proteins, and fresh vegetables for increased absorption of nutrients.

One of the strongest energetic properties of all the whole grains is their self-preserving nature. In the times in which we are living, self-preservation is of utmost importance. Keep on eating those grains!

32
Beans/Legumes

Legumes are seeds embedded in pods belonging to the leguminous family of plants. *Legume* is derived from the Latin *legumen,* which means, "seeds harvested in pods." Legume seeds, more commonly known as beans and peas, are vegetable protein foods dating back to prehistoric times and are thought to be among the earliest food crops cultivated by humans.

In Europe and the Near East, legumes (*pulses*) were once regarded as "poor man's meat." Today they rank as the second most important food crop in the world, after cereals. Legumes have played an important role in the history of human food. They helped diversify and satisfy our deep-rooted instinct to nourish ourselves with a wide variety of foods. Traditional diets based on starchy staples had a tendency to be monotonous, and legumes were often made into sauces and various other preparations. This not only added flavor to traditional diets, it also increased the meals' nutrition and thus helped to create a more balanced diet.

Most traditional cultures did not include beans for children younger than one year of age. After that point, legumes were considered crucial in children's development. Today, legumes are often advocated in the prevention and treatment of malnourishment, particularly among children.

Traditional cultures prepared beans by first soaking them to reduce phytates, then cooking them extensively, sometimes whole and sometimes finely ground into powder. A common method of bean preparation, and one that made them easily digestible (especially for children), was to germinate and ferment them. After being fermented, the legumes were combined with a portion of sprouted grain; both were then ground together and the mixture cooked into a soup. Legumes, while only approximately 25 percent protein, are also valuable sources of calcium, thiamin, and iron and when combined with small portions of animal products, become valuable sources of protein.

The world's three most important beans are soybeans, which have been cultivated for more than four thousand years and are now grown in greater abundance in the United States than anywhere else in the world; the American haricot bean, which has been found in excavations dating back to 7000 BC; and the European broad bean, which has been found in compost piles of prehistoric Swiss lake settlements.

Many beans can be traced back to ancient civilizations. The cultivation of kidney beans in Central America goes as far back to at least 5000 BC, and pea seeds have been found in the tombs of pharaohs. Recent archaeological discoveries dating back nine thousand years have shown that several varieties of beans had long been under cultivation in parts of Central Mexico. With the exception of soybeans, most beans and peas have experienced little evolutionary change under domestication from their original ancestry. The fact that beans have maintained their original constitution through thousands of years of environmental adjustments is a strong energetic quality and speaks volumes in support of this nutritious and adaptable food.

The Physical Properties of Beans

Legume seeds vary in size and are somewhat varied in shape, yet the basic structure of these seeds is pretty much the same as it was thousands of years ago. The two solid halves, called *cotyledons,* serve to store the energy, starch, and protein necessary for the legumes' growth. These are joined to a central embryo consisting of a root, stem, and a pair of leaves; these, in turn, are surrounded by protective seed coats with a small opening at the *hilum*—the place where the legume was once attached to its pod. It is at the hilum where legumes absorb nutrition, both from their native soil and from the water in which they are soaked and cooked.

A legume is a single seed; however, the plant it produces forms a pod, which in turn encloses and protects not one, but two or more seeds. The pods eventually dry and leave individual seeds (beans and peas) with the potential to store large volumes of protein, starch, and iron. Soybeans and peanuts are legumes, yet unlike other legumes, they store oil instead of starch.

Legume pods are the result of the ripened ovaries of the plant and can range in sizes from three to eight inches long. Legumes can be eaten in three different ways at three different stages of their development. Before fully grown, they are eaten whole, pods and seeds together; this form is commonly known as *string beans*. They can also be eaten just before fully mature, when the seeds are still tender; these are called *flageolets*. In Asia and other parts of the world some beans are consumed as sprouts. Or they can be dried, stored, and later soaked and cooked.

Research has shown legumes to be beneficial in relieving depression and regulating glucose metabolism—like whole grains, they produce a slow, steady rise in blood sugar. Their principal defense (immune) compounds are *cyanogens* and *lectins,* also called *protease inhibitors;* these help to protect their reproductive abilities. While protease inhibitors can interfere with digestion, these compounds present a problem only if legumes are not first soaked and then thoroughly cooked until soft, or in the case of cyanogens, if raw bean sprouts are eaten in excessive quantities. Not only do soaking and heat help to disable protease inhibitors, so too does more alkaline water.

Legumes are a nitrogen-fixing group of plants and have the ability to assimilate nitrogen directly from the air. The presence of bacteria in their roots acts as a stimulus to their growth. Nitrogen fixation occurs by bacteria accumulating in the nodules of the roots, causing enlargement of tissue that in turn produces a rounded swelling in the roots.

The nitrogenous molecules provided by beans are not only used by humans and animals as food; the nitrifying bacterial symbionts in root nodules also play an important role in the buildup of humus in the soil for the needs of other plants. Their concentrated protein, when combined with other protein sources of amino acids, has the potential to create a dense and solid foundation for human muscle and body tissue.

Although not complete in their essential amino acid profile, most peas and beans combine well with other proteins found in grains and animal products.

Bush and Vine Types

Bean plants grow in one of two ways: bush beans grow in clusters on a central bush; vine beans grow by using the stalks of some of their leaves as tendrils to spiral around poles in an upward direction. Whether bush or vine, these edible seeds are nourished by short, thin tendrils that supply a steady stream of filtered nutrition to the seedpod.

Beans are one of the easiest vegetables to grow and are among the most productive. The large seeds germinate rather quickly and the plants grow fast. Bush varieties grow an average of one to two feet tall; they mature about two weeks earlier, and do not bear as much or as long as pole varieties, yet they usually give two to three good harvests over a four-week period.

Vine or pole varieties grow an average of five to ten feet long and will continue to grow and produce new pods all summer, often until fall temperatures drop below fifty degrees.

Although beans are sensitive to temperature extremes and do require a moderate amount of moisture, they are very adaptable and can tolerate a variety of soil types. In ancient Oriental medicine, the shape of many beans and the way they hang suspended from the plant (particularly bush varieties) led to a corresponding association with the kidneys. Climbing peas and beans (vine varieties) were associated with the liver. Here is a partial list of bush and vine beans.

Chickpea

Also called *garbanzo beans,* this annual forms an erect, bushy herb that is drought-resistant with long taproots. Chickpeas are higher in fat content than most pulses; they are hard peas with a high energy concentration. Once considered to be antibilious, they also were thought during the sixteenth century to be aphrodisiacs. Chickpeas originated in the eastern Mediterranean region, northeast Africa, and southwest

Asia; they need well-drained soil with cool, dry air and bright sun-
shine in order to grow.

Soybean

This annual originated in China as a cover crop; it is a bushy, rather
coarse herb, usually erect with some twisting varieties. Because of soybean's high toxin content, it needs elaborate traditional methods of
preparation. Soybeans grow mainly in regions with good rainfall and
warm sun.

Lentil

Another annual, lentils form an erect, bushy herb, its lens-shaped seeds
existing in many varieties and colors. Lentils originated in the eastern
Mediterranean region and western Asia; they need well-drained soil and
are not hardy to frost but tolerant of cool temperatures. Lentils are easily digested; in the sixteenth century, people viewed lentils as having
properties opposite to chickpeas' aphrodisiac qualities, which is why
lentils were included in monastic diets on meatless days.

Lima

The lima bean is cultivated as an annual, biennial, or perennial
and grows in various colors. This climbing vine is native to tropical
America, grows best in hot, humid tropics and is tolerant of high temperatures, poor soil, and drought. Its pods and leaves are often eaten
as a vegetable.

Scarlet Runner

This vigorous climber is a perennial vine, usually grown as an annual.
Originally from Central America, the scarlet runner is grown at high
altitudes, tolerant of cool temperatures but susceptible to frost and
drought; it also requires rich soil.

Fabaceae

This is actually a family of beans, its most well-known member being
the kidney bean. Its other family members include haricot beans,

navy beans, snap beans, red peas, pinto beans, and northern beans. Fabaceae are generally vine-type beans, but some can be grown as bush beans. Kidney and pinto beans are annual climbing vines with dwarf varieties.

Fabaceae have their origins in tropical South and Central America. They are susceptible to frost, drought, and high temperature and need moisture during their growing season, along with warm temperatures for seed ripening. The fabaceae family of legumes has long been used as folk medicine for acne, bladder and kidney disorders, eczema, rheumatism, and sciatica.

Green Pea, Garden Pea

Green peas are the leading processed vegetable in the world. Thought to be an ancient Egyptian plant, this is an annual climbing vine or bush with many varieties. It requires a cool, moist climate and is susceptible to drought and high temperatures.

Broad Bean (Fava)

This annual, bushy herb with coarse upright stems has been cultivated since ancient times around the Mediterranean basin, as well as in Egypt, Ethiopia, and the Near East. It is the least drought-resistant of beans and cannot tolerate high temperatures, though it can tolerate acid soils more than most beans.

Mung

The mung bean is an erect, rather hairy, and shrubby annual bushy herb with origins in tropical Asia. It thrives in hot temperatures and adapts well to light soils. They are easily digested and have low flatulence factors; they tend to have a cool and damp effect on the body, particularly on the kidneys.

Adzuki

This annual, erect, bushy plant with numerous varieties has been cultivated for centuries in China, Korea, and Japan, where it often is used for cakes or confectionery. Adzuki is useful as an antierosion crop. More than sixty varieties of adzuki have been recorded, with colors including maroon, straw yellow, black, and brown. Adzuki, like mung beans, are prolific seed producers; they tend to have a warm and dry effect on the body, particularly on the kidneys.

Black-Eyed Pea (Cowpeas)

This annual climbing vine is thought to have originated in India, but wild forms have been found growing in Central and West Africa; it is drought resistant and tolerant of high temperatures.

The Energetics of Beans

Once dried, all of these self-preserving plant foods have the ability to store for long periods, and this makes legumes one of the most important and nourishing vegetable foods available.

When cooked, dried beans and peas generally have a warm and damp effect on the body, except for adzuki beans and lentils (which have a warm and dry effect) and mung beans (which have a cool and dry effect).

Their ability to adjust the soil through nitrogen fixation, their adaptability to their environment and high tolerance, and the support they give to other plants empower legumes with energetic qualities of presence, durability, and generosity. These qualities can impart to the consumer a deep sense of compassion for humanity.

The protein derived from peas and beans is qualitatively calming and soothing, compared to animal protein, which is more stimulating in effect. This is due to the high carbohydrate content of beans and the fact that the amino acid profile is that of an incomplete protein. The swelling of the root nodules, along with their fat and protein content, give beans a subtle expanding and muscle-building quality unparalleled in any other plant food, except perhaps nuts and seeds. The two cotyledons or paired halves that store the protein of legumes correspond to the paired organs of the human body—the brain and the heart, as well as the lungs, kidneys, ovaries, and testicles, and thus have a tendency to resonate in these areas.

Other energetic qualities imparted by these plants include a calm and relaxed nature, a warm and easygoing personality, and a smooth, soft, and pliable skin tone.

Beans and peas are unique among plant foods in that overcooking does not reduce their nutritional value. In order to be well digested, beans and peas first must be soaked, then the soaking water must be discarded, as it contains much of the dissolved sugars that contribute to gas. They then must be thoroughly cooked and properly seasoned before eaten.

There are many theories on how beans should be cooked—with pork rind, with kombu (a sea algae), with bay leaf, with spices, and so on. Which theory is right? It comes down to this: any and all these theories are fine if the beans get thoroughly cooked, and they are all useless if the beans do not get thoroughly cooked. *Cook your beans well!* Traditional recipes are the most reliable methods of bean and pea preparations. The common wisdom that beans cause flatulence is quite true—when one of the following factors occurs:

- the beans are not cooked enough
- the quantity consumed at one sitting is excessive in relation to the other foods in the meal
- they are eaten alone without any other foods

Any of these situations is enough to make that old wives' tale more than just hot air.

Bean Products

Soybeans have traditionally been processed in some special way, usually fermentation, whenever used for human food. This practice goes back at least two thousand years in Asia.

Today, however, soy products are marketed to the masses as a "health food" in myriad forms, including soy milk, soy hot dogs, and numerous other difficult-to-digest meat substitutes that have little to no health benefits. Dry roasting beans (of any type) does not render them digestible, by either animals or people.

Some additional by-products of soybeans include lecithin, which is derived from the residue of soy sludge, and soy margarine, which is derived from soy protein isolates obtained from defatted soy chips. Most of these nontraditional soy products are processed with hexane and other toxic chemical solvents.

Research has shown that animals fed on a diet of raw soybeans lose weight and develop pancreatic problems. Soybeans are extremely difficult to digest. It takes more effort on the part of the digestive system to break down soybeans than the energy derived from the beans. The body will often overproduce pancreatic enzymes in an effort to compensate. It makes you wonder about all those people who eat those disgusting "soy nuts" and fake soy foods that line the health food store shelves. Don't they ever sense that the stuff they're eating is actually yielding a net *loss* of energy?

With the exception of dips, spreads, sprouts and salads, which can be made from just about any well-cooked bean or pea, most commercially processed bean products are made from soybeans.

When consuming soy it is best to use small amounts of traditional products (soy sauce, miso, tempeh, natto) and avoid other mass-marketed soy junk foods, including soymilk.

Tofu

Tofu, bean curd, and *soy cheese* are names given to a soft, sometimes slightly firm, white and watery food made from soybeans. Tofu is one of those rare foods that has little personality by itself, but when combined with animal products, as has been the norm in traditional uses, with the addition of soy sauce, vegetables, or miso, it quickly comes to life. Its basic character is that of a blob that awaits stimulation through the medium of other foods with well-defined characters.

An adaptable food, tofu combines well with almost any animal product and vegetables. Alone, tofu has cold and damp effects. However, when fried (or especially, if deep fried), it has warm and damp effects. Dried tofu has a cool and dry effect. Tofu is not a substitute for balanced protein sources and should not be used as a protein substitute, but rather used in small quantities in combination with animal products to add variety to one's diet.

Soy Milk

Another product derived from soybeans, soy milk is the dairy-free health food advocate's answer to cow's milk.

Theoretically, soy milk is a great idea. Alas, being a great idea doesn't make it digestible, especially when substituted for milk. I cannot begin to tell you the scope of damage I have witnessed, both in children and in adults, from reliance on this so-called health food product. Alone, soy milk has a cold and damp effect.

Soy Sauce, Shoyu, Tamari

Soy sauce, shoyu, and *tamari* are all names used to describe a fermented salty liquid made from soybeans and salt. The difference between shoyu and tamari is that tamari is a liquid by-product from the making of miso. Shoyu, on the other hand, is a liquid made from fermented wheat, soybeans, and salt. Both are salty liquid condiments with a bitter taste, and both are used to flavor many Oriental vegetable and grain dishes.

There are various types of soy sauce; to the connoisseur, they all have very distinct flavors. Both tamari and shoyu are liquid products of a rich, fermented carbohydrate and protein mash with warm and damp qualities. Once the mash has been strained, however, the rich and damp quality takes on a more flat and dry quality in the remaining liquid.

Both shoyu and tamari create a dry and cool condition. Most traditional Oriental preparations that call for soy sauce as a seasoning also have added fat in them to help alter its qualities of dry and cool to damp and warm.

Miso

Miso is a fermented soybean paste made of soybeans and salt, with or without the addition of a grain, such as barley, corn, wheat, rice, or millet. Some American miso makers have produced additional varieties containing dandelions, leeks, chickpeas, lentils, peanuts, black soybeans, and numerous other ingredients. There are red, yellow, brown, sweet, short-term fermented, and long-term fermented varieties of miso, each with its own unique flavor and energetic properties.

The whole idea of miso is fascinating: a barrel of carefully controlled fermentation, a slow symbiotic process that results in one of the most nutritious and satisfying plant food combinations possible. This rich, robust food/seasoning is without a doubt the most beneficial way to consume soy—yet each person's relationship with it is so different. Some find it difficult to handle because of flavor or salt content, while others cannot go a day without it.

Miso has a wide variety of uses, and its rich combination of protein and fat give it the potential to create warm and damp effects. Additionally, miso has powerful cleansing qualities and can assist the body in eliminating toxins.

Sprouts

Although many types of seeds can be sprouted, the bean family historically has produced the sprouts most widely and commonly used as food. In sprouting beans, a common culinary custom of ancient Asia, the seed is germinated by first being soaked until it absorbs enough water to swell and burst open. The seed coat is shed and roots and leaves begin to develop. How big and how well the sprout develops is determined largely by the stored nutrition in the bean or pea seed itself, for this will be its only food supply unless planted in the soil. When planted, it would then receive added nutrition and sunlight, enough to develop into a full-fledged plant.

Sprouts are plant children and possess many of the characteristics of a growing child. Full of vibrant energy, the plant sprout relies on its stored reserves of carbohydrate and protein until these are depleted. It then seeks a nourishing medium for continued growth and development. If it does not get this, it will wither and die.

Energetically, sprouts induce a sudden burst of youthful and cooling energy that can be especially beneficial to sluggish and heavy individuals. Digestion is a process of cohesive organization between an eaten food and digestive enzymes. Sprouts represent the breaking away from an organized structure toward the unfolding of the plant from the seed. This rapid release from a solid structure can be controlled by heat through cooking or other traditional preparations that serve to temper and calm the dispersing energy of sprouts.

Sprouts are commonly eaten raw by many who believe that "live foods" give life, or because of the high nutritional profile of sprouts. These beliefs, regardless of their possible validity, do not guarantee the digestibility of this food, especially bean sprouts. However, individuals with very hot temperaments may not immediately recognize this, because sprouts are very effective in cooling the body.

Some types of sprouts are hardier than others and can withstand the effects of short-term cooking; these include most bean and grain sprouts.

One great advantage of sprouts and sprouting is that just about anyone can sprout seeds at any time of the year at home; and sprouted grains, beans, or seeds are the closest thing to fresh vegetables when a variety of the latter are not available. While many seeds are sprouted today, it is best to consider the time-honored traditions of sprouts and consume, in traditional ways, those that have been historically used for food.

Sprouts tend to create cold and damp conditions.

33
Nuts and Seeds

According to botanists, nuts are single-seeded fruits with tough, inedible coatings as opposed to fruits with fleshy sweet coatings. *The Oxford Book of Food Plants* defines nuts as "any seed or fruit containing an edible and usually rather hard and oily kernel within a hard or brittle shell."

The only true nuts are the sweet chestnuts, acorns, hazelnuts, and beechnuts, all of which belong to the family of trees called the *fagales*. The rest of what we usually think of as nuts are either relatives of various tree fruits, or seeds. Nuts grow on trees and are a food source that has been around for a very long time, possibly longer than sixty million years.

Nuts are used universally as garnishes and snacks; or they are ground into meal, to be used as fillers for breads and many other food products, including the extraction of nut oils for a wide variety of food preparations and body care products.

Nuts and seeds are important food plants for various reasons. They are excellent sources of protein and fat. They are plentiful and easy to gather, and they store for a long time. Like beans and grains, nuts (when unshelled) are self-preserving and do not require any modern methods of preservation. In countries where nuts and seeds are staple fare, they are thought to be good for cleaning the teeth and strengthening the gums.

Shelled nuts and seeds have a high fat content, which makes them

susceptible to rancidity if exposed for extended periods, especially walnuts, pecans, Brazil nuts, and sunflower seeds. They also tend to absorb
odors from other surrounding foods. They are best consumed within a
few days after being shelled.

Nuts on Fire

When I was in the second grade, every so often we had show-and-
tell, an entertaining and educational game where each student would
bring something from home or nature and give a little talk about
it. I remember one particular show-and-tell because of two unique
presentations.

The first presentation of the day was by a kid who was my best friend
at the time. He got up and proceeded to talk about the Brazil nut. He
told the class how Brazil nuts had a high concentration of oil and protein. Then he stuck three toothpicks into the bottom of a shelled Brazil
nut, forming a tripod. He then asked the teacher to light the top of the
nut with a match. She did so, and my friend then set the nut down on
its tripod base. The Brazil nut burned like a candle through three more
presentations.

I was amazed and sat staring at the Brazil nut candle until it completely burned out. I thought this was just great. The rest of the class
proceeded as usual, with nothing else that particularly burned itself
into my memory. That is, until the last presentation of the day, when
another friend of mine got up and spoke about his father. He said his
father enjoyed reading the rolled-up magazine he held in his hand. He
then revealed the centerfold of the magazine for all to see. Needless to
say, the teacher was shocked and quickly confiscated the magazine. It
wasn't until I became a teenager that I realized the poetic symmetry of
the day—both presentations had something to do with "nuts."

Now, setting nuts literally on fire is not the most common way of
preparing them—but it does take some sort of cooking or soaking to
render them not only edible but digestible as well. Many people who
eat natural foods think it ideal to eat nuts and seeds in their raw form.
While this may be philosophically ideal, it is not physiologically practi-

cal, since nuts and seeds become rancid from the outside toward the inside when shells are removed. Roasting not only crisps the outer tissue by drying it and further intensifying the flavor, it also seals the seed or nut and temporarily stops oxidation and rancidity. The nutritional content remains the same.

Roasting seeds and nuts also render these highly indigestible foods digestible, and unless your stomach and intestines are made of iron (which they aren't), you'll be better off roasting seeds and nuts. If you are eating them as a snack and would like to ensure that they are digested, roast them with a little sea salt or soy sauce and masticate them thoroughly.

Another method for aiding digestion of these wonderful and healthful foods is to soak them for several hours or overnight. This method of preparing nuts activates dormant enzymes and reduces phytate content. Once soaked and rinsed, they can then be slow-roasted at a low temperature for several hours.

Another method is to soak nuts overnight in water, then rinse and grind with water in a blender; then strain the liquid through a fine strainer to experience the most delicious milk you ever had. The most common nut milk is made from almonds; however, the same process can be used for macadamia, Brazil, hazel, pecan, and several other nuts as well. Additional ingredients of dates, vanilla, cinnamon, cocoa, and natural sweeteners are often added to the blended nuts for taste and variety.

High Anxiety

Nuts and seeds are well protected by their hard outer coat and, as with grains and beans, this signifies a high concentration of stored energy. Each nut has the potential to become a whole tree. Some of these trees are quite impressive: the chestnut, up to 115 feet tall; the walnut, up to 100 feet tall; the pecan, up to 150 feet tall; and the Brazil nut, 150 feet tall with a trunk as round in circumference as four men standing in a circle with arms extended and hands held together.

Years ago I recall awakening early one morning and out of the corner of my eye catching a glimpse of a little gray squirrel perched on a branch not more than two feet from the window where I stood. So as not to startle him, I froze in my position. So did he (perhaps so as not to startle me). We stared at each other for a moment, I in my underwear and he with an acorn stuffed in his mouth.

I didn't move—but the squirrel did, in a most unusual manner. He shifted in sharp nervous jerks, never taking his eyes off me for a moment. He was busy gathering a reserve food supply for the coming cool weather, and I couldn't help but think how high-strung and nervous squirrels seem, whether desperately gathering or not.

At first I thought squirrels are this way because they are small and have fast metabolisms, and they need constantly to be aware of any predators that may be near. While this is all true, I thought some more. I thought of that little, tiny body . . . and of the tiny acorn, with its potential to grow into a one-hundred-foot tree. This was the squirrel's preferred food, a highly energized food for such a small animal. The squirrel's food contains a tremendous energy reserve, yet the squirrel needs a large supply to last through the winter. This must mean not only that the animal metabolizes these nuts very quickly, it also means that the nuts must contribute in some way to the energetic qualities of the squirrel.

Since there was no "scientific verification" for my strange thoughts, I decided to experiment with eating a variety of nuts on a daily basis. Preparation of acorns in such a way as to make them fit for human consumption proved to be a long and tedious task (although this was certainly done by Native Americans and others throughout the world). So I resorted to the convenience of almonds, walnuts, pecans, and filberts, knowing that they too contained a similar, huge tree-containing potential.

Needless to say, the experiment was a success. Naturally, neither you nor I have the digestive equivalency of a squirrel, and my vain attempt at trying to be one proved disastrous on that level. However, my energy level did pick up—yet it was a strange kind of energy. According to the observations of a few close friends, I seemed more nervous and edgy than usual. They said it seemed like I felt the need to be doing something all the time, and it really didn't matter what it was.

A rather astute student of mine caught me off-guard one day and actually said "Steve, have you been eating large amounts of nuts?" I replied, "What makes you think so?" So he said, "You talk much faster than usual, you seem to be less receptive, and you seem to have a hard time listening. I can hardly get a sentence out of my mouth before you start talking."

Well, I was floored. Either my friend was being honest with me by letting me know what an ass I really was, or those nuts were actually contributing to my nutty behavior. I opted for the latter conclusion, and drastically reduced my consumption of nuts again. It wasn't long before I was back to my somewhat normal, cynical-yet-ready-to-listen self. Relieved that I could once again be accused of *being* nuts, yet not be accused of *acting* nuts, I continued to learn about my relationship with nuts.

Their place in relation to meals, and in diet in general, are as healthy snacks, garnishes, and condiments, yet they also do make a wonderful and satisfying white milk that can be used as a dairy substitute on cereals, or thickened for sauces and desert fillings. Those are just a few of my personal preferences, with which I have established a nice rapport.

That is, except for sunflower seeds—talk about an abusive relationship.

Seedy Memories

In the spring of 1981, I was driving west across country, starting from Massachusetts. After more than twelve hours of driving with an overheated cassette deck (you know, when no matter what tape you play it comes out sounding like heavy metal), hunger pangs were getting the better of me. I was bored and tired and after even more driving, I reached the flatlands of the Midwest. It was there that I decided to acknowledge the messages of hunger my stomach was sending me.

I was famished and had nothing to eat except a two-pound bag of roasted sunflower seeds. I knew I could have stopped somewhere out there (have you ever driven though unpopulated areas of middle America in the spring?), but for what, fake foods and Coke? I proceeded to eat the sunflower seeds, and I kept eating them—not a difficult thing to do when feeling very hungry. Nuts and seeds are like that: once you get started, those tiny crunchy morsels can become quite habit-forming.

Before long I had consumed most of the sunflower seeds in my possession. That ol' hunger void was satisfied—and while I wasn't sick, I wasn't exactly well either. My stomach lay in a state of dormancy, wondering what to do with this lump of semiground seeds. I wavered between the options of pulling the car over and taking a nap or stopping to get some exercise. The latter idea didn't excite me at all, yet I certainly didn't want to go to sleep for two hours, either, nor for the rest of the season. After a short jog, with some deep breathing exercises and a few jumping jacks, I resumed my position behind the wheel for another six hours of driving.

Feeling somewhat rejuvenated after the exercise, I sat while my stomach churned and gurgled as it proceeded to move those seeds through the remainder of their journey. I won't bore you with details, but by the time those ground-up seeds had settled in the intestines, I was regretting my choice. I drove the remainder of the trip with the car windows open and my mind preoccupied with strange thoughts like, "Maybe I should pick up the next hitchhiker I see and leave the windows rolled up." Naw, I might be nuts, but I'm not cruel!

That experience destroyed my relationship with sunflower seeds. I could care less if I ever saw them again as long as I lived. The sunflower experience is one that has helped me to clarify and understand my relationships with foods, and I cite it as an example of what *not* to do with food. It is just as easy to fall into the trap of abusive food relationships as it is with people relationships—and abuse in either will contribute to a similar adverse effect.

I have met many people who believe they cannot eat a particular food because of similar experiences of indulgence and abuse. Often this belief is the result of quantitative abuse, and needn't always be the grounds for avoiding a particular nourishing food. A so-called "bad experience" with a particular food does not necessarily mean it will always be bad every time you eat that food. (I'm still telling myself that about sunflower seeds, but so far, no dice.)

These kinds of experiences can often limit the almost unlimited possibilities in our food relationships, sometimes to the point of physical, mental, and social deprivation. Nuts and seeds are common foods that many people feel they cannot eat, and this is more often than not the result of a lack of a balanced relationship to these foods and other dietary factors. It is not about whether one should eat nuts or not eat them, or any food for that matter—it is about establishing relationships with foods in such a way as to know how, when, and in which way to eat them.

Nutty Cravings

People often ask me if it is okay to eat nut and seed butters, and I usually respond by asking them how they would like to eat them. Most people like to spread nut and seed butters on bread or crackers. While this method of eating nut butters may be a simple and tasty way of eating them, it is generally not conducive to healthy digestion, unless some fresh raw vegetables are added.

The most digestible and satisfying use of nut and seed butters I've found is to combine a butter with a small amount of either umeboshi (pickled) plum or paste, or miso, and a spicy vegetable such as chopped scallion, watercress, chives, or black or white pepper or other spices. Add enough water to produce a creamy paste, and mix the ingredients well. This combination can be used cooked or uncooked as a spread for breads and crackers, or as a satisfying sauce for grain and salads and cooked vegetable preparations. Sweeteners can also be added, depending on the combinations, for variety. The fermented flavoring and the spice help to render nut and seed butters digestible. Again, it is just as important *how* we eat something as it is whether the food can or should be eaten or not.

Many people have strong cravings for seeds and nuts and the butters derived from them, particularly those who follow strict or limited plant-based diets. These fat- and protein-rich foods do tend to fill the void for those in need. When people exclude traditional high-quality fats from their diets, they develop a tendency to crave them, and will often compensate for this by eating copious quantities of seeds and nuts, or seed and nut butters. This eating practice often results in digestive and respiratory problems that could easily be avoided if the individual used moderate quantities of a variety of traditional fats on a regular basis.

Another reason people crave these foods is because of a basic lack of protein in their diets, and this is often due to their belief in unfounded theories that label all protein as bad, especially animal protein.

While an excess of any nutritional element may contribute to health problems, some dietary approaches suggest a protein source of a mere 5 percent daily, and sometimes even less. There is no need to go from one extreme to another, especially regarding one's protein intake. In these extreme cases, one might experience extreme weight loss and a reduction of muscle tone. The addition of a moderate amount of traditional protein sources in one's diet can reduce these extreme cravings dramatically.

While nuts and seeds can take up to three hours to digest, they are a satisfying and important energizing source of nutrition and an essential part of a healthy diet.

Energetics of Nuts and Seeds

Most seeds and nuts have a hard outer shell that serves to protect the easily oxidized kernel. Once it is removed, the kernel quickly absorbs oxygen and, as I mentioned before, begins to become rancid.

Most nuts and seeds, with their protein- and oil-rich contents, also contain ample moisture, and it is this dampness that encourages oxidation. Energetically, this rapid absorption of oxygen manifests in the human body as a need for increased oxygen intake in order to metabolize these foods. If one is physically active, the digestion and metabolism of nuts and seeds is usually not problematic; however, if one is not physically active after eating seeds and nuts, there may be a tendency toward an increase in respiration, which in turn can contribute to anxiety and feelings of restlessness.

In general, nuts and seeds create a warm and damp effect in the body, with the exception of pumpkin, sunflower, and sesame seeds, which tend to create a warm and dry effect. They are also high in trace minerals, can contribute to the regulation of blood sugar, and many contain a high polyunsaturated oil content that is best consumed in the whole nut or seed, as opposed to being extracted and used as oil. For the most part, the health benefits of polyunsaturated vegetables oils are highly overrated and only a few should be used with any regularity.

As with all foods, each nut and seed has its own unique energetic properties. Convoluted nuts (pecans and walnuts), because of their shape, were traditionally thought to have positive effects on the brain and reproductive organs. Modern research has confirmed that walnuts are a rich source of omega-3 fatty acids and thus do indeed have a beneficial effect on the brain and nervous system.

Pistachios belong to the cashew family and possess a truly unique flavor. Filberts, also called hazelnuts, are perhaps the sweetest of all nuts. Sesame seeds have been cultivated for some five thousand years in the Middle East and are now grown in more than fifty tropical countries. The sesame plant can store large quantities of water and its seeds are highly stable. Pumpkin seeds contain zinc, and are sometimes used for their role in helping to balance blood sugar metabolism.

The unique and concentrated combination of fat, protein, and carbohydrate in seeds and nuts gives them a slow release of energy into the body, a time-release effect that feeds rather than floods the bloodstream. Use them regularly and in combinations to enhance the nutrition of any meal.

34
Fruits

Fruits are usually classified in different categories according to their nutritive value. The most nutritious fruits are more commonly known as cereal grains and beans; then come what are commonly known as nuts and seeds; and last are the *succulent fruits,* the sweet sugary fruits.

This last group of fruits has long been touted as especially healthy foods; researchers in the latter part of the twentieth century even went so far as to claim that fruit may help to reduce your chances of developing cancer and heart disease.

The word *fruit* is derived from the Latin *frui,* which means "to enjoy or to delight in." How true it is, too, for many are so delicious.

From a nutritional perspective, fruit contains the following ingredients: water, fiber, vitamin C, enzymes, phytochemicals, vitamins, some minerals, and lots of sugar. Additional properties of fruit can be understood through *what each fruit is* in relation to the environment it grows in and the potential effects it can have on the human body.

Fruits, because of their energetic nature and the ingredients they contain, have a cooling effect on the body. One of the express purposes of fruit is to cool organisms that have become excessively hot. This is why most of the more luscious and juicier fruits grow in hot tropical environments, and most fruits grown in temperate and colder climates grow mainly in the summer months.

Paradise Lost

Fruits are eaten as a primary food source by many herbivores, birds, and nonhuman primates. Historically, the use of fruit in human diet has been mostly as a supplemental food within a broader based diet, rather than as a principal food.

Numerous examples of fruit in mythology link it both with times of ripeness and with periods characterized by the disintegration of mental, moral, and spiritual values.

The 1960s through the early 1970s ushered in a wave of alternatives in health and spirituality in the United States and Europe. The cultivated seeds of Catholicism and the mid-twentieth-century version of the Protestant work ethic, strongly linked to the materialism of previous generations, left a sour taste in the mouths of a new generation of budding flower children. It was a time ripe for change, and the sweet fruits of Hinduism and Buddhism, along with some of their dietary practices, served to satisfy the need for physiological expansion from the confines of materialism. They also offered escapism through foreign yet appealing views on spirituality.

These Eastern approaches to spirituality offered Westerners the opportunity not to fear the wrath of God, as they had previously been taught, but to actually "be God." Moreover, this God, unlike the God of the Old Testament, would be peaceful, humble, and loving to fellow humans. Regardless of whether or not it succeeded in establishing the fruits of peace and godliness through its unique mix of Eastern cultural influences, Western middle-class affluence, abundant drugs, and free love, this era—one of the most unusual and interesting turning points in American history—helped to lay the foundation of a new way of viewing life and living that would influence generations to come.

Above all else, this era and the people associated with it desired *expansion*—and fruit, along with vegetarianism, drugs, and Eastern mysticism, helped to fulfill this desire.

While the sixties were a fairly recent manifestation, the themes of escape and ripeness for spiritual change—and their association with fruit—echo through the pages of history. The story of Adam and Eve, their relationship to ripe fruit and subsequent decline, is only one famous example. In its mythic depiction of good and evil, innocence and decadence, this allegory interestingly uses a people-fruit relationship to establish its point.

The "innocents" of the sixties might maintain that their Eden was *found,* not *lost,* through this more recent episode of escape. In any case, fruitarianism, a remnant of our more recent past, lingers as a "spiritual" lifestyle, and undoubtedly will continue to do so until the dangerous effects of this practice are realized among its followers.

The Big Chill

The "dangerous effects" I allude to stem from fruit's strong tendency to promote an *emptying* and *cooling* of one's inner fire and vitality. People who choose to eat or drink copious quantities of fruit and fruit juice must have enough internal heat reserve in order to consume fruit in large quantities. In other words, they need to have eaten large amounts of heating foods, such as animal products or fried or trans fat–heavy foods, or they must presently be eating these foods, in order to balance the cooling effects of large quantities of fruit.

Naturally, it is easier to eat large quantities of fruit more regularly when one lives in a hot, tropical climate, where one would naturally want to stay cool to create physiological balance between his body and the environment. However, if an excessive quantity of fruit sugar is introduced into the bloodstream (and the person is not physically active enough to discharge the accumulated excess), it can easily result in fatigue and weakness, even in a tropical climate.

The high sugar content of fruit can also contribute to weight gain, especially for inactive people. The human liver has a limited storage capacity for sugar. When one's sugar intake exceeds the liver's capacity and the sugar is not burned off through activity, it is converted to fat (triglycerides) in the body.

Fruit and Blood Sugar

A slightly more detailed view of how the simple sugar of fruit is converted and effects the body is as follows:

Once carbohydrates are consumed, they are converted to glucose in
the body; *insulin,* a hormone produced by the pancreas, causes glucose
to enter cells, where it can be used by hemoglobin, the iron-carrying
part of red blood cells. In order to be used by the body, glucose must
enter the cells—and insulin is the key that unlocks the cell doors and
allows the precious fuel to enter.

When too much glucose enters the bloodstream, the excess is carried
to the liver, where it can be held up to a capacity of about 150 grams,
and stored there in the form of large storage molecules called *glycogen,*
which the body can use when it needs sugar. When the liver's 150-gram
capacity is full, a second sugar-storage mechanism comes into play.

Insulin, in addition to unlocking cell doors to allow sugar to enter,
also has the ability to pull excess sugar out of the bloodstream and
convert it into fat for storage in body tissue. This accumulated storage
form of fat is called *triglycerides.* Once in this form, unfortunately, it
becomes far more difficult to convert the substance back into usable
glucose.

All carbohydrates must be broken down into simple sugars before
being absorbed by the small intestine. In fact, personality in many
ways is defined by one's ability to transform complex sugars (grains,
beans, vegetables) into simple sugars. These complex carbohydrates are
the kinds of carbohydrates that support physical and mental stability.
Refined sugar, along with other simple sugars such as the fructose from
fruits and juices, forces insulin into an emergency mode until the blood
sugar level is balanced and stable. Unfortunately, high insulin levels lead
to more fat storage and less fat removal from storage.

For example, let's look at three variations of the effect on blood
sugar of the fructose in apples. 1) Chewing a raw apple causes a peak
insulin level in the bloodstream that measures twenty-four units. 2)
Consuming the same apple processed in a blender, where the fiber is
broken down and sugar released, raises the insulin peak to thirty-three

units. 3) Consuming the same apple juiced with its pulp removed raises the peak insulin level to forty-five units.

Most Westerners have been overworking their livers and pancreases since they were children, starting out with diets loaded with orange juice, bananas, and other fruits, and large amounts of refined sugar products. Because of this, converting to a more complex-carbohydrate-rich diet can be difficult, and the effort can easily produce strong cravings for simple sugars. It would be far healthier if these cravings could be satisfied by fresh fruit—but for the most part, they are not.

It is interesting how easily things can be misconstrued through advertising. I recently saw an ad supporting the low-carb diet that claimed a baked potato raises the blood glucose faster than a bowl of (whatever their brand name was) ice cream. The real reason for this, of course, is that the ice cream has such a high level of fat (cream), which buffers the high sugar content. Throw a generous dollop of butter and sour cream on the potato, and suddenly you wouldn't be able to make the same claim!

Botanically, a fruit is the fleshy organ that surrounds either a single seed or numerous seeds, and is derived from the ovary of a flowering plant. Grains, beans, and nuts are called "simple dry fruits," and sweet, sugary fruits are called "fleshy fruits." While both are sources of carbohydrate, energetically and nutritionally they have little in common.

Fleshy fruits can be eaten raw, cooked, or dried and supply the body with sugar, energy, and fiber. Of the three ways fruit can be eaten, raw is the most cooling to the human body. Dried fruit contains little water, yet a stronger concentration of sugar, as well as high fiber. Dried fruits will tend to absorb more internal fluids when consumed. This is not surprising, since like any dried food, they have the strong tendency to rehydrate.

For people with cold dry conditions, cooked fruit with added cinnamon would be more beneficial than plain fruit, as this preparation adds both moisture and warmth to the fruit. Cooking fruit helps to break down the fiber and further concentrate sugars; cinnamon has a warming effect on the body. On the other hand, dried fruits could be helpful for those who are water retentive and tend to bloat easily.

How one chooses to eat fruit is best determined by one's individual condition. While it is not in any form a *building* food for the body, it does assist in the breakdown of excess mass for those who might need it.

Primates (monkeys, apes, etc.) do well with fruit as a primary food because their intestines are designed to accumulate and ferment large quantities of plant matter, which they eat continuously. Fruit-eating primates also exist naturally in hot climates, where cooling fruits help to keep them comfortable. The larger primates move slowly though life and spend most of their time relaxing and eating.

Individuals with strong digestive abilities and those who are physically active have less difficulty digesting fruit in any form, compared with those who have weaker digestion and are inactive. Climate is also an important consideration when deciding how much fruit to consume. Humans can easily consume more fruit when living like primates. Living like primates? Yes: if and when you should happen to be in a position where you are living a lifestyle that requires continuous eating, along with little physical activity and absolutely no thinking.

It is interesting to note that traditional cultures from hot climates consume moderate amounts of fruits as a regular part of their varied diets—but not exclusively.

The sugar content of temperate-climate fruits can range from 10 to 15 percent sugar, while tropical varieties range from 20 to 60 percent sugar. The lemon is unique among tropical fruits in that its sugar content is an average of only 1 percent.

Tropical Fruits

Semitropical and tropical fruits (orange, papaya, mango, grapefruit, banana, etc.) all have similar characteristics that energetically place them in the same group, due to environmental factors. These particular fruits all have a thick outer peel that protects a soft and juicy inner flesh. The sweet, fleshy inside is the part that is eaten and the peels are usually discarded. In contrast, the majority of nontropical or temperate-climate fruits can be eaten with their peels.

Tropical fruits are more fragile than most temperate-climate fruits, as they cannot adapt well to extreme climate changes. There have been numerous instances where an early or sudden cold spell has devastated entire groves of oranges and grapefruit. (With the current drastic changes in climate afoot, this is happening with increasing frequency.) Their attempt to grow tough outer coatings to protect their delicate insides does little good for tropical fruit when the environment makes a sudden shift.

The citrus varieties of tropical fruits (orange, grapefruit, tangerine, etc.) are composed of sectioned compartments. These individual compartments are called carpals and are actual portions of the plant's ovary. The diversification of a sectioned ovary in citrus varieties of fruit can adversely affect fertility and sex drive when eaten in excessive quantities.

The potential effects of large quantities of tropical fruits on our psychophysical bodies include: a tough yet pale exterior with a soft inner core, a fragile and delicate physiology, a self-protective attitude, perishable (easily bruised) and swollen muscle tissue, thin and weak blood, often with low iron levels, fatigue, and body coldness.

The energetic effects of the banana on the male reproductive organs may be obvious, but I had better clarify them by pointing out that shape is only one of many characteristics. Notice how soft, flaccid, and prone to rapid spoilage the banana's substance is? A little imagination, and you get the point. The same energetics of bananas, applied to the female reproductive organs, can contribute to menstrual irregularity, sexual frustration, and certainly minimal satisfaction. Very cooling, indeed, are bananas, for both male and female.

While it is true that citrus fruits have ample amounts of vitamin C, the largest amounts of this vitamin exists in the *peels* of these fruits, with only small amounts actually existing in the fruit's flesh. Vitamin C is one of the most fragile vitamins and is easily destroyed when heated. The fruits of this group are highly acidic and quite high in sugar, and when consumed beyond moderation or as an extreme dietary program may contribute greatly to the depletion of our internal mineral balance, resulting in kidney weakness.

On the other hand, for conditions of excessive heat that often manifest as anger and elevated body temperature, these are the most effective fruits for producing a cooling effect. Like one's environment, one's individual condition is an important factor in determining which tropical fruits to consume and how much.

Temperate-Climate Fruits

Temperate-climate fruits (apple, pear, peach, plum, berries, etc.) are fruits that grow in the summer and late summer months of a four-season climate. The majority of these fruits are categorized as members of the *rose* family.

The rose family consists of numerous subcategories, one of which is called *pome* fruits. These fruits contain a compartmented core that holds the seeds. Pears and apples are two examples of this group.

Another group is the *drupes,* or stone fruits. Each fruit in this group contains a single seed surrounded by fleshy fruit. Peach, apricot, plum, and cherry are examples of this group and represent some of the most luscious and sensuous nontropical varieties of fruits.

Still another group or subspecies of the rose family is the *rubus,* which includes raspberries, blackberries, and boysenberries. Actually, these "bramble berries" are aggregates of numerous small stone fruits or drupes, each tiny section being a drupe in itself. The strawberry is often called the "false fruit," because it is derived from the base of the flower, as opposed to other fruits, which are derived from an ovary. Blueberries, currants, and cranberries are drupes, and are considered by botanists to be true berries, as they are single fruits derived from an ovary.

The squash family includes still another family of fruits, and these are the melons. They fall under the genus of *cucumis,* which also includes the cucumber. Each of these fruits has specific energetic characteristics as well. We can discover the energetic potential of all fruits first by categorizing them according to their growth patterns.

Fruit from the Trees

These fruits tend to grow up high and have an energetic effect on the upper part of the human body, particularly the lungs, heart, and throat. They include semitropical and tropical varieties: orange, grapefruit, avocado, mango, papaya, and so forth; and temperate varieties: apple, pear, peach, plum, cherry, apricot, and the like.

Upon ripening, a tree fruit will detach from its stem and fall to the ground, where it rapidly decomposes—that is, if animals do not eat it first. Although this image of ripened fruit falling from a tree might seem to suggest the energetic qualities of detachment and freedom, it is quite the contrary.

The stem by which the fruit hangs is what directs the nourishment from the tree to the fruit. When the fruit detaches from its source of nourishment, it will continue to ripen and eventually decompose. This need for tree fruits to accumulate nourishment from the tree actually reveals a characteristic of attachment—for without their source of nourishment, these fruits would gradually decompose.

This is true of all foods, yet among plants there exist many stages of decomposition, as well as different means of nourishment. You can observe an interesting contrast between fruits and vegetables in the way that each grows and develops.

The leaves, stems, and roots of many vegetables can be eaten at just about any time during their growth and developmental stages. A fruit, on the other hand, is ready to be eaten when the seed is fully mature and the fruit has reached its final stage of ripening. The ripening of fruit is the beginning of its rapid decay. The disorganization of the fruit's cells and tissue becomes more obvious when a fruit is bruised or punctured; due to its high sugar content, it will then change color and decompose very quickly, as compared to most vegetables.

Fruits that grow on trees have the extra burden of weight from water buildup in their tissue, causing them to fall to the ground if not picked first. Falling from grace, separating from the source, and increased heaviness of mental gravity are some of the energetic properties that accrue from a diet high in tree fruits.

Among tree fruits, there exist two types: stone and multiseeded. Both types affect the upper part of the body, and because of their high sugar content, can adversely affect blood sugar; and therefore one's mood and thinking.

Stone fruits (peaches, plums, cherries, nectarines, dates, mangos, etc.) each have a single seed surrounded by a soft, fibrous, and fleshy tissue. Their ability to organize tender flesh around a single seed gives them energetic qualities that differ from multiseeded fruits.

For example, stone fruits tend to affect the fibrous tissue of the body, thus increasing the circulation of sugars throughout the body and brain. These fruits affect one by cooling the blood vessels and deeper body tissue, and this effect is most noticeable in the upper part of the body, where the lungs and heart reside. Also, the flesh of these fruits tends to be soft when ripened, and this contributes to cooler as well as softer muscles and damp skin.

Psychologically, stone fruits tend to concentrate and organize their energetics toward the center of the brain. Suppose, for example, you are writing, painting, or drawing. The sugar in any fruit, once it reaches the bloodstream, will flow to the brain. If you are unable to stick to or concentrate on a particular idea during an artistic endeavor, stone fruit will tend to have a more organizing effect on your thought processes than other fruits. On the other hand, in the same situation, multiseeded fruits (orange, apple, pear, etc.) will tend to have a more diversifying, dispersing effect on your thoughts. Multiseeded tree fruits have the tendency to connect thoughts loosely with other thoughts. This could be helpful for the individual who might be stuck on one idea.

Multiseeded tree fruits consist of two types: multiseeded fruits with a porous flesh, such as apples and pears; and multiseeded fruits with sectioned compartments, including oranges, grapefruits, and tangerines. As mentioned above, these fruits tend to diversify thoughts and ideas. Apples and pears have a porous flesh that gives them energetic properties of superficial expansion and cooling. These tend to affect the surface of the body, the skin, and extremities (the hands and feet). Sectioned multiseeded tree fruit (especially citrus) tend to affect deeper organ tissue and glands with a deep, cooling effect that causes internal heat to rise to the surface of the body and dissipate.

There is a wide variety of tree fruits because nature has given them all the unique characteristic of natural genetic mutation. When a seed from a tree fruit is planted, it will result in a slightly different variety than the parent plant. Most tree fruits are propagated for consistency of type by grafting.

Unusual Fruits

A few unusual tree fruits are the avocado, the banana, the fig, and the coconut.

Avocado

Evidence for avocado consumption from Mexico goes back as far as twelve thousand years. There are three distinct varieties of avocado and all are excellent sources of nutrition. Ample quantities of potassium, vitamins A, C, B_2, and B_6 are just a few of the many vitamins stored in the creamy rich flesh of avocados.

The avocado is a green, pear-shaped fruit and a member of the laurel family. The word *avocado* comes from *nahuatl,* an Aztec term that means "testicle tree." This fruit grows in pairs, and a number of historical references praise the avocado as having aphrodisiac qualities.

Unlike most other tree fruits that are juicy and sweet, the avocado has a soft, creamy flesh, a mild flavor, and a large quantity of mono-unsaturated fats. Also, while most other fruits ripen and soften while on the tree, the avocado matures on the tree but does not ripen and soften until it has been picked.

An anomaly among fruits, the avocado has twenty times the fat of other fruits; also, cellular division in the flesh of the avocado continues throughout the life of the fruit. In tropical and subtropical climates, the avocado grows all year round, offering a continuous supply of food.

It is a delicate fruit, highly susceptible to oxygenation and chilling injury. Most are hand-picked to avoid bruising. If deprived of oxygen they will not ripen, and once oxygen is restored they will spoil quickly.

Energetically, the avocado has a cool and damp nature. The creamy flesh is easily digested and soothing to the digestive system. It is high in protein and its high fat content contributes to healthy skin color and tone.

Banana

Cultivating the bananas we are familiar with today was indeed a remarkable accomplishment for our ancestors. The suggested forerunner is a giant herb with soft stem and fruits that are hard and full of seeds. Once domesticated, it became seedless and is now grown as a *rhizome* into a tall green plant.

The banana is a berry, botanically speaking, and is an exception to the rule that all staple foods are either root crops or cereals. Bananas have been the staple food of many tropical areas in the world for thousands of years. These traditional bananas, however, were not like what most people in developed counties eat on their breakfast cereals or as a snack. For one thing, they were not very sweet. They were more like the *plantain,* a starchy plant typically eaten cooked and still used as a carbohydrate staple today in many tropical environments. In fact, starchy, nonsweet bananas were cultivated in the Indus Valley six thousand years ago and are mentioned in the Indian historical classic *Ramayana.* Ancient wall inscriptions seven thousand years old found in Assyria depict banana cultivation.

In modern times, man has managed to rid the banana of seeds and alter the flavor. Shoots from an underground stem now propagate them. This cultivated version is sterile and unable to reproduce without human assistance; when assisted, however, a banana plant can grow to the height of an average man in three months. It takes six months for the fruit to begin to form and another four before it is ready to be harvested. At this point, the plant will bear only one bunch of fruit, but this one bunch may contain more than one hundred bananas. To get more bananas, the remaining part of the plant must be chopped down and a new one planted.

Almost all fruit experience fertilization of the female ovule by male pollen, a process that initiates the production of growth hormones that cause expansion of the ovary wall. The banana plant is one exception: it is one of the few fruit plants that carry the genetic trait of developing fruit without fertilization.

With the exception of people from countries where bananas originate, Americans are the world's most avid consumers of this unusual fruit. To most Americans, bananas represent a "source of potassium," a topping for breakfast cereals, or a snack. In fact, they are much more than this. Sweet bananas, more than almost any other fruit, are energetically influenced by a tremendous flow of centrifugal energy—upward, unwinding, dissipating energy. A food with this much centrifugal energy, combined with an extremely high concentration of sugar, has an exceptionally strong, deep, cooling effect on the human body, especially on the bones. This may very well be the single most cooling fruit there is.

For an excessively hot condition, bananas can sometimes be helpful, especially for individuals with an excessive sex drive.

Plantains, on the other hand, have a different effect than sweet bananas. Plantain can be eaten when hard and starchy or after they have ripened to become soft and sweet. Either way, they are traditionally cooked, usually fried and served with beans and other traditional foods from South and Central America or with traditional Asian foods. For that matter, plantains, like other bananas, have adapted nicely to regional diets in tropical and subtropical locations around the world.

These bananas are a healthy source of starch and have a warm and damp effect when cooked. They also have a soothing and relaxing effect on the middle organs of the body (spleen, pancreas, and stomach).

Fig

There are hundreds of varieties of figs; one of the most popular and unusual is the Calimyrna fig. These figs bear fruit by a process called *caprification,* which is one of the most fascinating "mating" rituals in the plant kingdom.

First, a tiny *blastophaga* wasp grows inside an inedible male fig. When the female wasp is hatched and begins to crawl out of the fig, she picks up pollen on her wings. The goal of the wasp is to lay eggs inside of another male fig, but she ends up inside one of the more numerous female figs, where she tries to lay her eggs. However, the structure of the female fig makes this virtually impossible—but while inside the female fig, the wasp introduces the pollen of the male fig to the female fig, and this results in pollination of the female fig. This bizarre transspecies soap opera repeats itself in endless cycles—and is the natural way the Calimyrna fig can pollinate.

Figs are native to Asia Minor and, like dates, have been valued primarily for their sugar by Egyptians and Greeks for thousands of years. They were also used to tenderize flesh foods. This "fruit," actually the swollen flower base of fig, contains both male and female flowers. Anatomically, the fig resembles an inverted strawberry: the flesh surrounds, rather than supports, the true fruits. They develop without the fertilization of their flowers, and their seeds contain no embryos. Growers of the common fig must tie caprifigs (male figs) containing wasp eggs to the branches of the female fig tree in order for pollination to occur.

Figs have a higher concentration of sugar than other common fruit and are easily susceptible to deterioration. Fig trees produce no blossoms, as the flowers grow inside the receptacle of the fig itself.

Like many other foods, the fig is steeped in mythology. The Bible tells numerous stories of the fig, and many other stories abound throughout western Asia and the Mediterranean. To some, the fig stands for veiled fertility, while to others it is a symbol of infertility.

Energetically, figs are very weak fruits. The female fig is edible while the male is not. The need to be pollinated by a wasp (and only one specific type) via the caprifig gives the fig qualities of consistency in species; yet at the same time, its deeply intimate relationship with the insect world gave it special qualities to ancient Egyptians.

It is a private fruit, unwilling to expose its flowers or fruit (the seeds are the fruit) in reproduction. Human reproduction is also an internal and private affair and the eating of figs can have a strong influence on this process.

When used to tenderize meats, figs have a strong ability to weaken and soften ligaments and flesh. Figs have dark and secretive qualities, combined with cold and damp energetics that primarily affect the fleshy tissue of the reproductive organs.

Coconut

Not only is the coconut an unusual fruit; it is in fact an amazing fruit with astounding natural healing qualities.

How coconuts came to be, no one really knows. Like so many other superfoods, its origin is shrouded in mystery, although some botanists suspect an origin in the Malayan archipelago. For those traditional people who live where coconuts are plentiful—and that includes many coastal and island locations around the world—the coconut tree is recognized as "The Tree of Life." This well-entrenched belief is due to the fact that the coconut tree can produce more than one hundred useful products. Bowls for food, jewelry, fibers for bedding . . . then there are the nutritional benefits of the fruit. The water inside the coconut has the same level of electrolyte balance as human blood and is so pure and clean it has been used as intravenous fluid to save lives in some South Sea islands. The water is in fact quite similar to the blood plasma that makes up 55 percent of our blood. As a food, it is a blood purifier, rich in minerals and vitamin C.

The products made from the meat (kernel) of coconut have supported the health of traditional peoples in many obvious ways. Healthy hearts, regulated metabolism, smooth and silky skin tone, strong and pliable muscle tone, and healthy teeth and gums are just a few of the benefits derived from coconut milk and coconut oil.

Coconut milk is made by first drying and shredding the white kernel (called *copra* when dried) and then pouring boiling water over the copra. The resulting thick liquid is coconut milk and is one of the most metabolically satisfying foods one can eat. Traditional uses of coconut milk include sauces, broths, desserts, and marinades.

It is almost impossible to heap too much praise upon coconut oil. It is often considered a functional food—a food that provides health benefits over and beyond basic nutrients. In other words, it has many energetic properties. Here is a list of a few of these benefits:

- The oil is easily absorbed into tissue and cells, making it very good for cellular repair. Unlike polyunsaturated fats, which drive cholesterol into cells, making them rigid and inflexible (while giving the false impression of lowering cholesterol in a healthy way), coconut oil is mostly saturated fat and causes no damage to cells or tissue. Its medium-chained fatty acids are easily absorbed into cells, making them strong and flexible.

- It is the perfect fat for regulating metabolism while nourishing the body and increasing strength.
- It contains medium-chain fatty acids in the form of *lauric* and *capric acid*. Lauric acid forms into *monolaurin* in the body. Research has shown that yeast problems (*Candidiasis*), ringworm and *giardia* (a parasite) have been inactivated or killed by monolaurin. It has been recognized for its antiviral properties, which occur through its ability to disrupt the lipid membranes of viruses, including the HIV virus and herpes. It is also antibacterial and antimicrobial. Monolaurin is not found in the human body and must be supplied by diet. Capric acid, which forms into *monocaprin* in the body, is another medium-chain fatty acid with additional supporting benefits.

We can learn about additional energetic properties of coconut by observing some of the tree's unique characteristics. The coco palm is a tree that can grow from sixty to one hundred feet tall over a period of nine months. It is a natural water filter that filters water by drawing it up through a complex network of fibers to the coconut, where it is stored in a completely sterile state. Nine months is of course a prominent human cycle of conception to birth; this correspondence underscores the fact that this unique food is supportive to pregnant and nursing mothers.

The coconut tree prefers light sandy soil and has shallow, widely spread roots that allow for a much needed air supply. It also tolerates and filters salty water. These functions closely mimic the functions of human kidneys, making foods from coconuts supportive to kidney and adrenal functions. Coconuts (milk, water, and kernel) can help with the regulation of minerals and sodium levels, assist in the maintenance of urinary tract health by helping to reduce infections, and enhance sexual functions by helping to increase sperm quantity and vaginal lubrications.

The coco fruit takes from eleven to fifteen months to reach maturity; while one coconut is on its way to maturation, another may be just beginning to sprout. All stages of fruit are bearing life at all times on the coconut tree, from the youngest to the oldest. The whole process is truly a family affair and makes the "Tree of Life" one of the most fascinating and nutritionally supportive food crops of the world.

Vine Fruit

Vine fruits include watermelon, cantaloupe, honeydew, and others.

Melons have their origin in Persia, except for watermelon, which supposedly is native to Africa. Melons grow low to the ground on sprawling vines and are related to squash and cucumbers. All belong to the same species, *Cucumis melo*.

Melons are very social among their own genus. They tend to interbreed when grown together. If different varieties are not grown far enough apart, insects will cross-pollinate them, producing a new variety.

Watermelons differ from other melons in that the flesh of the watermelon is placental tissue, while in other melons the flesh is derived from the ovary wall. Energetically, they tend to affect the lower part of the human body. Melons tend to be water-heavy and can affect the soft tissue in the intestines, bladder, and reproductive organs. Historically, they were purported to have anticoagulant properties.

Vine fruit do not fall from high altitudes as tree fruits do, nor do they have the intricate filtering system of nourishment found among tree fruits. In addition to sunlight and other external environmental influences, tree fruits get their nourishment filtered through the trunk of the tree; it then continues to be filtered through the branches, followed by the stems, and finally to the fruit itself. The vine fruit (melons) appear to have a single long siphon hose that rapidly feeds water and other needed nourishment to the developing fruit.

Unlike tree fruits, melons become larger as the greater water content causes a swelling of the fruit's tissue and cells, thus making it larger and heavier than other fruits. Melons can grow more than five cubic inches a day and are over 90 percent water. This type of stem-to-fruit feeding also accounts for the fact that melons have a short growing season. This, in addition to the fact that they grow at the hottest time of the year, reveals the plant's insatiable need to drink and store water in order to produce fruit.

When fully ripened, a melon will detach itself from the vine with ease.

The seeds of melons are not usually consumed as food, except for a chosen few who persist in the belief that it best to eat the whole food. The lightly textured inner flesh is the portion of melon eaten, and unlike other fruits, melons begin to lose their characteristic sweet taste the closer one gets to the skin (rind.)

Grapes are vine fruits, but do not grow on the ground. They are climbing vines, and energetically tend to affect the lungs and respiratory system.

Shrub Fruit

Shrub fruits include raspberry, blackberry, blueberry, strawberry, boysenberry, and others. These berries grow on shrubs or bushes and usually are small, sweet, and tart fruits. There are hundreds of varieties of berries, including both edible and poisonous types. Berries tend to grow at a height between that of tree and vine fruits; thus, they affect the middle region of the body, the liver, gallbladder, spleen, pancreas, and stomach. Another correlation with this section of the body is shrub fruits' uniquely sweet-and-sour taste combination.

Fruit plants of the bush variety occur in various sizes, some large (up to four and five feet) and others smaller, anywhere from six inches on up. These plants all have similar mechanisms in terms of feeding and nourishing their fruit. Their structures consist of numerous branches, sometimes accompanied by protective thorns that make some berries unapproachable, especially for small children. Nevertheless, blackberries, raspberries, and others of this sort have such an appeal, particularly the wild varieties, that it doesn't take long before most children—and adults—will submit themselves to the pain and irritation of cuts and scratches wrought by the bramble and thorns of these plants in order to get to that single perfect berry or group of unreachable perfect berries. The thin, firm, and wiry stems of the branches give berries a sharp infusion of concentrated nourishment that results in their characteristically tart flavor.

Berries are easily the most charismatic of fruits, and they tend to have this effect on people. I like to call them the "shy exhibitionists" of fruits because of their uncanny ability to attract attention, and to keep it. They exhibit strong qualities of both feminine and masculine natures. Berries like to reveal their ripened splendor for all to see. Many types of berries have this characteristic, and it is developed early on in bramble varieties (unlike other fruits) as they begin to group their seeds in clusters around a central core.

Berries can also be shy; some will hide behind the plant's leaves. You may recall a time while berry picking when it seemed as if you had picked the last of the ripe berries in an area—and you suddenly lift a leaf, or ever so slightly move a branch, and there before you is the best clump of berries you have ever seen. A child will usually express herself with a surprised or astonished yell. Some adults do, too, but most adults respond to the situation mentally with a silent "ah hah!" or "wow!" The more serious adult might address the berries personally with, "You thought you'd get by me, didn't you?" And they *did* think that, didn't they . . . or were they just being coquettish?

Berries, the ones with seeds on the outside, are communal fruits and have energetic properties that can assist an individual in expressing his or her character. They can help introverts come out of themselves a little more. They can help to add color to a flat or boring personality by attracting attention.

Physically, they push excess to the surface of the body. Strawberries (one of the most popular fruits in the world, and grown almost everywhere), raspberries (the most perfumed of fruits), blackberries, and the others have long been associated with hives or skin rashes. Many foods may contribute to hives or rashes, but it is the natural tendency of these types of berries to move their energy (and yours, when you eat them) from the center to the periphery.

Other berries, such as blueberries or loganberries, have similar characteristics, yet they do not have their seeds on the outside. People tend to be more particular about blueberries, in that they either despise them or they are the only fruit they really feel comfortable eating. In my experience with people and their relationships to fruit, I have frequently been told how blueberries are the only fruit that seem to satisfy and sooth the tension in the middle organs. This does not surprise me, considering the soft, juicy texture and cool, blue color of blueberries.

Blueberries are a Swedish folk remedy for digestive disorders. Blueberries and black currants are high in therapeutic agents called *anthocyanosides,* substances that have proven lethal to bacteria and pathogenic viruses.

The above categories of fruits and their energetic properties may be applied to common problems. For example, a person with a tendency to retain water in the lower abdomen may desire to eat fruit. This may not be the best food to eat while having such a problem. However, if he wishes to do so, it would be wise for him to choose a tree or shrub fruit, rather than a vine fruit, because vine fruits tend to be heavier, contain more water, and thus have more of an accumulating effect on the lower body.

Since this condition is one of excess fluid retention in the abdomen, melon would not be the best choice, since melons contain lots of water. Any of the smaller and less watery fruits would be a better choice. On the other hand, if an individual was experiencing constriction and heat in the lower abdomen, melon might be an appropriate choice, since it has the tendency to resonate in the lower body and has expanding, relaxing, and cooling properties.

Again, note that simply because a food, whether fruit, vegetable, or animal, has a tendency to affect a certain part of the body, it does not necessarily follow that it is "good for" that part of the body. What is important to determine is not simply that a food will resonate in a particular part of the body, but specifically what kind of effect that food will have on that particular part of the body.

As with all other categories of foods, each fruit is unique in its own characteristics. It is important to get to know fruits, as it is all traditional foods, some intimately and others more as casual acquaintances.

35
Condiments and Seasonings

Condiments and seasonings are used to enhance the flavor of food
preparations and to improve their digestibility. They can include a variety of raw or cooked herbs and spices, seeds and nuts, vinegars, oils, vegetables, and products made from combinations of grain, salt, beans, sea
vegetables, animals, and fruits. Though various types of fats have been
used in ample quantities as a macronutrient among traditional peoples,
for convenience and ease of access I will include the energetics of fats
and oils at the end of this section, as they are also used to enhance and
flavor food in much the same way as other seasonings and condiments.

Any of these ingredients, when used in small quantities to enhance
a particular food preparation, can be considered a condiment. Generally
speaking, the stronger or more intense the flavor of a particular condiment, the smaller the quantity needed to enhance a preparation. The more
mild the flavor, the greater quantity needed to enhance a preparation.

Condiments act as *carriers* of other foods. In addition to enhancing
the flavors of foods, condiments energetically can help carry foods and
preparations in the human body in one of the following four directions:

- upward and outward
- downward and inward
- upward and inward
- downward and outward

Ginger root, for example, has a *downward and outward* energy. When added to sautéed dandelion greens (upward-growing vegetables with an *upward and inward* energy), the greens are enhanced by the *downward and outward* quality of the ginger. Sautéed dandelion greens, without added ginger, will tend to strongly affect the upper body, yet the addition of ginger can bring these qualities down to the middle or lower organs of the body. Ginger root grows under the ground and outward, so it carries the energy of whatever it is combined with in that manner.

If the same sautéed greens are seasoned with black pepper instead of with ginger, then the preparation, rather than having an *upward and inward* effect on the upper part of the body, will now have an *upward and outward* effect. The upward vine-growing pepper is spicy and dispersing and adds these qualities to the sautéed vegetables.

How much a condiment carries a preparation or a food in a particular direction through the body is based largely on the quantity of the condiment used. If the sautéed vegetables mentioned above are prepared with very little oil, the vegetables will maintain an *upward and inward* effect. However, if they are sautéed with a large amount of oil, the vegetables will have less of an *upward and inward* effect and more of a *downward and sinking* effect.

These energetic directions of foods and condiments have been observed and applied to food by people for thousands of years throughout the world.

Another example of how a condiment might carry a food preparation in a particular direction would be a kidney bean stew prepared with carrots and onions, and garnished with chives. Once cooked, this stew would have a *sinking, downward and slightly inward* energy. However, when garnished with chopped raw chives, which have an *upward and dispersing* energy, the stew would retain its *downward* energy, but the addition of the chives will carry energy of the stew *slightly upward and outward*. While spices and herbs can have extreme effects, they can also help to balance other extreme foods.

Many condiments serve the dual purpose of being both a seasoning and a vegetable or animal, while others are single-purpose condiments and are used purely as seasonings. The onion is a vegetable, yet when finely chopped and used as a raw garnish, the onion becomes a condiment or seasoning. Tiny fish and shrimp are animal foods, yet when dried and ground into powder and made into a paste with hot peppers (a common seasoning in Thai and other Asian cuisine), they become condiments.

The mustard seed is an example of a single-purpose condiment. Unlike the onion, mustard seed has far too strong a flavor to be eaten as a vegetable. Therefore, it is used as an ingredient to flavor other foods, or as a spread.

Dual-purpose condiments consist primarily of vegetables that can be eaten as vegetables or can act as seasonings. These include scallions, onions, garlic, watercress, radish, turnip, chives, and so forth.

Single-purpose condiments consist primarily of seeded or small leafed spices and herbs used primarily for seasoning, and include pepper, mustard, cumin, cinnamon, nutmeg, oregano, thyme, sage, etc. Many of the seed spices can increase metabolic rate and promote circulation.

Prepared condiments, a third category of condiments, consist of numerous combinations of seasonings and whole foods, prepared through various cooking methods or processed in some way. They include miso, tamari soy sauce, kuzu, corn starch, vinegars, umeboshi plum or paste, fish sauce, shrimp paste, and the like, as well as simple home preparations using seed and nut butters, and vegetables.

To write about the energetics of every condiment would be virtually impossible. Herbs and spices alone would fill a book. Therefore, I have chosen a few examples of what I feel to be some of the more commonly used condiments essential to a healthy diet.

Garlic

Garlic is a member of the onion family that includes onions, chives, leeks, shallots, scallions, and other pungent-flavored plants—yet garlic is more potent in flavor than most of its family members. It is unique among the onion family in that it consists of a bulb neatly wrapped in a delicate papery tissue that contains additional individually wrapped cloves joined together at a root base.

Both garlic and onions were among the first foods cultivated. The ancient Greeks, Egyptians, and Chinese are just a few of the many cultures who revered garlic as an important plant food. The historical shroud of mystery and contradiction surrounding garlic is as prevalent today as it was in times past.

On the one hand, it has a reputation for making people who eat it smell bad and for being overly dispersing and stimulating. On the other hand, garlic is one of the oldest antibiotics known and has proven to have beneficial antiviral, antibacterial, and antifungal properties; to detoxify excess bacteria produced from meats and seafood; to purify and cleanse the blood; to eliminate intestinal parasites; to stimulate the immune system by reducing oxygen depletion; to destroy free radicals; and to reduce high cholesterol.

Garlic has the broadest spectrum of any natural antibiotic substance known. Recipes for healing potions of ancient Sumeria, dating as far back as 4000 BC, state that both garlic and onions had been used for centuries as antiseptics, diuretics, sedatives, poultices, and aphrodisiacs. These qualities have led to the belief that garlic is more suited to medicinal uses only, or as no more than an occasional seasoning. While these are certainly appropriate uses for garlic, it also holds a vaunted position as a true vegetable in many places throughout the world.

The bourgeois of eighteenth-century Europe, while acknowledging its strengthening properties, thought garlic fit only for laborers and the poor. In Asia, the Koreans, Chinese, and others have enjoyed the health benefits of garlic for thousands of years. For a long time the exceptions to Asian garlic lovers were the Japanese, who now use it creatively in much of their cuisine.

In fact, Japanese scientists have done much of the scientific work proving the therapeutic benefits of garlic. Their research has shown that cancer patients undergoing chemotherapy and radiation experience reduced side effects when eating garlic. Among alcoholics who consume garlic, there have been reduced fat deposits on the liver. Garlic also proves helpful in the treatment of jaundice, hepatitis, and yeast infections.

The shadowy relationship between garlic and vampires reveals the powerful effects of this food on the dead—or should I say, the undead.

The symbolism of the vampire—who has an insatiable thirst for fresh new blood, who cannot leave his grave or coffin if surrounded by garlic, and who cannot harm the living if they are protected by garlic—is but one of many mythical homages to the blood-purifying, life-enhancing, and cleansing qualities of garlic.

A Spicy Controversy

Garlic is generally thought to have a hot temperament, meaning it is purported to make one hot. However, just because garlic is hot to the taste does not necessarily mean that it generates heat in the body. This rule holds true for most other hot-tasting spices as well.

Throughout the world, the people who consume the largest quantities of spices and spicy foods are those who dwell in hot or tropical climates. People living in hot environments certainly would not want to increase their body temperatures.

In fact, people in hot climates traditionally eat spices in order to keep themselves *cool*. This effect occurs because spices first stimulate blood circulation, which induces heightened perspiration, allowing for a greater release of body heat through the surface of the skin.

Spices tend to have a *cooling and drying* effect on the body.

There are three categories of spicy foods, and as with other foods, variances in temperaments exist among them. There are the *seed spices,* which include black and white pepper, cumin, cayenne, and mustard; the *leafy spices,* which include watercress, chives, scallions, basil, and arugula; and the *root spices,* or underground spices, which include radish, ginger, garlic, and onion.

Many of the leafy and root categories can be prepared as vegetables, while those of the seed category tend to be used only as seasonings for other foods.

The heating and cooling temperaments of any spicy food or seasoning can be determined by two factors: 1) with what other foods the spice is combined and eaten, and 2) the internal reserves (fortitude) or lack of same within the individual choosing to eat it.

The nature of spice is to stimulate and disperse accumulated energy. This causes a release of stagnation in the blood and body. If a person has a hot temperament and a strong inner reserve of energy resulting from an excess consumption of fat and protein, then spices and spicy foods will affect him in one of two ways.

Should this individual drastically reduce his consumption of concentrated foods, the spices will eventually assist in cooling his hot temperament by breaking down his concentration of inner reserve. However, if the person with the hot temperament continues to consume large quantities of fats and animal proteins in addition to using spices, then the hot temperament will not only continue to remain hot, it can become even hotter. Spices stimulate the stored reserves of heat-producing foods (meats, eggs, cheese, and so on), thus increasing body temperature.

In other words, it is not the spice per se that heats the person. It is the stimulating action of the spice on the concentrated foods or the individual's stored reserves that makes the spice appear to be heating. The simulating action of spice on dense or concentrated foods also helps to balance these foods by assisting in the breakdown of the food and the regulation of metabolic functions.

An individual with little inner reserve, with a cold temperament, or one who is very depleted, thin, and weak may experience a temporary warming effect from spice, due to its stimulating properties. However, the effect will quickly change to one of greater cooling if the person does not include more substantial, nutrient-dense foods in combination with the spice.

If people with cold temperaments choose to eat spices with the intention of increasing their body warmth, they also must increase their protein and fat consumption (richer, more dense foods) in order to produce the desired effect.

The quantity of spice one eats and the regularity of use is best determined by what one has eaten in the past and what one is presently eating.

Pepper

Pepper (*Piper nigrum*) has historically been the most important and most widely used spice in the world, and still is today. In the United States, we use more pepper than all other seasonings put together. It is, without a doubt, the "king of spices." It is native to southwest India and bears no relationship whatsoever to the nightshade family of capsicum peppers.

Pepper grows on vines that thrive in tropical climates. The vines, complete with tendrils, will cling to any tree that may be convenient to them. Once attached to the needed support of a tree, pepper vines grow an average of fifteen feet; they have been known to climb up to thirty feet. Each vine contains hundreds of flower spikes, and each one of the spikes will produce a cluster of about fifty peppercorns.

The optimum growth requirements for pepper are found close to the equator. However, environments with high temperatures, long rainy seasons, and partial shade will encourage pepper vines. Pepper vines begin to bear fruit after two to five years, and will continue to bear fruit for forty years or more.

Black and white peppers are the same species. The small fruit, called peppercorns, are green when full grown. As they begin to ripen, they turn a yellowish-red color. Black pepper comes from peppercorns picked when ripe, then sun-dried until they turn black. White pepper comes from ripened peppercorns that are soaked in water to loosen the skins; the skins are then rubbed off and the peppercorns are dried. White pepper can have a stronger flavor than black pepper; however, this can vary, depending on the type of pepper and where it is grown.

Pepper has a strong dispersing nature; when added to hearty food preparations and animal foods, it can induce a deep, sensuous feeling of warmth. When added to lighter fare, it stimulates the blood and produces a deep cooling and dry effect. It has a strong ability to disperse deep internal heat in the body and, because it is a climbing vine, it tends to disperse heat centrifugally. Because it is a seed, it also disperses heat rapidly. Seed spices tend to have a more explosive release of energy than leaf or root spices.

In ancient times, pepper was used to slow down spoilage of other foods by inhibiting microbial growth. It also has powerful antifungal properties and can be helpful for those with unhealthy bacteria in their digestive systems. It can also be beneficial for upset stomachs due to food poisoning and stagnant blood due to inactivity. If stored properly, in a cool, dry environment, pepper can keep for up to one hundred years.

Mustard

After pepper, mustard is the second most important and widely used seasoning in the world. It is native to Eurasia and belongs to the cruciferous family of plants, a family that includes radish, cabbage, turnip, mustard greens, and cress. This family includes approximately two thousand species, none of which are poisonous.

Mustard was cultivated in many areas of Europe during the Stone Age. It is a highly productive plant, so much so that the ancient Indians regarded it as a symbol of fertility.

Not only was mustard traditionally regarded as an important table condiment, it was also used as both an external and internal medicine by the Romans and Greeks. Internally, it was used to relieve toothaches, and externally, it was ground to make mustard plasters, a remedy applied directly to the body for the relief of aches and pains as well as inflammation in deep tissue. Mustard also is an age-old remedy used in footbaths to relieve tired and aching feet.

A unique quality of the mustard seed is that it contains a good amount of oil, up to 35 percent. This oil is used widely as a seasoning in much of Asia, particularly to flavor meat and fish dishes. Although the mustard seed is high in oil, the seed is very dry and the distinctly pungent flavor of mustard is not released until the seed is broken and wetted. When moistened, a chemical reaction takes place between an enzyme and a glucoside in the mustard seed, producing spicy oil.

The two most common types of mustard are black mustard and white mustard. Both are often used together, and both plants contain edible leaves that make fine additions to salads and soups.

Like pepper, mustard is a natural preservative and can retard the growth of bacteria in certain foods. It also has an emulsifying effect on fats through the action of binding and thickening.

Unlike pepper, which releases deep internal heat, mustard has a more surface level or peripheral cooling effect on the body. It stimulates the skin and superficial blood flow, especially around the reproductive organs. When eaten with oily or fatty foods, it can assist in the storage of internal heat, yet when eaten with lighter fare (salads), it tends to have a dispersing, cool and dry effect. Mustard is especially effective in dissolving excess mucus and helping to rid the body of common cold symptoms. It is also well known as an appetite stimulant.

Ginger

Though native to tropical Asia, ginger has also spread to many other tropical areas of the world. Records show cultivation in China as early as the sixth century BC. An underground stem often thought to be a root, ginger is actually a rhizome (like the potato), producing new stems and roots from the mother stem. Ginger is a deciduous perennial plant that needs long, warm, humid summers to grow.

One of the most important ingredients in Asian cooking, this knobby fibrous "root" adds a moist pungency to a variety of animal and vegetable preparations. It is also used as a spice in baking throughout much of Europe.

The medicinal use of ginger has a long history in Asia, where it was used either alone or in combination with other herbaceous plants to treat a wide variety of illnesses.

Ginger grows underground in an irregular pattern. Unlike most other root plants, it grows horizontally outward rather than vertically downward. Its pungent, dispersing quality primarily affects the middle organs, the pancreas, spleen, liver, and gallbladder. It has a tendency to create hot conditions by causing an influx of peripheral blood flow into the organs. In addition to producing heat, it stimulates the production of bile and pancreatic and other digestive enzymes.

Like other spicy seasonings, the effects of ginger can be determined by what it is combined with and the condition of the individual using it. Even though it is of tropical origin, ginger, more than any other spicy seasoning, has the strongest ability to produce heat in the body—heat derived through stimulation of stored reserves in the middle organs. It has long been considered helpful in ridding the body of toxins and is well known as a remedy for vomiting, coughing, abdominal distension, and fever. In Africa, a tea made from ginger root is used as an aphrodisiac.

Horseradish

Horseradish is a cylindrical taproot that is a member of the cruciferous family of plants. Its origins are vague, yet some historians believe it originated in or near Germany, which historically is the area where it has been most widely used. Many consider it the most pungent of all the cultivated edible roots.

Horseradish tends to grow vertically downward, with many small branching roots extending from the main root. Some horseradish roots have been known to grow as large as a human infant.

While it is used in many of the same ways that ginger is used, it is also used either straight or with added salt and vinegar as a table condiment for hearty meat preparations. Its downward growth is indicative of how it primarily affects the organs of the lower body—the intestines, bladder, and reproductive organs. Historically it has been known for its many healing and cleansing properties relative to the digestive system, where it is helpful in ridding the body of accumulated wastes and stimulating intestinal peristalsis.

Cinnamon

True cinnamon is native to Ceylon (Sri Lanka). It grows as a bark on a tree that can reach heights of up to sixty feet. Another cinnamon, properly called *cassia,* which is more highly scented and has a dark reddish brown color, is the plant most widely used as cinnamon in the United States and Europe.

True cinnamon is tan colored, more slender, and has a milder flavor than cassia. Cultivated cinnamon comes from a dense bushy plant that does not reach its natural height, but grows only to about seven feet in height.

The first-known reference to cinnamon is in a Chinese treatise on plants from about 2700 BC; however; there is evidence of its use in Egypt several hundred years earlier.

Both genuine cinnamon and cassia consist of the inner bark peeled from the tree's inner shoots during the rainy season. Once dried, the bark rolls up into quills. These brown spiral whorls are warm and spicy to taste and emit a pleasant and soothing odor.

Energetically, cinnamon tends to have a warm and dry effect on the body. It tends to focus its energetics on the kidneys, bladder, and spleen. When used in cooking, it contributes slow, smooth, and calming warmth to the body. It is especially beneficial for those suffering from stagnant cold conditions.

Vanilla

The vanilla plant is an orchid native to Central America, more specifically to southeastern Mexico. It is the world's most popular flavor and is now grown in a number of tropical countries with high rainfall, including Madagascar, the world's largest producer. There are three grades or qualities of vanilla, and Mexico produces the best, exporting about one hundred thousand pounds annually to the United States.

A climbing vine that attaches itself to the sides of trees, the vanilla plant is capable of reaching a length of 350 feet. The vanilla orchid is a species of the decorative orchid flowers commonly used to make corsages. A vanilla pod in its natural state is virtually odorless until it goes through a process of fermentation. During this process it sweats for hours and begins to release its familiar odor and distinctly pleasing flavor. Vanilla is used in many parts of the world to make perfume.

The fruit of the vanilla plant consists of a long thin pod between four and twelve inches long, filled with a multitude of tiny black seeds imbedded in a sticky liquid. The pods are picked when ripe, yet not if fully ripened because the pods will split open by themselves and dry out. The harvesting of vanilla pods is therefore a bit of an ordeal: each one must be picked individually at precisely the right time.

The vanilla plant is hermaphroditic, that is, it contains both the male and female organs of generation; yet it cannot pollinate itself. A tonguelike protrusion between the anther and stigma of the pod is set up in such a way as to permit only one insect (the *melipona* bee) or one small breed of hummingbird to extract and later deposit the pollen. Man now does artificial cross-pollination—and it is not an easy task. It is a delicate operation that must be done by hand. This is one reason vanilla is so expensive.

The word *vanilla* is a diminutive of the Spanish word *vaina,* meaning "sheath" or "pod." *Vaina,* in turn, comes from the Latin *vagina,* for "sheath." Apparently, the shape of the vanilla bean suggested this name and at the same time inspired vanilla's reputation as having aphrodisiac qualities.

The sweet and mildly aromatic qualities of vanilla give it energetic properties of being slightly warm and damp. It has a sultry, sensuous quality and tends to slowly relax and soften the reproductive organs, thus causing a slow and gradual filling of the blood vessels.

Vinegars

Vin aigre is French for "sour wine," and that is actually what vinegar is, or at least what it starts out being. The making of vinegar is an ancient process that goes back before the days of the Old Testament. Historically, vinegars have been used to season both raw and cooked vegetables, as a marinade for meats, for pickling, and in some parts of the world, as a folk remedy for a variety of ills.

We can classify vinegars into two groups, the first being *fruit vinegars* made from fermented fruits (including apples, grapes, berries, and so on), and *grain vinegars,* which are less acidic and tend to be milder in flavor; these latter are made from fermented grains, such as rice, barley, or wheat.

While both grain or fruit vinegars make fine complements to salads of all sorts, one's choice of vinegar is more or less determined by the type of preparation one is using it for. A Chinese stir-fry just doesn't seem right when made with sweet and tart balsamic vinegar. On the other hand, a marinated Italian bean salad just wouldn't be an Italian bean salad without a fruit (balsamic or wine) vinegar of some variety.

Most European styles of cooking lean toward the use of wine or fruit vinegars and most Asian or Oriental cooking styles lean toward the use of grain vinegars. A variety of high-quality vinegars certainly deserve a space in any creative chef's kitchen.

Vinegars of all types are sour with varying degrees of acidity and sweetness. Energetically, they create a cool and dry effect in the body. They are astringent and have the tendency to empty full and hot conditions. The effect on body tissue can be likened to a wet sponge being squeezed dry.

Being fermented, vinegars affect rising blood flow in the body, particularly in the liver, where large quantities of blood are stored in order to rise to the heart for circulation. For people with empty conditions, those who are cold, thin, and weak, the excessive use of vinegar can contribute to wrinkled skin, depletion of energy, and weakened muscle tone. For people with hot and full temperaments, vinegar can have an all-around cleansing and soothing effect.

Olives

Although olives are in a sense pickles, for many they are much more, and thus they deserve a separate mention. They are indeed a food of great historical significance, and one that has played a vital role in shaping the character of Mediterranean, Middle Eastern, and other peoples, gracing many of their poetic legends and myths. They also are a food of great importance to the West, since Mediterranean cuisine, more than any other, once represented the heart of Western civilization.

The cultivation and processing of olives for food and oil goes as far back as the fourth millennium BC with roots in Syria and Palestine. The versatility of the olive made it indispensable to the ancient world. Not only was it an important food, its oil was also used as a base for soaps, perfumes, and medicines.

The olive tree possesses a unique personality and has become known as the most deeply loved of all trees. It has been said that the olive tree can live for centuries, some even beyond two thousand years; however, botanists claim that the average life span of an olive tree is anywhere from three hundred to six hundred years. In the beginning, the tree is slow to bear fruit, and if cut down it will sprout new branches. Olive trees possess deep, penetrating taproots, do not tolerate shade, thrive in full sunlight, and have an uncanny ability to rid themselves of excess water and moisture.

This civilized tree with its vital fruit has long been a symbol of peace, as exemplified in one of the most commonly read stories in the Bible. When Noah sent a dove from the ark to see if the flood had subsided, the dove first returned empty-handed. On the second try, the dove eventually returned with an olive branch, a symbol of peace that announced the endurance and constancy of trees and the hope of peace through the rebirth of civilization. The olive tree and its fruit have long been associated with revitalization, regeneration, wisdom, continuity, longevity, and even immortality.

Green olives are unripe, while black olives are ripe. There are numerous varieties, some having a rich, tart flavor and others having a combination of sour and bitter flavors. Whatever the flavor, they are a fresh, cleansing, and sensual food. Depending on the type, they can have a cooling and dry effect or a cooling and damp effect on the body. Olives and olive oil can be beneficial for congested lymphatic conditions and lung congestion, and are soothing to the stomach.

Olives are a sophisticated, civilized, and respectable food, one of the few foods that have always been able to bridge the gap between the most decadent of the rich and the poorest of poor. One of the world's original pickles, the olive is a healthy digestive aid to any meal.

Salt

Salt is the most assertive and dominant seasoning of all. It is this basic substance, sodium chloride, that makes plant and animal food coherent for human digestion and assimilation.

An essential dietary element in one form or another, salt is the ultimate catalyst of transmutation and biological transformation. Some Native Americans did not use it, and neither do Eskimos—but that does not mean they did not and do not *get* it in their food.

The Romans considered salt a valuable commodity: the word *salary* comes from the Roman word for salt. One who was deemed not "worth his salt" was worth not much indeed. History abounds with such references to the inherent value of this quintessential mineral and to its pivotal role in shaping our physiology and human destiny as the "salt of the Earth."

Salt brings out the flavor of food by penetrating it. No other seasoning has the penetrating power that salt does. It has the power to draw out flavor as well as lock it in. It can create the coldest of cold conditions or it can contribute to the hottest of hot conditions.

However, salt is capable of doing little in and of itself. Salt is a team player—indeed, it *needs* a team (consisting of fat, protein, and cardohydrates) in order to accomplish anything. Too much salt, and the team becomes overly aggressive and arrogant. Too little salt, and the team becomes confused, lost, and lacking in endurance and focus. It is the only ingredient in the world of food and cooking that can fit in and play with any food and any preparation—yet it cannot be consumed by itself.

How much? Only you know for sure. "Take it with a grain of salt"— but take it, and preferably with a grain of high-quality sea salt!

Other Essential and Supportive Supplements

While condiments and seasonings are essential to any healthy diet, additional supplementation with high-quality food-grade supplements can help to replace the need for stimulants, drugs, and junk food including "natural junk foods." They can also provide supportive nutrition to the declining quality of your daily foods.

When choosing your type of supplementation, it is important to have your macronutrition in order first. In other words, consider how well balanced your daily consumption of carbohydrates, proteins, fats, and minerals is before choosing supplements. Well-balanced diets will require less supplementation—and no supplementation can replace the essential nutrition found in healthy foods.

Minerals
In sea salt, Na (sodium) and K (potassium) are the two *cations* (positively charged ions) that seek balance and regulate water economy in the body. Other forms of mineral supplementation may include calcium and magnesium. However, remember that minerals need fats to help them metabolize properly, and fats need proteins to help them metabolize, and proteins . . .

Many of our foods today are mineral deficient, so first seek foods high in minerals, such as sea vegetables and wild plants. The body can tolerate a vitamin deficiency more readily than a mineral deficiency.

Herbs and Spices

We have already discussed a few herbs and spices, but it is important to add them to your diet, even if you are not used to them.

Many herbs and spices have powerful healing qualities. For example, leaf cilantro (also called *coriander* when in seed form) has been shown to help release heavy metals such as mercury from the body; it is also helpful in clearing infections and viruses.

Enzymes

There are three basic types of enzymes:

- Metabolic: present in every cell, tissue, and organ; responsible for maintaining body system balance
- Digestive: the body secretes these from the salivary glands as well as in the stomach and pancreas to help digest macronutrients
- Food enzymes: found naturally in fresh raw foods and fermented foods; a supplement of plant-based food enzymes can be helpful to aid in digestion

Superfoods

Many superfoods are *biomodulators*. Biomodulators are substances that affect many functions and systems of the body in a synergistic manner. They can help to restore, maintain, and optimize normal body functions.

Some of these superfoods transcend boundaries, while others have more specific functions.

Blue-green algae, chlorella, wheat grass, bee pollen, maitake mushroom, reishi mushroom, cordyceps mushroom, and *mangosteen fruit* are just a few of many superfoods that are not vitamin supplements but can be used in a similar way, in small quantities, to naturally enhance nutrition. Some have natural medicinal qualities, while others have a combination of high nutritional components with additional medicinal qualities.

For example, *bee propolis* is a resinous substance collected by bees from the leaf, bud, or bark of a tree. It is used as an adhesive for structuring their hives. Because this resin represents the lifeblood of the tree, carrying protection to every part of the tree, ancient Egyptians regarded it as a source of eternal health and life. Today we know it as a natural antibiotic with many health benefits.

Royal jelly is another ancient superfood involving bees—in this case, not simply collected by bees, but actually produced by them. Royal jelly is secreted from glands of young female bees and is the only food used to nourish the queen bee—and while other bees have life spans of six to eight weeks, the queen lives on average five to eight *years*. The queen is also significantly stronger and larger than the other bees.

Many superfoods have ancient origins and long traditions behind them and can be very supportive to good health.

Sweeteners

Other supplemental foods to use in small quantities include various natural sweeteners. Honey is pehaps the most ancient sweetener used in human diets. Other healthy sweeteners that may be used in moderation with a healthy diet include: raw honey, agave syrup, rice or barley malt syrup, raw cane sugar, maple syrup, and fruits.

Fats and Oils: Misunderstood, Mistreated, and Misrepresented

Fats of all types consist of three basic elements: carbon, hydrogen, and oxygen. They are concentrated forms of energy with strong thermogenic properties. Fats can be considered building foods, especially those fats containing a greater quantity of saturated fats. Most polyunsaturated fats are liquid; fats with more saturated fatty acids tend to be solid at room temperature. Fats with ample amounts of saturated fats are those derived from animal meats, dairy products, and some tropical plants, including palm oil, palm kernel oil, and coconut oil.

Olive, sesame, walnut, almond, hazelnut, soy, safflower, sunflower, and canola are examples of plant oils high in polyunsaturated and monounsaturated fatty acids, yet not all of these are suitable for human consumption. Almond oil has such a fine viscosity that it has actually been used to lubricate the detailed mechanisms of watches.

Whether unsaturated or saturated, fat in some form is an essential ingredient to human metabolism. Fat is essential to metabolic integrity and is required by the body for helping in the assimilation of the fat-soluble vitamins A, D, K, and E. The essential fatty acids found in some fats are also necessary to hormone synthesis and are important for maintaining the membranes that surround each cell. Fat also forms a protective layer around nerve tissue that helps to insulate nerves from shock. This is why people deficient in fat are often irritable and unable to withstand strong environmental stimuli.

How you digest and process fat in your body depends on your individual metabolism. How you metabolize fats, in turn, is largely dependent on your consumption and absorption of essential vitamins, minerals, and protein, along with the quality of fats you choose to eat or not eat. As a macronutrient, fat is both dependent on and essential to the digestion and assimilation of carbohydrates, proteins, vitamins, and minerals.

The Saturation Point

No diet will remove all the fat from your body because the brain is entirely fat. Without a brain, you might look good, but all you could do is run for public office.

GEORGE BERNARD SHAW

Contrary to prevailing popular thought, saturated animal fats are not necessarily "bad" for people. Consumption of excessive hydrogenated (artificially solidified) saturated fat has been linked with numerous health disorders. However, while the *excessive* consumption of saturated fat (as with anything in excess) can be unhealthy, for many people the *total elimination* of saturated fats can contribute to even more serious problems than they had in the first place.

For individuals eating a diet based on vitamin- and mineral-rich whole foods with little or no animal foods, fats can be one of the most challenging and difficult foods with which to establish a balanced relationship. It is unwise and even dangerous to eliminate all types of fat from one's diet, even if one has overconsumed fats in the past.

Fats dissolve in fat—not in water. Fats will also dissolve in alcohol, and the high trans fat intake of many Americans—about 30 to 40 percent of average diets—may be a strong yet still undiscovered link in alcohol abuse. The drastic reduction of fats from your diet can contribute to both a hardening of previously accumulated trans fats and intense cravings for additional fats.

Linolenic acid, found in high-quality palm and coconut oils, is said by some researchers to actually help discharge aggregated deposits of saturated fats and cholesterol in body tissue. Research has shown that fat consumption of less than 5 percent of total caloric intake inhibits the absorption of the fat-soluble vitamins A, D, E, and K, and can lead to nutritional deficiency.

Research has shown that polyunsaturated plant oils should not be heated or used for frying, because the oils react to heat and thus produce *free radicals.* Free radicals are the result of oxidation that occurs when oils are subjected to high temperatures (hence the value of antioxidants in that they can help to prevent this damage), and they can in turn cause destructive chain reactions in the oil molecules. An excess of free radicals can lead to tissue degeneration, early aging, hardening of the arteries, and cancer.

It is true that the production of free radicals is an important and normal biochemical function of the human body. It is only when free-radical production gets *out of control* that they become harmful.

The real danger lies in the types of fats and oils used for cooking. All food molecules change when they are cooked; fat is not the only food that is subject to producing adverse chain reactions in molecules. An individual eating a diet low in vitamins and minerals and high in processed dairy products, meats, and other processed foods stands a good chance of developing problems from heated oils and the free radicals produced from them, because of the diet he or she is eating. Heated oils, if they are high-quality, heat-stable, organic oils, are not the cause of these problems. Rather, it is a toxic diet combined with poor-quality fats that results in the excessive accumulation of free radicals, which may then adhere to cell membranes already sticky with excess refined polyunsaturated fats, hydrogenated fats, chemicals, and fake foods.

For thousands of years our ancestors ate both unsaturated and saturated fat and were relatively free of these problems. However, diets high in *never-before-eaten polyunsaturated* oils, *processed* saturated fats, and *processed* foods is a relatively recent phenomena.

It is well worth noting that Tannenbaum, the man who did the original work on dietary fat and cancer nearly forty years ago, in fact, *did not use animal fat* in his experiments—he used hydrogenated and processed cottonseed oil and soybean oil. His experiments did show severe hardening of the arteries—and this shoddy research led to oil industry propaganda that all forms of saturated fat are created equal and thus dangerous.

Animal Fat or Vegetable Fat?

Another interesting piece of perspective here is that animal fat consumption has not increased in the last sixty years, during which we have seen the incidence of coronary artery disease climb so drastically—but the consumption of processed polyunsaturated and saturated fats (margarine, soy, canola, safflower, cottonseed oil, and pasteurized and homogenized dairy products) *has*. There is indeed an international epidemic of heart attacks, hardening of the arteries, and all the other problems associated with "saturated fat"—but its dietary causes are not what the popular press has led us to believe they are.

Moreover, dietary cholesterol overall has only increased by about *1 percent* in the last eighty years. It's funny how our nation quickly becomes a nation of believers when the "experts" claim a statement of truth. There is an issue concerning *quality* here that I don't expect large oil companies with profit-only concerns to address, but you and I had better address it, and we need to do it now!

From an energetic perspective, the oil in a plant seed serves as an energy reserve and a catalyst that the seed uses to become a seedling. Just as the eggs of animals store fat as energy to develop into full-grown animals, so too do the seeds of plants need enough stored reserve energy to become full-grown plants. It is the oil contained in the seed that nourishes this unfolding metabolic process of growth and development. Likewise, the quality of fat or oil you choose to eat will affect your metabolism and your process of growth and development, on many levels.

Hydrogenated and partially hydrogenated plant and animal fats will accumulate, harden body tissue, slow metabolism, and make you fat. These types of fats also contribute to low tissue oxygenation, and this interferes with your cells' ability to use oxygen to the point where cellular membranes become defective and cells become weakened and disorganized. This can further lead to depression, neurosis, and finally degenerative disease.

On the other hand, nonhydrogenated, naturally occurring organic plant oils and animal fats do not produce the effects of the trans fat group of fats and some of the polyunsaturated fats. Rather, these fats and oils assist metabolic functions by contributing to the flexibility and permeability of your cells. They also contribute to physical and mental flexibility, and they do not make you fat.

Simply put, the best sources of animal fats include fat from all animals used traditionally for food, such as butter, ghee (clarified butter), chicken, cow, pig, lamb, goose, duck, and so forth.

The best and most healthy sources of plant-based oils for daily food preparations include coconut, palm, palm kernel, olive, hazelnut, and sesame oils. Although olive, hazelnut, and sesame oils cannot withstand the higher temperatures that the others can, they are still traditionally used oils and are beneficial to health. Small amounts of some raw, high-quality seed and nut oils for marinades and dressings are also fine to use. Oils to avoid include (but are not limited to) flax, soy, corn, sunflower, canola, and safflower.

Each type of oil has unique qualities. For example, sesame oil, when used exclusively, will tend to contribute to dry skin, especially if used for frying, sautéing, or baking. Sesame oil traditionally was used in Asian and Middle Eastern cooking more as a seasoning and added after, or near the end of, sautéed vegetables. Sesame has a dry and cool effect.

Olive oil may well be one the most digestible and healthiest monounsaturated oils because of its high levels of monounsaturated fats. It certainly has a history of varied uses, including as an external lubricator for beautifying and toning the skin, and as a lamp oil that supplied illumination for the ancient Greeks, Egyptians, Romans, and others.

Like other quality oils and possibly more so, olive oil has the vital properties of penetratiing, softening, strengthening, and nourishing. Incorporated into human cells, olive oil has proven to increase their stability and protect them from free radicals already present in the body. Traditional peoples throughout the Mediterranean region believe olive oil keeps the cells alive longer and thus retards the aging process. Walnut and almond oils are also easy to digest but are best eaten raw, as the high polyunsaturated fat content makes them more susceptible to oxidation and they are unable to withstand heat.

Some plant oils can withstand higher temperatures than others. Those with low saturated fat content do not like light or warm places, and they therefore should be stored in a cool, dark place.

Quality plant oils, when used for cooking, generally have a warm and damp effect on the body. Cooked oil also helps to build a metabolic foundation from which one can better absorb and assimilate protein, carbohydrates, vitamins, and minerals. When plant oils are used raw, as in salads, marinated vegetables, and pickles, they have a cool and damp effect on the body.

Cooked oils have a sinking nature that tends to affect the middle and lower organs of the body. Raw oil has a rising nature that tends to affect the middle and upper organs of the body.

Animal fats tend to have a warm and damp effect on the body, more so than plant oils. Many plant foods contain fat; the amount of fat contained in a particular food is precisely enough to balance that food's other components. However, a meal containing foods with already existing fat (beans, grains, and so on) does not necessarily mean the meal contains enough variety of fat to digest and process the meal. This is why some form of additional animal or plant fat was added to meal preparations throughout the world.

Fats and Oils, Revised:
Awakened from Blind Belief

Back in 1987, when I was preparing the first edition of this book, I was in the midst of a very busy seminar schedule and had not given a great deal of thought to the issue of fats and oils. After all, it was accepted "scientific fact" that saturated fats, including those of animal origin as well as tropical oils—palm, coconut, and palm kernel—were just about the deadliest food products one could eat. Sure, one could eat them—but according to the research, one would face the very serious threat of heart disease and cancer if you did.

At that time, I was more strongly in support of a semi-vegetarian/macrobiotic diet, so the current scientific research on fats happened to fit my own agenda rather well, and therefore, the fats and oils issue for my book was pretty much a done deal. The verdict was in, the science was there to back it and it was clear: saturated fats were bad, unhealthy, and downright dangerous to your health.

Just like everyone else, I bought this agenda-driven science completely. Why did we all buy into this saturated fat myth?

Science, yes, in part: scientific research said it was true, so it must be true. Not only true, but true based on highly credible sources.

Years later, as more information and resources became more readily available (in large part thanks to the Internet and its epic capacity to democratize information), it turns out that the "science" behind the fats-and-oils research for the most part simply does not wash (is not water-soluble!)—and that saturated fat was not the enemy it had been presented as being. Hell, ten years ago I was not aware of the American Soy Association (ASA) propaganda campaign to rid the market of tropical oils like palm and coconut oil.

The idea was to replace tropical saturated fats with inferior polyunsaturated trans-fatty acids in order to help support the vegetable oil's several-billion-dollar industry. The best way to do this was to create a health crisis where there wasn't one. Saturated animal fats and tropical oils equal degenerative disease. Sure, that will work—and in the minds of most people, it did work, and quite convincing it was.

That is, until it backfired—and the new inferior replacement products proved to be the real contributors to the health crisis. It is sad to see that some of the very people we are taught to trust for solid nutritional information, the experts in the field, can be bought by multinational companies with one agenda: to profit, even if it is at the expense of our health.

Let this serve as a lesson for all of us who need it. Had I carefully researched traditional peoples' use of tropical oils, instead of blindly accepting the scientific literature, I would have realized that so many island peoples and other traditional cultures where coconut and palm oils were and are consumed are generally healthy people with great skin and low incidence of heart disease and cancer. After all, these oils, along with traditional animal fats, have a long and strong history, having been used for thousands of years by peoples with very positive results.

By contrast, the scientific methods used to condemn tropical oils and traditional animal fats are in their infancy, a point that speaks volumes when it comes to the energetics of any aspect of food and diet. How a food was eaten and how long a food has been used by indigenous peoples is critically important—and in many ways, far more important than scientific or technical research. Whenever a food has a long history, we can ascertain that its many properties have been well understood—through experience, not theory—by the people consuming it. If a food with any historical relevance did not provide health benefits, then traditional peoples would not have continued to eat it—or if they did, it would show up as having been to their detriment. Tropical oils have long provided tremendous health benefits, and the very same method of scientific inquiry used to originally condemn them can now be used to prove their exceptional health benefits.

As natural product consumers, what many of us need to come to terms with is that there are two general sources of scientifically derived information on nutrition.

The first is the genuine science of linear dissection commonly used to find the answers we all want to know. One example is the old saying that "fish is brain food" and the modern scientific discovery of omega-3 essential fatty acids found in some fish and this substance's benefits to brain tissue. Many positive steps in nutrition have been made through this approach to science and will continue to be made through the sincerity and dedication of its researchers.

The second source of scientific information incorporates the same methodology and is perhaps best termed *agenda-driven science.*

While as convincing as any good science, agenda-driven science is just that, scientific activity driven by a specific agenda. Often the people behind it will spare no expense in enrolling and enlisting the media, scientific journals, the medical profession, case studies, and anything else necessary to pound their square pegs into those round holes.

It is not unusual to find blatant examples of the use of good science to support an agenda to make something unhealthy look healthy. As an example, the omega-3 fatty acids that occur naturally in the tissue of some fish have been given equal status to the omega-3s in flax oil, a decidedly inferior source. While the omega-3 fatty acids from fish have been eaten for millennia, the omega-3 fats found in flax seed oil cannot be credibly compared to the traditional source. Flax oil is a substance that no one has eaten until fairly recently. Does the sheer fact that both sources are high in omega-3 fatty acids automatically mean that these two are equally healthy choices? Nothing could be further from the truth.

Saturated and Unsaturated Fats: Differences

To gain a better understanding of the fat controversy, let us consider some basic science-derived information on the nature of fats.

All fats, whether of plant or animal origin, contain a mixture of saturated, monounsaturated, and polyunsaturated fats. The essential differences between the various fats and oils lie in their proportions of these three basic types of fatty acids, and each has its unique effect in the body owing to its unique proportion of these three basic fats.

- Saturated fats contain the most hydrogen of all fats, and therefore have little room on their molecules for any additional hydrogen atoms. This property gives them a solid consistency at room temperature.

- Monounsaturated fats are missing one pair of hydrogen atoms. Olive oil is the most commonly known monounsaturated fat; it contains omega-9 fatty acids from oleic acid.
- Polyunsaturated fats are missing more than one pair of hydrogen atoms and thus are less stable than either saturated or monounsaturated fats. Polyunsaturated fats can be filled with hydrogen atoms; the result of this process is called trans fats.

While most vegetable oils consist of mostly polyunsaturated fats, there are three common exceptions: olive oil, which is largely composed of oleic acid and is mostly monounsaturated fat; and coconut and palm oils, both of which consist of mostly saturated fats—even more so than beef tallow and lard. Coconut oil is up to 92 percent saturated fat.

Within these three types of fats, there are also three types of fatty acid chains: long, medium, and short. Long-chain fatty acids are found in abundance in polyunsaturated fats, while medium- and short-chain fatty acids are found mostly in saturated fats.

When medium-chain fatty acids are utilized by the body as energy, the efficient burning process does not produce body fat or negative cholesterol. Medium-chain fatty acids also help to break down accumulations of the long-chain fatty acids that have a tendency to accumulate in the body. If more people were aware of this simple fact—that fat dissolves in fat—there would be far less interest in low-fat diets, which can be damaging in the short run, and certainly do not work in the long run.

In today's world, obesity is caused mostly by an excess of trans fats and polyunsaturated fats—in other words, the wrong kinds of fats—and refined carbohydrates, which turn to fat in the body. In order for fat to help dissolve fat for the purposes of weight loss, one simply needs to replace poor-quality fats with the right fats: natural animal fats, coconut oil, and palm oils. Yet we have all been conditioned to believe the opposite.

Long-chain fatty acids from polyunsaturated vegetable oils require special enzymes to pull them through our cells' double membranes, which causes the process of converting fat to energy to be slow and taxing on our enzymes reserves. Polyunsaturated fats also force cholesterol into body tissue, giving the impression that they lower cholesterol—when in fact the whole process is extremely taxing to the system, especially the pancreas, which is overworked by having to secrete a large amount of insulin.

This process is exemplified in the biochemical reactions of popular low-fat diets so prevalent today. For example, low-fat diets are known to lead to nutritional deficiencies, and dieting in general causes a decrease of oxygen to cells, thus slowing metabolism. Fat, especially saturated fat, is essential for regulating metabolism. When the only types of fats being consumed when dieting consist of polyunsaturated fats, the polyunsaturated fatty acids end up replacing the natural saturated fats in cell membranes, causing the cell walls to become weak and inflexible. Blood cholesterol is then driven from the blood into tissue and cells to help them regain structural integrity. This is why polyunsaturated fats *appear* to reduce cholesterol.

Medium-chain fatty acids from saturated fats, on the other hand, easily permeate both cellular membranes without the need for enzymatic support, where they are then sent directly to the liver and converted to energy, resulting in increased metabolism.

Insulin is not involved with medium-chain fatty acid absorption. When our metabolism is increased, our cells function at a higher rate of efficiency. Polyunsaturated fats, with their long-chain fatty acids, slow metabolism and decrease cellular efficiency.

Dr. Mary Enig, one of the foremost experts on lipid research, states in her book *Know Your Fats*: "... the practice of calling animal fats 'saturated' is not only misleading, it is just plain wrong." She then enlightens the reader with examples such as beef fat (which is 54 percent unsaturated), lard (60 percent unsaturated fat) and chicken fat (about 70 percent unsaturated)—all of them *less than half* saturated. Dr. Enig's book is essential study material for every fat-fearing fanatic and for anyone interested in eating a healthy balanced diet.

Trans-Fatty Acids

Most of the fat-causing disease today is the result of trans fats derived from polyunsaturated refined vegetable oils that have been either fully or partially hydrogenated.

Hydrogenation, a process introduced in the 1930s, involves removing the fat-soluble vitamins A and D from plant oils and, under high temperatures, bombarding the oils with hydrogen molecules to force-saturate the fat. The purpose of hydrogenation is to prevent spoilage, and it turns out to be less expensive to produce and market these force-saturated fats than traditional tropical oils and animal fats.

Current evidence linking trans fats to disease is undeniable, while evidence for any adverse effects of unrefined tropical oils and natural animal fats is severely lacking.

Trans fats have different structures from naturally saturated fats. Unlike saturated fats, trans fats are not found naturally in the body. They cannot be recognized as nutritional sources by the human body, nor can the body utilize them in a constructive way. They have been shown to adversely affect the genetic blueprint, leading to degeneration of human tissue. The consumption of trans fats can lead to premature aging, immune depression, and the destruction of white blood cells. Trans fats also cause tissue to lose omega-3s, while interfering with and reducing the conversion rate of omega-3s to the prostaglandins EPA and DHA (prostaglandins are hormonelike substances that help to regulate normal cellular processes). In fact, natural saturated fats are needed to help the conversion process of omega-3 fatty acids.

When cooking with fats, the fat's stability is of utmost importance. A fat's stability is determined by its degree of saturation. This is important because saturated fats and monounsaturated fats are capable of withstanding varying degrees of heat. For cooking purposes, saturated fats are the most stable, and unrefined vegetable oils the least stable.

Stability also has to do with a fat's ability to store at room temperature. Most seed and nut oils are relatively unstable; the most unstable are flax and hemp. Because they are more susceptible to oxidation and rancidity at room temperatures, especially in warm weather, most seed and nut oils should be refrigerated after opening.

The best uses for polyunsaturated oils are in salad dressings, marinades, and other raw preparations. It is best to use the time-tested olive, hazelnut, macadamia nut, and sesame oils for these purposes and for various types of light cooking. The best and most healthy fats for general cooking purposes are coconut oil, palm oil, palm kernel oil, butter, ghee, lard, and other types of animal fats (such as goose, duck, chicken, and pork).

Some Fats to Avoid

Soy, like flax oil and many other vegetable oils, has a very short history as an edible oil—and for very good reason: it is very difficult to extract oil from the soybean. Because of this, modern equipment uses high pressure, chemical solvents, and high heat to do so. This in turn destabilizes the already heat-sensitive polyunsaturated oil.

More than two-thirds of the vegetable oil used in the United States today is soy oil, and most of that is hydrogenated with trans fats. It has been estimated that about two-thirds of the fat that clogs the arteries, causing arterial plaque and giving rise to heart disease, is from unsaturated vegetable fats (polyunsaturated oils). The reason for this is that saturated fats do not oxidize as easily as polyunsaturated and monounsaturated fats.

Oxidation of vegetable fats occur mostly from processing methods that remove the important fat-soluble vitamins A, D, and E, and also subject the oils to heat, which produces free radicals. It is this type of oxidized fat that tends to end up as artery-clogging plaque and contributes to a host of other health problems as well. Although soy oil is high in EFAs (it is sometimes used as the model against which other sources of EFAs are measured and compared), this does not make it a healthy oil to consume.

How are we supposed to know this, when all the scientific research on the soybean makes it look like nature's perfect food? Many people naturally assume that if the bean is so good, then the oil from the bean should be pretty darn good, too. The truth is, neither the oil *nor* the soybean that produces it offer all those health benefits they are said to possess. And as far as processed soy products go, the only ones fit for human consumption are those processed in the traditional manner of aging and fermentation, such as naturally brewed soy sauce, tempeh, miso, and natto. Even then, it's a good idea to use them sparingly, for this is how they were used traditionally—and certainly not as substitutes for more reliable healthy and balanced sources of protein.

Canola oil is one of Canada's major exports, its largest market being the United States. The oil is produced by gene transfers from the laurel plant, a toxic weed that has been known to cause considerable damage to livestock when used in feed. Originally used as a lubricant, canola oil tends to form a latexlike substance called transisomers that have been shown to cause red blood cells to clump together. Like most of the other oils mentioned in this section, canola depletes vitamin E (an antioxidant) and blocks enzyme function. It has also been shown to contribute to vision and respiratory problems.

Safflower oil is like canola in that when heated, it produces *polymers*, latexlike substances that are damaging to blood cells. Left at room temperature, it becomes sticky; this is why it is so highly valued as a base for paint in India.

Flax was also used for this same purpose (as a base for paint), but never consumed as part of any traditional diet. Flax oil has a history of use in textiles and paints that reaches back thousands of years. This fact of history is often misquoted as meaning that flax oil has been *consumed* for thousands of years. If it were a healthy oil to consume, then it certainly would have been—but it was not, and for very good reasons.

The same is true of safflower oil. The flowers of safflower were used in China to make a tonic tea to treat menstrual problems, pain, and swelling from trauma . . . but otherwise, the oil was nowhere consumed as part of human diets.

Some Healthy Fats and Oils

Olive oil is composed mostly of monounsaturated fat and it contains substances with pharmacological properties. *Oleuropein,* one substance found in olive oil (and in many medicinal plants as well), can stimulate blood flow in the heart, has antispastic properties, and can be helpful in reducing blood pressure. Olive oil is a versatile oil that has been consumed by Middle Eastern and Mediterranean peoples for thousands of years.

Butter, while being about 80 percent saturated fat (the rest being milk solids), is another healthy fat that simply cannot be substituted with margarine or any other modern imitation-butter product.

Ghee, or clarified butter, is 100 percent saturated fat. In India, it has long been recognized as a food that "regenerates life by satisfying internal fire." It was called the "golden fire" for its even consistency of metabolic burning in the body, and was also used externally as a body lotion.

Coconut oil is about 92 percent saturated fat and one of the healthiest—if not the single healthiest—fat one can consume on a regular basis. It is a clean-burning fat that leaves no residue. It is especially supportive to glands and the production of body fluids.

Palm kernel oil is a relative of coconut and is quite similar to it, though from a different species of palm tree. Palm kernel oil is derived from what look like white mini-coconuts.

Palm oil, on the other hand, comes from the husk surrounding the palm seed and is reddish-brown in color, due to its high carotenoid content: natural palm oil is high in vitamins E and A. Refined palm oil, unfortunately, has these antioxidant vitamins removed. In tropical countries, palm oil has a red color; in nontropical countries, it is orange. Both varieties have high levels of the antioxidant vitamin E and only moderate amounts of omega-6s. They also have low levels of polyunsaturated fats, are stable at high temperatures, are resistant to rancidity, and are nature's most abundant source of vitamin A. Palm oils, along with coconut oil, have been used in India, Southern China, and Africa for thousands of years.

These tropical plant oils, high in stable saturated fats, help to keep food fresh while increasing shelf life. They are sometimes called "low-fat fats" and have antiviral and antibacterial properties. They are also called "functional foods" because they provide numerous health benefits beyond their basic nutritional contents.

Unhealthy hydrogenated or partially hydrogenated varieties of these tropical oils are best avoided and should not be confused with healthy unrefined tropical oils.

While polyunsaturated fats are generally best consumed as whole foods in the form of nuts, seeds, and so forth, there are some that have long been used for various preparations throughout history and are healthy oils to use on a regular basis. For example, western Mediterranean countries have long recognized the healthy qualities of olive oil and walnut oil, while other peoples have used hazelnut and sesame oils.

The Importance of Fats in Physiology

Fats, especially saturated and to some degree monounsaturated fats, have important effects on all body tissue, skin, bones, muscles, and organs. The brain is 70 percent fat.

Fats help protect and cushion vital organs from impact and trauma.

Fats are essential for proper nerve functioning; fats insulate nerves by supporting the myelin sheath that surrounds them. Fats' role in nerve regulation can in turn have stabilizing effects both physically and emotionally in conditions of increased stress.

Fats supply healthy cholesterol to cells that help them to form properly. It also determines the flexibility and permeability of cells. Cholesterol is a fundamental element in all cells and plays an extremely important role in metabolic functions. Minus water content, about half of our adrenal glands are pure cholesterol, while 10 to 20 percent of the brain is made up of cholesterol.

Our bodies also need cholesterol to produce sex and stress hormones and vitamin D. The nervous system and immune system are also dependent on cholesterol. There are two types of cholesterol, often referred to as "good cholesterol" or HDL and "bad cholesterol" or LDL. Many people panic at the mere word *cholesterol,* but it is important to recognize the essential role that good cholesterol plays in health.

Fats help to regulate hormones and glandular function. Without an adequate amount of fat in the diet, vital organs suffer and hormone problems become prevalent.

Fats help to balance and regulate the absorption and assimilation of other macronutrients and micronutrients, including the fat-soluble vitamins A, D, K, E and carotenoids. Having less than 5 percent saturated fat in one's diet inhibits absorption of these vital nutrients.

Fat is the primary energy source for the heart and kidneys. It is essential for healthy skin and the regulation of metabolism that helps to control blood sugar and curb eating disorders.

36
Algae

Algae are nonflowering water plants, unique in the world of food for a variety of reasons. Algae occur in numerous varieties, forms, and sizes. Out of the approximately eighteen thousand varieties of algae, most are *marine algae.*

Marine algae, commonly called *seaweeds* or *sea vegetables,* are saltwater algae. Unlike flowering land plants, marine algae do not have roots, leaves, flowers, or stems; however, their basic structure does closely resemble that of flowering land plants.

The structural delineations of sea vegetables consist of: *holdfasts,* rather than roots; *stipes,* instead of stems; *fronds,* in place of leaves; and *spores,* instead of seeds. The holdfast, for example, closely resembles the root system of land plants, but serves an entirely different purpose: its primary function is to anchor the plant. It does not absorb water and nutrition the way the roots of land plants do.

Unlike land plants with roots, leaves, and stems, where each section plays an individual role in the life cycle of the plant, every cell in the entire algae organism takes on all the roles required of the individual sections of land plants. Each part of an algae organism performs the same function every other part does.

In many ways, sea vegetables are like photonegatives of land plants. They are constantly in motion, flexibly swaying with the rhythms of the sea, whereas land plants have a stiff, rooted structure with little movement except under strong prevailing winds. Unlike many depleted and unproductive land masses, where plants may suffer from drought or crop failure, virtually all of the sea is rich in minerals: a lush, uncultivated garden capable of growing a thriving population of sea vegetables. (However, our oceans too are becoming increasingly polluted due to oil spills, medical waste, toxic agricultural and industrial runoff, and numerous other human causes.)

In hot tropical climates where the sea has warmer temperatures, sea vegetables tend to be smaller and less plentiful. This again stands in contrast to land plants, which are more abundant and larger in size in tropical climates. Colder waters contain larger, longer, more rapidly growing, and more abundant sea plants, whereas land plants from colder climates tend to be smaller and less abundant.

The reproductive process of marine algae is either asexual, wherein algae can regenerate from any part of its structure through cell division (*mitosis*), or sexual (allowing them to reproduce sexually through the emission of spores). Photosynthesis occurs in algae just as it does in the leaves of land plants—except that with algae it occurs throughout the whole plant. It is during photosynthesis that algae release large quantities of oxygen into the surrounding waters, thus supporting the life cycles of other marine creatures.

These ancient plants (if one can really call them plants) basically consist of a stem with a variety of fronds that absorb light and nutrients from the sea and give off abundant oxygen.

Of the four basic types of marine algae—brown, red, green, and blue-green—light of different colors and intensities are absorbed in varying degrees, depending primarily on the depth in which the algae grows. The phyla of algae is uniquely high in chlorophyll, and their ability to literally eat light is what determines their color makeup. The green and blue-green varieties absorb more light of longer waves, while the browns and reds absorb light more in the form of shorter waves.

Their high chlorophyll and mineral content are two of the primary reasons for algae being powerful life-enhancing foods. Algae also contain natural antibacterial, antifungal, and antiviral ingredients. Most of the brown varieties of algae contain *alginic acids* and a substance called *fucoidan* in large amounts; both of these are natural immune defenses

that help to protect algae from bacteria and fungi. Fucoidan has also ·
been shown to be effective in retarding the growth of cancer in laboratory experiments.

Marine algae also contain a sodium compound called *sodium alginate*
(though they are actually quite low in sodium chloride). Sodium alginate's
claim to fame is that it binds to and allows us to eliminate the radioactive
elements that find their way into our twenty-first-century bodies.

Seaweeds are also generous with their prodigious regenerative powers. They are a rich source of organic compost material for farmers;
research on marine algae has shown that when liquid seaweed extract
or dried seaweed is added to the land used for growing vegetables, the
planted vegetable seeds reveal an increase in speed of germination and
increased respiratory activities. In the classic O'Flaherty documentary
Man of Aran (one of cinema's earliest masterpieces), Irish settlers are
shown transforming barren, rocky seaside cliffs into fertile soil, solely
through applications of seaweed compost. If marine algae can do all this
in the soil, imagine what they can do for your interior!

Sea vegetables do not grow well in polluted waters—an interesting
point, when you consider their ability to strongly influence the fluid
and mineral balance (osmosis) both inside and outside the body cells.
Algae contain large amounts of all the vital minerals and trace elements
needed for the maintenance and important functions of the nervous
system and immune system. These vital water plants have proven themselves many times over in terms of their ability to assist the body in the
elimination of toxic wastes of many kinds.

Developing a close relationship with marine algae can be both
invigorating and at times trying and difficult, but there is no question
about it: any human being would benefit greatly by establishing a physiological bonding with algae on a regular basis. Energetically, algae have
incredible regenerative powers and buoyant characters—just a few of
the wonderful gifts available to us from these ancient organisms.

Preparing Marine Algae

Most marine algae are purchased in dry form. Many can be baked and ground into a powder for use as a condiment. When used as one would use vegetables, marine algae are first reconstituted by soaking in water, where they increase in size and actually come back to life. At this point, if it were placed in its original environment this single-celled organism could continue to reproduce. If left to soak, it simply continues to circulate water and the ingredients it has released into the water through its simple structure.

The tougher brown algae, particularly hiziki, arame, and sea palm, when soaked, release a blackish-brown tanninlike substance that turns the soaking water brown. The soaking liquid may also contain other toxic substances that may not be conducive to health, so it is best to discard the soaking water before using the sea vegetable. These particular sea vegetables generally require a longer soaking time than most others, and discarding the soaking water along with a thorough rinsing of the hiziki, arame, or sea palm before preparation not only helps to eliminate potentially toxic substances, it also renders the sea vegetables more palatable, thus making this unique food accessible to more people who otherwise would not or could not eat them. I have yet to encounter any evidence showing a reduction of nutrition in sea vegetables caused by soaking and rinsing thoroughly.

Another way to turn seaweed cooking from an unappetizing obligation into a wholly satisfying experience is to use *oil* in their cooking. These same tougher seaweeds also manufacture large amounts of the oil-soluble vitamins A and D, and preparation with a high-quality stable oil, which has been the rule of thumb in many of the world's seaweed cuisine traditions, greatly assists in their digestion, thus ensuring that you receive the maximum benefits of absorption.

Aside from vitamin absorption, I also suspect that a much wider spectrum of the algae's minerals are also made more available to the modern, weakened intestinal tract when the foods are cooked with some oil. Likewise, experience suggests that other seasonings can greatly assist your absorption of the seaweed's essential treasures. Grain vinegars, *mirin* (a rice-based cooking wine), sea salt, shoyu, umeboshi vinegar, and spices all play a role in making seaweeds both delicious and more physiologically useful.

Regarding the use of sea salt (or shoyu, umeboshi, etc.), it is important to note that while marine algae live within a salty environment, they (like ocean fish) actually absorb very little of that salt. Algae cells maintain an osmotic balance with their environment, keeping potassium ions within the cell and sodium ions out. So don't hesitate to add salt seasonings to seaweed dishes, remembering that consuming too little salt is as unpalatable as using too much!

The Benefits of Eating Marine Algae

Once ingested, algae begin to go to work like a janitor, cleaning, purifying, and strengthening the internal environment. Lighter, more free-floating waste materials are detoxified and easily discharged, but those dirty, stubborn, and deeply stored old toxins and trans fats: the algae works away at scrubbing and washing them out too, and eventually, through regular use and time, they finally let go and are eliminated.

Now, a few things happen during the cleansing process of internal toxic waste by algae.

Bodies starving for minerals and trace elements (which means more or less all of us) begin to feel renewed and vitalized. Many of us also have additional bacterial and yeast populations thriving either in the bowel or throughout the system. It is here that the algae will often upset the status quo. Where the more peripheral and lighter toxins are eliminated through the normal discharge channels of the bowels and urinary tract, the deeper, longtime storehouse of wastes often put up resistant barriers in the form of headaches, nausea, taste repulsion, and other adjustment symptoms.

Some energetic characteristics shared by all marine algae include adaptability, regenerative power, flexibility, ancient and primitive memory restoration, physiologically and psychologically cooling (preparation not considered), elimination of toxins, and internal environmental balance. Nutritional qualities include high levels of minerals, trace elements, iron, iodine, and protein.

Sea vegetables have a cold and dry effect on the body, although these can be altered through various forms of preparation.

Here are some individual energetic qualities of specific marine algae.

Brown

These include hiziki, kombu, wakame, alaria, arame (commonly used Japanese names), and sea palm.

Hijiki

This is an erect sea vegetable with tight branches accompanied by twig-like extensions that make it resemble a land bush. When soaked, it absorbs water and expands about four times its original size, at which point it resembles a blackish-brown pasta.

Hiziki requires longer soaking and cooking time (as well as more thorough rinsing) than other sea vegetables. It is a low-growing algae and is especially strengthening to the intestines, where it has the ability to assist in the absorption and assimilation of other foods.

Kombu

Kombu is a flat, slimy, and long sea vegetable with the potential to grow up to 1,500 feet. Kombu is a rubbery and flexible plant, smooth, strong, and durable, with the tenacity to withstand the rougher and deeper waters of the sea. It is especially supportive to the reproductive system and kidney and adrenal functions.

Wakame

Wakame, a tender, serrated leafy sea vegetable, is supported by a durable and flexible spine. It is especially supportive to the liver and nervous system. Wakame also contributes to physical and mental flexibility.

Alaria

This is an East Coast version of wakame, a bit tougher, with similar characteristics to wakame.

Arame

This is a two-branched sea vegetable with long, flat, leaflike appendages. Since it is tough in its original form, it is shredded into fine threads for easy use. Arame is a somewhat small, low-growing algae with a mild flavor and relaxing nature that is especially supportive to the middle organs (spleen, pancreas, and stomach).

Sea Palm

This is a low-growing, bulbous, and ribbed sea vegetable with a central stalk accompanied by ribbed leaflets; it resembles a palm tree (hence its name). It grows on rocks along the rocky shores, where it endures the constant thrashing of waves. If torn from the rocks, sea palm will set spores in the same place where it stood and a new one will grow to replace it. It probably endures more hardship than any other edible marine algae. Because of this, it contributes greatly to physical and mental stamina. Sea palm is also supportive to glandular functions.

Dulse

Dulse is a soft and delicate sea vegetable with flat leaflets resembling a glove or mittens. It is high in iron and has a rather strong but pleasant, salty taste. It is especially supportive to the heart and spleen. Research on marine algae has shown dulse to be the easiest to digest and assimilate.

Agar Agar

Called agar agar or just agar, this is a sea vegetable with a trunklike stem accompanied by tubular thorny leaves. It grows in deep waters.

Agar is processed into flakes, powder, or bars and is used to thicken soups, desserts (sometimes called *kanten*), and other preparations. It has a very cooling effect on the body and acts as a lubricant to the digestive tract. The tubular structure of agar makes it especially supportive to blood vessels and arteries.

Irish Moss

Irish moss is a spiky sea vegetable with dichotomously branching leaves resembling kale. It contains *carrageenan*, an emulsifier and stabilizer with many uses. Irish moss has calming and soothing effects on the stomach and contributes to healthy, shiny hair.

Red Laver (Nori)

Laver is a low-growing, fragile, and delicate broad-leafed sea vegetable (similar to leaf lettuce) that grows in shallow waters. One of the most popular marine algae, laver is commonly known as *nori,* a pressed sheet of algae used for rolling sushi. Nori is stimulating to the heart and circulation, where it can contribute short and quick spurts of energy. It is also helpful for fatigue and laziness.

Ao-Nori

This variety is quite similar to nori, except that it has more ruffled and clustered leaves. It is found around shores and is more abundant in warm waters. It has similar effects as red laver.

Freshwater Algae

Like marine algae, freshwater algae has been eaten by numerous ancient peoples, including the Aztecs, Maya, and Africans. Many of the general descriptions of algae above apply to freshwater algae as well as to marine algae, but there are also some unique properties specific to the freshwater varieties, too.

For one thing, many of the freshwater species predate the increasing salinity of the planet's oceans. In other words, compared with marine algae, they are more ancient still.

Given their affinity with less saline water, freshwater algae correspond energetically more with the human being's lymph than the saltier blood. The lymphatic system, which networks the body's immune system, is managed energetically by the spleen and pancreas. The spleen, aside from storing red blood cells, assists in the production and regulation of lymphocytes (white blood cells) and other immune cells.

The pancreas, occupying a central position in the torso, is responsible for a wide range of digestive and hormonal balance levels and was considered by ancient traditional medicine to be the central coordinator of balance. (The word *pancreas* itself means "all creation.")

Thus, while marine algae are powerful janitors and cleansers, freshwater algae fulfill these functions but also tend to carry out a more fine-tuned, delicate role of regulating the entire metabolism in perfectly coordinated harmony.

Freshwater algae is a single-celled organism that does not form a plant-like structure as marine algae does. The best-known varieties are *chlorella*, a green algae, *spirulina*, and *aphanizomenon*, both varieties of blue-green algae.

There are two radically different categories of freshwater algae: the wild, uncultivated type and the farmed, cultivated type. I have pointed out throughout this book that foods in their wild and natural state have stronger energetic effects on the body than their cultivated counterparts. As with farmed vegetables versus foraged plants, or with domesticated animals versus wild game, algae in their wild and natural state have stronger energetic effects on the body than do their cultivated counterparts.

The wild uncultivated algae *Aphanizomenon flos-aquae* is a single-celled organism. It is nourished by large quantities of minerals from its surrounding environment and thus can be absorbed rapidly, requiring minimal digestion. Because of this and its fast-growing nature, along with its phenomenal capacity for photosynthesis—the ability to literally eat light—this freshwater algae has a revitalizing and rejuvenating effect on the body.

Many people who eat freshwater algae have experienced a renewed sense of clarity and renewed energy in addition to improved digestion and absorption. Both marine and freshwater algae have a bright and promising future as some of the most important foods for ensuring our health and well-being.

Algae's "Hidden Agenda"

Much has been written about the nutritional benefits of algae. Very little is written or taught on their *quality* and energetic effects, whether on the body or on the mind and overall characteristic—yet the benefits here are, in my opinion, far more dramatic than those on the sheerly physical level of *quantity*.

The ancient and primitive *qualities* of algae—the most ancient plants on the planet—resonate not only with our blood and lymph but also with anything having to do with our biological and psychological past. These adaptable, flexible, and regenerative plants greatly assist in the unfolding of stuffed, hardened, accumulated experiences and issues pertaining to one's darker, hidden past. Negative memories often come to light and surface with new and refreshing ways of perceiving and evaluating past problems and conflicts.

For many, this can be a difficult process, and psychiatric buffers are often used to express and cope with these problems. While this may be helpful in some cases, the regular use of algae, which has the natural inborn *quality* of the ancient past, offers a challenging but powerfully effective approach for the adventurous individual willing to confront issues of his past. Where deep emotional and psychological issues are concerned, algae can assist us in bringing them to the surface where we are forced to face them head on.

More than just about any other food, algae often seems to be especially challenging for people (particularly non-Asian people) to relate to. However, through persistence and flexibility (another energetic property of algae), there comes a time when the person making this transition soon becomes very comfortable eating algae and will often enjoy it to the degree where a day without some kind of algae just doesn't seem right.

Algae's central purpose, which it has pursued successfully and tirelessly for billions of years, is to generate, animate, and inspire life on earth. When you eat this organism, you consume that global healing agenda too, and it becomes a part of you.

Toward a Global Consciousness

The study of algae—both intellectually (through research) and experientially (through using them as food)—offers a fascinating and revealing lesson in humility. It also holds extraordinary promise for our future on this planet.

Why "humility"? Let me explain.

It is common with the various natural foods, natural healing, and other related movements to speak of human beings' capacity for "global consciousness" and higher levels of awareness.

However, while there is no doubt that among animals, we humans do represent the pinnacle of biological development, our vaunted position at the "top of the scale" may not be so absolute as we might like to imagine. In many ways, plants and other animals exhibit some traits that are far more civilized than those common to our human societies.

We are the earth's most *recently developed* life-form. Algae are one of the planet's *earliest and most ancient* life-forms. Given their position at the opposite end of the evolutionary spectrum from us, looking into the "time mirror" of algae clarifies some surprising observations about our own true nature.

Homo Not So *Sapiens*

The first observation is that we human beings are in a way the organisms *least* naturally suited for global consciousness.

"Primitive" one-celled creatures such as algae have an extraordinary ability to act together as a community, yet also to behave independently. (Remember what they did to those sheep in Scotland?) Blue-green algae, in particular, exhibit these traits, since they are classified not only as plants but also, based on their cellular structure, as *bacteria*.

Bacteria have the unusual characteristic of sharing genetic information freely with one another. In fact, bacteria—including blue-green algae and the various other "food bacteria" found in traditionally fermented foods such as good-quality miso—can "learn" a certain behavior, such as the ability to adapt chemically to a new toxin in the environment—

and then share that ability with other bacteria *throughout the globe* in a matter of months! (It has been calculated that this same feat of communal genetic adaptation would take human beings roughly one million years.)

Aside from their capacity to communicate with each other, bacteria and algae also excel at adapting to their environment. As creatures develop from one-celled organisms to multicelled aggregated creatures, several things happen. One is that each individual cell becomes more and more specialized and less independent—in other words, more dependent on its neighboring cells. It also becomes less willing to adapt to its environment by changing itself, and begins to adapt more by altering conditions with the group's internal environment.

At the extreme of sophistication, we have warm-blooded mammals. Now, we seem to be highly adaptable. But look at *how* we adapt. When the weather around us cools, we don't adapt by *changing,* we adapt by maintaining our internal temperatures *to stay the same.* We don't survive by following the changes around us—we survive by resisting them.

Ninety-eight-point-six, you might say, is an example of how biologically opinionated we are.

In short, the way humans "adapt" is to *resist change as much as possible.* It is our constitutional, species-wide nature to resist change. Many of the perverse behaviors demonstrated by masses of people, such as greedy corporations, monolithic bureaucracies, and the unthinking mass media, are not so much borne out of conspiracy as they are simply examples of the human tendency to resist change and maintain the status quo—no matter what it takes!

It's a simple fact of human character: when forced to change, we'll change as little as possible. The truth is many would rather *die.* If you don't believe that, just take a look at the latest figures on terminal heart disease.

A second trait that develops with biological "progress" is that more "evolved" species become in many ways *less automatically integrated* with our surroundings. We become more aware of ourselves as separate entities but less immediately aware—biologically—of the world around us. We develop skins, then clothing, homes, and ultimately the trappings of technological civilization, not to attune ourselves more intimately *with* the environment, but to insulate ourselves more effectively *from* the environment.

While bacteria and blue-green algae are busy sharing biological information around the globe in the twinkling of an eye, we are having a hard time just learning how to say "Hello" in a nice way to our next-door neighbors.

Combine our fierce biological and psychological resistance to change with our staunch, cloistered biological individualism, and you can see why I say we are the least naturally suited to global consciousness.

"Voiding Our Differences"

Yet while bacteria naturally manifest this "global consciousness" automatically and constantly, we *imagine* it and *aspire* to it.

As much as we are set up to resist change, over the past ten thousand years of history, we have slowly and painfully taught ourselves to behave socially and as equals. We have gradually pulled ourselves up by our social and spiritual bootstraps to transcend the pecking order of poultry, the slavishness and docility of sheep and cattle, and the aggressiveness of fish.

We have begun to learn hard-won lessons of adaptability, and have developed to the point where, as we step into this new century, even as we stand at the very brink of reaping the horrendous harvest of all our social and environmental folly; we are also embracing the possibility of positive change on an epic scale.

Our relationship with algae is profound—because we are as different from each other as possible. We humans are the most complicated, most self-oriented, and most recent animal species to have booked a ticket on the food chain. Algae stand at the very beginning of the food chain—and they are the most ancient, most essential, and most biologically gregarious organisms.

Algae offer us an opportunity to participate in the dignity of the earth—her beauty, grandeur, roughness, and wildness—and to reconnect with those *qualities* within ourselves.

Algae and the Promise of Food Energetics

"Voiding our differences" is not only what this century is all about—it also describes the core promise of food energetics.

Birds of a feather *do* flock together! It takes *effort* to unite with your opposite. The less you consciously involve yourself in that effort, the more you will tend to eat foods that are *just like you already are*. It's not only that you are what you eat—the truth is, you tend to *eat* what you *are*! It's easy to eat what you already are. Remember Bob, Billy, and Jim?

But wouldn't it be more interesting to stretch ourselves a little? I hope you just said "Yes" to that question, because as much as we've stretched in the past ten thousand years, the drama of People vs. Planet is just now reaching its climax.

The foregoing discussion of humans and algae, for me, puts the entire matter of food into an enthralling global and historical perspective. Learning to grasp the *quality* of foods and to choose them energetically is more than a matter of improving your personal health, raising your consciousness, and taking a stand for creating the highest possible *quality* for your life. It is all these things—yet it is also humanity making a statement at this teetering juncture of our history on earth.

The present and future health of our food and the environment depends on us—just as we depend on them for our existence. Getting to know our food intimately is a cultural imperative, and by doing so, we can clarify powerfully our vision of what we want for the future of the planet and the children who will inherit it.

PART V

A Forbidden History of Food and Agriculture

37
The Origins of Agriculture

In the distant past, a few *Homo sapiens* made a decision that altered the biological, psychological, and spiritual essence of humanity. That decision was to work in partnership with the land through the domestication of plants and animals. Researchers from numerous scientific disciplines have made great strides in attempting to explain the origin of agriculture. However, exactly when, how, and why this happened at all is still very much a scientific mystery.

The information gleaned from extensive research in this multidisciplinary pursuit has offered a range of insights into how humans adapt to social and environmental pressures, develop patterns of health and disease, and structure sophisticated forms of culture and civilization. These ideas about agricultural origin are rooted in the *cultural evolution* theory, which today serves as the basis upon which academic beliefs and ideas are formed and supported by scientific research.

Much of this research is based on fossil records, comprised of bones, seeds, and stone tools gathered from the caves and hearths of ancient settlements. These records help us to formulate possible circumstances for addressing the following questions:

1. Where and when were plants first cultivated and identifiably domesticated?
2. What evidence is there to support current theories, and what

alternative interpretations can we draw from the available evidence?

The Cultural Evolution Theory
and the Fertile Crescent

The earliest domestication of plants may have been in the Near East's "Fertile Crescent," an area that stretches from the eastern shore of the Mediterranean Sea and curves around like a quarter moon to the Persian Gulf.

For nearly two centuries, explorers and scientists from different parts of the world have traversed this area in search of the origins of civilization and agriculture. Einkorn and emmer wheat, barley, and lentils, goats and sheep all purportedly originated here between five thousand and ten thousand years ago. Religious texts, legends, and archaeological discoveries document the antiquities of Sumer, Ur, Babylon, and other thriving cultural centers. This part of the Near East housed a literal treasure trove of artifacts, bones, and seeds that were used to substantiate the cultural evolution theory. This archaeological evidence has helped to form a consensus that has become the basis of today's textbooks on ancient history, prehistory, and culture.

The most thoroughly researched area of the world for the advent of civilization, the Fertile Crescent, is held today as the model to which all other such research sites throughout the world are compared. The Fertile Crescent, goes the theory, is where it all began—agriculture, civilization, all of it. Indeed, this "cradle of civilization" idea is so entrenched a part of historical orthodoxy that its axiomatic status has served to discredit those pieces of evidence that seem to challenge it.

This sort of fitting fact to theory is not new in scientific methodology. Archaeological and anthropological researchers commonly revise initial testing results for findings; this is a normal part of scientific procedure whenever deemed necessary.

For example, South and Central America are still termed "New World" countries, the underlying assumption being that their development must postdate that in the Near East. However, increasing amounts of controversial data are being found both in the Americas and in parts of Asia. Such evidence is tested with a variety of technologies, including accelerator mass spectrometry (AMS), which is in essence an upgraded form of radiocarbon dating.

AMS can accurately date samples as small as a single grain while detecting and reducing errors from fossil displacement. This can be especially useful when a sample (say, of bone or seed) has a different date than that of the strata in which it is found. However, even with the latest technology, much of the plant remains found are so severely carbonized or decomposed that they make it extremely difficult to determine whether a sample is wild or domestic.

Carbonized seed remains are a common source of agricultural evidence. The process of carbonization occurs when organic compounds are subjected to high temperatures and converted into charcoal. While this process does preserve remains for reliable analysis as to composition, it also causes morphological changes that can make it difficult to distinguish wild varieties from their domestic counterparts. Among grass seeds, there is also the problem of trying to determine the relationship, if any, between the wild grasses (emmer, einkorn, and barley) of ten thousand years ago to those of the present. Wild stands still grow throughout the Fertile Crescent and beyond.

The Independent Location Theory

While ancient plant remains have been extensively studied in the Near East, such is not the case in the "New World." Plant domestication research in Mexico and South America currently involves about a half dozen cave sites.

In Mexico, samples of squash seeds and beans dating around 7000 to 9000 BP ("before present," meaning before the radiocarbon baseline of 1950[1]) have been found in the deepest strata in some of these caves. Domestic squash seeds found in a cave at Oaxaca, for example, were dated at 9790 BP—the oldest date of any domestic plant species found in the New World.

Testing was based on dating a charcoal sample found next to the seeds; because of the extreme antiquity of the date, the age of the seeds was immediately cast into question. It was suggested that the seed samples had somehow been displaced downward from the upper level of the cave, or that the charcoal sample had somehow been displaced upward from the deeper layer.[2] Both explanations are possible—yet one cannot help but wonder why experts feel compelled to resort to such elaborate reasoning when the discoveries occur in a location so far removed from the established Near East cradle.

Furthermore, the Mexican sites are not alone in this. The people of other ancient civilizations from the Peruvian highlands, China's Yangtze River valley, and parts of Egypt, India, and Papua New Guinea all may also have domesticated plants dating back as far as those of the Fertile Crescent. However, the excavations for evidence of agriculture at these locations are still in their infancy and cannot yet be compared to the extensive findings in the Fertile Crescent.

Another part of the world with a long history of agriculture is Southern Asia, where a wide variety of annual and perennial forms of "wild" or "free-living" rice survives today without human intervention. Not too many years ago, domestic rice was thought to have a history going back between one thousand to two thousand years; current findings have pushed its origin back much further. The recent discovery in the central Korean village of Sorori of a handful of rice dating back fifteen thousand years strongly suggests that an agricultural practice here coincided with or even preceded that of the Fertile Crescent—which is still nevertheless viewed by many researchers as the site of agriculture's origin.

> The age [of the Sororian rice] challenges the accepted view that rice cultivation originated in China about 12,000 years ago. . . . The region in central Korea where the grains were found is one of the most important sites for understanding the development of Stone Age man in Asia.[3]

After thousands of years of cultivation, it is difficult to establish the identity of the original wild progenitor of domestic rice. Researchers struggle with whether present "free-living" rice is truly wild, a cultivated escapee, or something in between: cross-pollination, genetic exchange, expanding landscapes, and shrinking natural habitats have distorted genetic qualities between wild and domestic species. "Weedy" forms of rice have also evolved over time, escaping into unmanaged natural habitats, flourishing at the edges of agricultural landscapes and exchanging genetic material with both wild and cultivated varieties.

Even as they wrestle with the problem of potential multiple domestication sites, researchers are also faced with this paradox of the origins of agriculture: Why did hunter-gathers begin domestication of plants in areas with ample resources of wild foods? Thus, experts today still cannot state conclusively where plants were first domesticated and agriculture began—and the very hypothesis that it began because of hunter-gatherers' need for a new food source is under challenge as well.

Classification, Morphology, and Genetic Testing

When determining whether or not a plant should be classified as domestic, scientists look for large and fast-sprouting seeds, *glume* (grain hull) adherence, and strong *rachises* (the part of the grain that attaches the seed to the stalk). These traits are considered markers of domestication because, since they are naturally selected against in wild species, they could evolve only under cultivation.

Large seed size, for example, is usually considered a marker showing an adaptive response to selective pressures relating to domestication. The hunter-gatherer's deliberate planting of slightly larger, preselected seeds from wild stands into seedbeds rather than into the plant's natural wild habitat is believed to eventually cause morphological changes in the plants, resulting in larger, domestic-type seeds. By selecting wild mutant seeds with thinner glumes and stronger rachises, early hunter-gatherers were able to build up a seed supply of mutant seeds from wild stands over time. It is from this supply of stored mutant seeds that domestic cereals are said to have originated.

It is important to know that, even with the multiple scientific disciplines used to study agricultural origin, the sources of evidence vary considerably in reliability. The three important founder grains from the Fertile Crescent—emmer wheat, einkorn wheat, and barley—are the earliest examples known to be located near their wild relatives. There are several species growing today in the same area that are viewed as possibly being the original ancestors of these domestics.

However, after intensive study of morphologies and genetics, including analyses of plant proteins and interfertility testing, we are often still perplexed by a wild progenitor to which the domestic species appears morphologically identical *but with which it has no genetic compatibility.* To illustrate this "looks can be deceiving" aspect, Daniel Zohary states:

> A special case of species diversity is provided by "sibling species," that is, taxa so similar morphologically that it is very difficult—or even impossible—to distinguish between them by their appearance; yet, crossing experiments and cytogenetic tests reveal that they are already effectively separated from one another by reproductive isolation barriers such as cross-incompatibility, hybrid inviability, or hybrid sterility.[4]

A well-known example of sibling-species relations is that of wild and domestic emmer wheat. *Triticum araraticumm,* one species of wild wheat, is morphologically indistinguishable from domestic emmer wheat. However, all attempts to crossbreed the two have failed, thus proving that the former was not in fact the progenitor of the latter. Furthermore, a true ancestor, morphologically different from emmer wheat *yet with identical chromosomes,* was found and successfully interbred, thus linking it credibly to emmer wheat as a potential wild progenitor.

Wild progenitors used to be classified as separate species from domestics but are now ranked along with the domestics as a separate subspecies. For example, domestic emmer, *Triticum turgidum,* is the subspecies *dicoccum.* Its suggested wild ancestor, once called *Triticum dicoccoides,* is now classified as *Triticum turgidum dicoccoides.* What are the most obvious differences between them? The domestic grain somehow got larger, and the rachis got tougher and less brittle.

But are these variations, together with the fact that interbreeding was successfully accomplished under laboratory conditions, enough to identify *Triticum dicoccoides* as the wild ancestor of domestic *Triticum turgidum*? Or is there a danger here of leaping to simplistic conclusions?

We must remember that numerous factors, such as changes in climate or animal and human intervention, have influenced genetic variations and diversification among the wild progenitors over thousands of years. While it is generally believed that the wild progenitors of most cultivated plants have been satisfactorily identified, many researchers recognize the need for more data.

> The simple identification of a morphological change does not, in itself, constitute adequate documentation of a plant species having been brought under domestication. Linkage must be provided between the observed morphological change and a set of causal behavior patterns. It is not enough simply to document phenotypic change. It is also necessary to explain why such change appears in response to a newly created environment of domestication.[5]

The example of wild and domestic emmer, *Triticum turgidum*, may fit most additional criteria for domestication: both the wild and domestic emmer could successfully interbreed and they have identical chromosomes. Yet is it not possible that the putative wild ancestor of emmer could in fact have once been a cultivated escapee itself, one which then adapted to a wild environment over thousands of years?

Another example is the fragments of emmer wheat dated 9500 BP from the southwestern tip of the Fertile Crescent at Jericho. Evidence as to whether the fragments are wild or domestic is still inconclusive. Other samples of emmer dated 9700 BP and found just north of Jericho near Damascus, however, are domestic.[6] Keeping in mind the fact that these specimens are thousands of years old and have been through extreme changes, is it not possible that, again, what are thought to be wild samples of emmer are simply genetically altered cultivars, that is, a once-cultivated subspecies that has since run wild?

In order to consider this possibility, we must reexamine the common assumptions about our earliest agriculture origins: could these "origins" in fact be examples of *reemergence* from previous cycles of civilizations?

Without giving this consideration due weight, we are left with the mysterious appearance of numerous species of grasses, some of which share similarities to cultivated grain species both genetically and morphologically. One could argue that the dates of our examples fit the conventional timeline (ten thousand years for domestication), yet these are only a few examples of what has been found.

The recent and totally unexpected find of several grains of morphologically domestic emmer wheat at the Palestinian site of Nahal Oren also raises the possibility that grain was under cultivation as early as 14000 BC.[7]

An archaeological site in Israel, called Ohalo II, reveals ninteteen thousand well-preserved grass grains. Among the specimens are pieces of wheat and barley dating twenty-three thousand years ago[8]—about seven thousand years older than the Nahal Oren samples cited above! In light of findings such as these, it seems quite possible that many wild progenitors could be cultivars from a civilization or civilizations *predating* the orthodox theory for agricultural origin.

What are often called wild progenitors of domestic grasses may be suspect for other reasons. Several other sites in the Fertile Crescent have combined specimens of wild and domestic emmer, einkorn, and barley. The mix of wild progenitor and domestic is often interpreted as signs of early cultivation from wild to domestic. However, these may simply be examples of separate food stores for ruminants and humans. And while animal domestication does not happen until around 8000 BC, according to orthodox timelines, it is still possible that a sufficient condition of an earlier animal husbandry existed to account for wild grass harvests.

Cultivars and Wild-Growing Domestics

Einkorn wheat represents another perplexing example of early wild and domestic plant research.

The present-day northern portion of the Fertile Crescent yields broad bands of wild einkorn, yet research has designated the wild progenitor of domesticated einkorn as being restricted to a small region near the Karacadag Mountains in southeast Turkey, far removed from the northern broad bands of wild einkorn.

If the northern stands of wild einkorn are not the progenitors of domestic einkorn, then what are they? Could they be a once-domestic species that ran wild at some distant period of prehistory, eventually having adapted to their present environment?

It is believed that hunter-gatherers living in permanent settlements were harvesting a species of wild einkorn along the Euphrates River eleven thousand years ago.[9] If hunter-gatherers were already harvesting by that time, perhaps they had been harvesting it for thousands of years before that time too. What species of wild einkorn was this? Was it the progenitor of domestic einkorn, the species found in the Karacadag Mountain region? Or was it another species, like the one representing the broad bands of the northern regions, a species that never became domesticated?

For that matter, what about the modern wild einkorn found in the area comprised of Israel, Lebanon, southwest Syria, and Jordan? This Palestinian variety has large seeds, often larger than those of domestic wheat.[10] Could these too be feral crops that were once cultivated in antiquity and have now adapted to the regions? Large seed size is considered to be a marker of domestication—yet this wild species has seeds larger than most domestic species.

As long as we are focused on the Fertile Crescent, let us consider the origin and introduction of barley, the third founder crop of this region.

Two types of domestic barley have been recovered here from early settlements. It has been suggested that hunter-gatherers harvested wild barley before domesticating two-rowed barley, followed shortly afterward by six-rowed barley. Between these two types, two-rowed barley shows more of the wild barley characteristics; both two- and six-rowed domestics have been found together in early settlements.

Wild barley, like wild einkorn and emmer, develops brittle rachises for dispersal when fully ripened. These rachises are segmented so that individual spikelets and grains can be shed from top to bottom when ripe. Only about 5 to 10 percent of the rachises are semitough in wild barley, and this small percentage represents the average amount of seed that is held to the stalk at the time of maturity.

According to theory, early hunter-gatherers selectively chose seeds from these specific stalks at an early stage before ripening, and they did so because even if the 5 to 10 percent of rachises held their seeds, at maturity they would immediately fall to the ground when pulled by the hands of humans. The hunter-gatherers (so goes the hypothesis) would have saved these partially ripened seeds for planting stock.

In order to have the motivation to do this, these hunter-gatherers would have had to believe that these wild grass seeds, after being planted in homemade seedbeds, would produce larger, more stable seeds and larger yields after a few generations. Are we to assume that they knew what the outcome would be before they tried it? And are we to further believe that these wild grasses could genetically morph into domesticates through simple cultivation and planting techniques, when it has still not been demonstrated today (nor is there any evidence that such a demonstration is possible) that a wild, mutated seed can be transformed into a domesticate through cultivation in a foreign seedbed?

As with emmer and einkorn wheat, it is not uncommon to find wild and domesticated barley fragments together in archaeological sites. In areas of the Fertile Crescent, fully cultivated emmer wheat and two-rowed barley have been recovered from ancient sites, accompanied by wild-weed einkorn, ryegrass, and other weeds considered preadapted to cultivation. It is still highly questionable whether or not the selective pressures imposed on wild grasses, as suggested by the cultural evolution model, caused the morphological changes that resulted in domesticated varieties of cereals.

Early hunter-gatherers were just as highly attuned to their food sources as are modern-day hunter-gatherers. With hundreds of thousands of years' experience in finding food, knowing which plants to eat, observing animals in their natural habitats, and incorporating some of these habitats into daily life, it is difficult to believe that these people, who hunted and ate ruminants, were ignorant about the wild grasses eaten by these animals. After all, countless generations of hunter-gatherers used wild grasses for bedding, basket-weaving materials and fuel. Could these tough, brittle, wild grains really have been food for these early people, as some leading specialists suggest?

While there is plenty of evidence for wild grain harvest, there is actually little evidence supporting human consumption. Evidence for the latter is restricted to a few Paleo feces found in caves. The location and lack of evidence would suggest that a famine or climatic disturbance may have been in effect, causing the humans to hole up in the caves until it was safe to venture outside. If this were the case, the usual foods may have become scarce, causing those people to eat whatever they could find. (We must also consider the possibility that Paleolithic peoples were able to process wild grasses, rendering them digestible and fit for human consumption, without the pottery to soak the grains or cook them, but this possibility is quite slim.)

Proteins can be useful genetic markers for distinguishing wild ancestors from domestics. Shared genetic characteristics, if found, can reveal the wild progenitor of the domestic. However, this methodology is difficult to apply if the wild progenitor no longer exists, as is often the case, leaving us with hypothetical ancestors because of some particular similarity between the two.

Cross-pollination, genetic exchange, and environmental changes have blurred the lines between wild and domestic varieties over thousands of years. Along the way, opportunistic weeds of many varieties have joined the mix and contributed to new gene pools.

Simply put, it becomes increasingly difficult to determine whether the domestics came from weeds or the weeds came from the domestics.

Which Came First: Teosinte or Maize?

A good case in point is *teosinte,* a diverse group of wild grasses native to Mexico, Guatemala, and Honduras.

Teosinte is suspected to contain the progenitor of domestic maize because the two are genetically compatible and successfully crossbreed through repeated hybridization in fields. They differ, however, in the morphology of the female ear. The few small seeds of teosinte husks look nothing like the large, fully seeded ears of maize. Teosinte has numerous branching stalks, each culminating in a few small, shattering seed spikes. Corn, on the other hand, is a single stalk containing an ear of tightly arranged, rowed seeds that cannot disperse naturally.

Because of its unique makeup, some experts believe teosinte is a descendant of domestic maize. Most agronomy books and relevant literature see it the other way around, presenting teosinte as the wild ancestor of maize. Yet regardless of which direction one subscribes to, teosinte-to-maize or maize-to-teosinte, how such an extraordinary transformation could have taken place in the remote past at all is an inexplicable mystery.

Many varieties and sizes of domesticated corn have been found in deep levels of caves throughout Mexico, revealing the extensive knowledge of plant genetics and breeding techniques among early inhabitants of Mexico and Peru. A comparison of proteins between teosinte and domestic maize reveals some similarities, and no species of wild maize has yet been found. Some teosinte types have been categorized as subspecies, yet there are no morphological indications or examples of their transformation into domestic maize.

With all our current technology, it seems reasonable that we should be able to create a domestic species from a wild one in a controlled environment, simulating an early hunter-gathers' planting methods—if that is indeed what happened. What would it take? And if this would prove the prevailing theory of wild mutant seed transformation, why haven't we yet done it?

Ancient Gene-Tweaking

Identification of chromosomal affinities between wild and domestic crops is another method for finding wild progenitors. If cultivated crops show full homology and interfertility with a wild species from the same genus, then that wild species could be recognized as the ancestor of the crop. This may be misleading, though, because chromosomal affinity does not necessarily determine ancestry. This is especially true when there are wide variations in morphology, as is typical with many grain progenitors and their domesticated offspring.

> An obvious advantage of domestication traits is that they evolved only under cultivation and are strongly selected against and absent in the wild.[11]

If this is true, it should be easy to reverse the process and produce wild, "shattering" crops from domestics once the specific gene sequence is found. ("Shattering" crops are those wild forms whose seeds drop to the ground upon ripening, rather than adhering to their stalks as do the seeds of domestics.)

> . . . . crosses between wild progenitors and the cultivars have shown that this shift is brought about by a recessive mutation in one major gene or (more rarely) by a joint effort of two such genes. In all these crops, breeders have also performed many intra-crop crosses (between cultivars). Except for barley, none of these within-crop crosses has been reported to produce wild-type brittle or dehiscent. . . .[12]

It would appear that our ancestors were able to "tweak" that single gene from wild grasses so that it could not be reversed. Only domestic barley, with its two independent recessive genes, has successfully produced wild-type, brittle grains and these are still different from the wild species.

Aside from wild chenopod pseudocereals that shed their seeds in a couple of days at maturity and can be husked by simple rubbing and winnowing, the idea of preagricultural peoples regularly consuming wild grasses (progenitors of einkorn, emmer, barley, rye, and spelt), as promoted by many researchers, may simply be an attempt to promote the cultural evolution theory. However, the premise that Paleolithic humans' eating of wild grasses may have led to the eventual domestication of the wild species also supports the gradual-step theory, which is not unlike the theory that seed plant cultivation followed other vegetable plants. Evidence for hunter-gatherers cultivating propagated vegetables before seeds is lacking, but the theory of a gradual-step process comfortably fits the current paradigm.

Could these grass species of einkorn, barley, and emmer, so often suggested as the wild progenitors of their modern day domesticates, be something other than wild?

Based on the hypothesis that over thousands of years a plant could experience numerous morphological changes, is it not possible for a once-domesticated plant to revert to some semblance of a wild version? It has already been suggested that wild grass species, once cultivated, could morphologically transform within three hundred years when transplanted into seedbeds. An example of this morphological change could appear as brittle rachises becoming "semitough" enough to be identified as cultivated.

While this may be possible, it raises another question: could other important markers (thinner glumes, larger seeds, greater adaptation to climate and soils, resistance to diseases and pests, etc.) that resulted from selection pressures and were found in domestic species also have morphed along with the rachises, or did some of these traits occur earlier and others later?

Some of these developments are major adjustments to a wild grass species involving genetic manipulation at some level in the process, and there is no indication these markers, not to mention increased nutrition and faster sprouting time, could have occurred consecutively or simultaneously over a few hundred years by being planted in seedbeds, even if the seeds were carefully selected, wild, mutant seeds. Granted, some hunter-gatherers from the Epipaleolithic period knew a great deal about the growing cycles of plants (and even about seed planting, and cultivation to some degree), but the genetic manipulation of a wild grass species into a productive, nutritious offspring is something quite extraordinary.

The question thus remains: who were these people and how did they know how to manipulate plants at the genetic level? Evidence at many archaeological sites indicates that the knowledge for plant domestication was already there and was not an evolutionary process.

Domestic Escapees Run Wild

The idea that many of these "wild" species of cereals are actually cultivars is a realistic consideration. Edgar Anderson addresses this important issue in his book *Plants, Man and Life*. He suggests that we consider previous cycles of cultivation when examining what we think are "wild relatives" of our basic food crops.

This is indeed a consideration for researchers, as it is now well known that some species were in fact cultivated before the time they were once thought to have originated. Corrections in origination dates, along with genetic mixing of wild and domestic crops, environmental pressures, and time can realistically contribute to deevolution of a domestic species.

An example Anderson gives of how one might encounter in a jungle a smaller version of a cultivated fruit, giving the first impression that it is a wild relative of the domestic version, is an all-too-common occurrence. While it is possible that what you are witnessing is a wild food, it has been repeatedly shown that many of these wild-appearing foods are remnants of refuse heaps, a seed spit out of a hunter's mouth after finishing his lunch from home where he cultivated the fruit, or a garden escapee. I have personally encountered wild-growing samples of cacao, coffee, papaya, avocado, and other familiar varieties while in the remote jungles, far from any agricultural base, of South and Central America.

Anderson also points out the great variations among wild-growing domestic avocados in Central America. Such variations appear to an even greater extent among avocados presently growing under managed cultivation. He brings to attention the fact that apples appear in pastures, forests, and fields throughout the country, yet none were here in America when the first European colonists arrived. Apples are likely from Asia, where various species are native. We do not know how much of a connection the wild-growing apples have with previous cycles of cultivation, but they are, without question, examples of cultivated apples that have run wild. The same is likely true for many "wild" relatives of cereal grains. When I lived in Vermont, we had three apple trees and two pear trees on our land. We were the first on record to build on this particular spot, yet, although we did not plant the trees, they were not wild fruit trees.

Wild weeds are highly successful plants that can easily overcome a disturbed habitat, as evidenced in most gardens by weed races commonly found among domestic annuals and perennials. Early hunter-gatherers, like their modern counterparts, are known for having collected and stored a variety of wild seeds. Most of these seeds are known for specific uses, such as food or medicine. But what evidence is there that preagricultural peoples actually used wild grasses for their own consumption?

Jack Harlan, an authority on agricultural origins, was able to prove that a small group of people, within a period of just three weeks, could harvest by hand enough wild grain to sustain themselves for one year. To some, this classic study suggests that our ancestors did the same. However, it does not prove that they did nor explain why they did it, if they did. Were harvests for predomestic ruminant consumption, or for some other highly useful purpose?

Recently, a team of international scientists found fields of wild einkorn wheat in the Near East that provides the closest genetic match to domestic einkorn. By obtaining DNA samples of sixty-eight separate lines of cultivated einkorn, all samples were found to be closely related. DNA profiles were also taken from 261 separate populations of wild einkorn in the same area. Of the 261 wild samples, nineteen from the volcanic region of the Karacadag Mountains in Turkey were distinct from the other wild einkorn lines. Further analysis showed that eleven of the nineteen samples had a close phylogenetic similarity to the culti-vated einkorn. As a result, these eleven wild samples could be identified as modern descendants of the wild progenitor for einkorn wheat.[13]

Note that these wild samples were identified not as wild progenitors but as *descendants* of a wild progenitor, based on their similarity to the domestics. But how can they credibly be seen as descendants of a wild progenitor if we don't know where or what the wild progenitor is? Phrases such as *similar to, related to, descendants of,* and so on imply a link to some long-lost original strain of wild grass that, through a series of mutations, became the domestic grain we know today. Yet, in many cases, there is still no known actual progenitor.

Evidence does strongly suggest an area for the earliest domestication of einkorn wheat, but, like so many other domestic plants, the wild progenitor remains elusive. What we have are suspected descendants of these elusive wild progenitors, much like the situation in the study of human origin with its search for the elusive "missing link."

What Really Happened?

The presence of grinding stones, sickle blades, and storage structures in many early hunter-gatherer sites indicates a long reliance on wild-seeded plants, particularly wild grasses. Refinement of harvesting and cultivation techniques by selectively choosing plumper seeds eventually transformed fields of grain into crops with thinner husks, stronger and less brittle rachises, stalks with increased seed clusters, larger and more dependable yields after harvesting and threshing, increased nutritional value, and spare seed for storage. These newly cultivated crops could have eventually replaced their wild counterparts in importance. After much trial and error, these once-wild grasses, first through careful selection of suitable wild seeds and later through repetitive cycles of sowing, reaping, and harvesting, became domestic crops fully dependent on human intervention.

Some archaeobotanists believe morphological changes, which include changes in size, shape, and form, could have taken place anywhere from one hundred to three hundred years after the first time a seed was planted in a seedbed by early hunter-gatherers. Others believe it may have taken longer, up to 1,000 years. This is an interesting hypothesis that appears to be based on sound evidence, albeit interpreted though the theory of cultural evolution. Nevertheless, it is a hypothesis—not a fact. The evidence is therefore open to interpretation from alternative perspectives as well.

In *Origins and Seed,* Gordon Hillman discusses cultivation as a precursor to domestication and suggests that cultivation in the Jordan Valley could have started as early as 12,000 BC. He further states, "However, detecting the start of cultivation will, as ever, be problematic." The reasons for this, says Hillman, are that "cultivation prior to domestication can be recognized only from indirect evidence, not from the remains of crops themselves" and "domestication itself is often difficult to detect." Further influences in the process would include unripe harvesting and genetic infiltration of wild genes from neighboring populations of wild grasses.

> Indeed, even with the most rapid domestication, it is inevitable that "modifier genes" would have ensured that the crops continued to contain an admixture of wild forms for many centuries. . . . This effect, combined with the inherent problems of distinguishing wild and domestic cereals from charred remains [archaeological records], ensures that detection of domestication in the archaeological record will continue to be extremely difficult.[14]

So why cultivate in the first place? Why spend centuries planting something that will not produce the desired result for generations? Furthermore, when the plant finally does reach its full potential, its product becomes a causal factor, according to many historians, in both the creation and downfall of civilization. Jack Harlan nicely sums up the scientific position on the question of cultivation:

> What does planting and reaping, planting and reaping, that is farming, do to the genetic architecture of annual seed crops? Most of our answers to this and similar questions have been intuitive or simple guesswork.[15]

Again, while there is no doubt that wild grasses played an important role in the lives of hunter-gatherers, it may not have been for food. What about those 261 "wild" samples from the Fertile Crescent, only nineteen of which have genetic similarities to domestics? Could these be additional examples of cultivars that have morphologically reverted to their present status after running wild some thousands of years ago?

Research has shown that some early hunter-gatherers from the Fertile Crescent practiced what is called *vertical transhumance,* wherein groups of people would seasonally move their campsites from low elevations to higher elevations in the spring to harvest ripening wild grasses and to hunt wild goats and sheep that followed these ripening grasses. If we remove the cultural evolution model as an interpretation for this scenario, we are left with typical pastoralists herding their flocks to ripening grasses. Admittedly, this would be at a time well before they are believed to have had domestic animals—but the truth of the matter is that, as with our inconclusive results concerning plant domestication, we really don't know when animals were first domesticated.

The majority of researchers still either hold to the Fertile Crescent theory or believe that plant domestication began independently in several parts of the world within the last five thousand to ten thousand years. Both perspectives depend on the cultural evolution theory for their basis. Either orientation posits a long period of experimenting by hunter-gatherers with wild grasses predisposed to domestication before agriculture appeared on a large scale.

But is it possible, at least in some of the major areas where agriculture began, that plant domestication did not happen through this evolutionary process of human experimentation? Although they specifically address contact between the hunter-gatherers and early farmers of central and northern Europe, the editors of *Last Hunters—First Farmers* offer another suggestion that could just as easily be applied to any number of other locations where agriculture began:

> The origin of agriculture involves only *a very few places in a few brief moments* of time. The spread of agriculture is the primary means through which farming has become the basis of human subsistence. It would seem essential to keep *both colonization and adoption,* and the kinds of evidence and questions that they involve, in mind in any discussion of the transition to agriculture [emphasis added].[16]

CONCLUSIONS

Agricultural origins cannot at present be conclusively proven to have begun close to ten thousand years ago when additional evidence for agriculture extends further back in prehistory. What can be unequivocally stated is that agriculture emerged several times in numerous parts of the world in the last twelve thousand to twenty thousand years, and perhaps as early as fifty thousand years ago, with the last six thousand years producing the most recent evidence for this cultural phenomenon.

Evidence, in the form of submerged ruins of fully developed civilizations (i.e., agricultural civilizations) in several parts of the world, is mounting. Once established, it will seriously challenge the hypothesis that humans first began as hunter-gatherers and later evolved to agriculturists some ten thousand years ago—a hypothesis that at present has no solid basis in proof, yet is still readily believed by many.

Genetic manipulation of plants, particularly cereal grains, occurred at some point in prehistory, enacted by people who already had the knowledge to do so. These same people created a vital and lasting human food source, no doubt for very specific reasons.

In each of the major areas of the world where plants and animals were domesticated, we find legends, both written and oral, describing the origin of agriculture as a gift of the gods, culture-bearers who taught indigenous peoples agriculture and the sciences of civilization. Could this possibly be coincidence, the accident of mere imagination?

Not one of the hundreds of worldwide legends nor the historical written records of our ancestors contains any allusion to agriculture's having begun by a trial-and-error process from selected mutant seeds being planted in seed beds over generations. Rather, what we do have is a consistent record of diffusion, migration, and colonization.

Our ancestors left us more than bones, seeds, and stone tools—they left us examples of extraordinary feats of engineering and architecture. They left us legends, myths, epics, and sagas. Isn't it about time we heard them out?

38

The Prehistory and Reemergence of Agriculture

Reconsidering Human Origins

More than ever before, new discoveries in the scientific fields of archaeology, astronomy, anthropology, geology, and genetics are challenging scientific theories that have served to shape and form our fundamental beliefs about who we are and how we arrived at our present position. Along with the theory of cultural evolution, as described in the last chapter, one of the most jeopardized of such theories is the famous theory of human evolution of Charles Darwin, the nineteenth-century British naturalist who has shaped scientific and academic thought for the past century and a half.

The Ascendancy of Darwinism

In 1859 Darwin wrote his seminal work, *The Origin of Species,* in which he theorized that simple life forms developed into more complex ones through gradual, ascending steps. These steps were the basis of evolution and were controlled by "the survival of the fittest," which Darwin referred to as the theory of natural selection. Through this process, a species improved or evolved by adapting to environmental pressures in order to survive. To most people it was known simply as the theory of evolution."

Shortly after publication, Darwin's theory rapidly gained the support of some intellectuals and educators. However, some of its controversial ideas were rejected by many critics. Among the detractors were fundamentalist Christians whose "creationist" views Darwin's theory flatly contradicted. But while believers in the biblical creationist model landed a few crippling blows to the evolutionists, their own acceptance of the biblical explanation of creation was based primarily on faith, not on science. For the most part, proponents of human evolution found nonscientific, religious beliefs to be of little relevance in discussions of human origin, regardless of whether the particular views represented Christianity, Judaism, Hinduism, or any other faith. The British-American anthropologist Ashley Montague made this succinct observation:

> Science has proof without any certainty. Creationists have certainty without any proof.

And writing a century earlier, Darwin's contemporary Mark Twain lampooned the advance of science with characteristic dead-on accuracy:

> There is something fascinating about science. One gets such wholesale returns of conjecture out of such a trifling investment of fact.

Over the years, some of the critics' more scientifically based attacks on Darwinism raised quite a few pertinent issues, causing Darwinism's supporters to be saddled with the burden of proof—something they have yet to produce. Still, the evolutionists' camp, increasingly viewed as a faith-based religion of its own sort, managed to dominate most facets of education under the banner of "righteous science." The media and most educational systems in Europe and America presented evolution to the public and students as though it were fact.

As we saw in the previous chapter, a conjunctive theory of cultural evolution also permeated our society so deeply that anthropology, paleontology, botany, and many other sciences based most of their findings on it. Cultural evolution even became the basic theory for rationalizing almost every dietary trend from raw foods and vegan diets to high-protein and low-carbohydrate diets.

One compelling reason for Darwinism's powerful hold over scientific and cultural thought has to do with the larger cultural context. The formative years of academic studies in human history were marked by the prevalence of racism and Eurocentric attitudes. Today, while these social conditions have markedly improved, many of the concepts they influenced continue to endure. In most universities throughout the world, students are still taught the theory of African genesis: that we evolved from the trees of the African savanna from ape to primitive African savage, and that all prehistoric peoples, whether simple hunter-gatherers or agricultural peoples, were evolving savages who eventually culminated into modern-day *Homo sapiens,* the epitome of creation. (The racist-culturalist implications of this scenario are impossible to miss.)

Although the term *savage* is no longer used to describe the often brilliant peoples of prehistory, only recently have our ancestors gotten the true recognition they deserved. Yet because of early biased viewpoints that defined our textbook perspectives of human prehistory, it is still often difficult for many to perceive our ancient ancestors in any other way than as primitives who evolved to the point of becoming "civilized" only around ten thousand years ago. For many, this colorless viewpoint still prevails today.

Dogma and Heresy

While there has been a wealth of information compiled over the past century on hunter-gatherers, supposedly the forebears of agriculture, confining agricultural peoples to the Stone Age ancestry of the Neolithic period has led to much confusion—for there is a vast amount of evidence that suggests otherwise.

This limited perspective is especially confounding when we attempt to study dietary traditions. Undoubtedly there have been Stone Age peoples, but to say that the majority of human prehistory belongs to a period defined as Stone Age, wherein all peoples are "primitives," may be focusing in blindly on but one part of a far greater story.

Evolutionists often point to the spurious fossil records as evidence that mutation and natural selection can prove how evolution happens. Examples include the transitions of single-celled organisms to fish, fish into amphibians, amphibians into reptiles, and so on to mammals— even though these particular models are no longer considered valid.

You may recall the grade-school history-book image of a series of creatures emerging through an evolutionary process into a man. Many people are unaware that this model is no longer recognized as valid by most scientists. Furthermore, while most people are aware that there is a "missing link" between the ancestral apes of chimpanzees and humans, and may even be aware that the search for this elusive link is ongoing, few realize that there are many such "missing" evolutionary transitions for animals and plants in the fossil record. These transitions, said to be the results of mutations or natural selections, simply do not show up in the fossil record with any kind of consistency.

This is rather strange: according to theory, there should be an abundance of transitional fossils revealing the transformational steps from one species to another. Instead, what the record shows us is fully formed species that seem to suddenly appear, remain consistent in makeup over long periods, and then eventually disappear. With the exception of a few species, such as sharks and crocodiles that continue to live as they were, living creatures are replaced by what appear to be entirely new and different species. This is true for both prehistoric animals and nonflowering plants, which are supposed to have evolved into flowering plants about one hundred million years ago. Here too we find a lack of intermediaries between the two types of plants.

Is it possible that this highly influential theory, one that so confidently explains who we are and where we come from, could be seriously flawed?

With new players, including the proponents of the "intelligent design," "lost continent," and "interventionists" theories in the human-origin field, the heated debate on evolution is rapidly coming to a boil. Never before in its short history has this theory faced such intense scrutiny as it is facing today, as the dedicated research of diverse groups of scholars and historians with multidisciplinary scientific methods is bringing about a genuine revolution in how we think and what we believe about human origins. Indeed, many believe that these new researchers are armed to the hilt with more evidence *against* the theory of evolution than those who support it have for its defense. Wielding such compelling evidence, many of these "alternative" historians claim a greater antiquity for civilization than most cultural evolutionists are willing to acknowledge.

Unfortunately, the lengths to which some evolutionists have gone to discredit alternative historians have been at times extreme. For the professional whose work is either directly or indirectly linked to the study of human origin, it is becoming clear that to challenge the theory of evolution is an extremely bold and politically incorrect position to take. Thus, despite the fact that free thinking and open-mindedness are the quintessence of genuine scientific inquiry, the theory of evolution nevertheless has a habit of closing the door to archaeological and anthropological finds that do not fit into its ideology. Just as faith is the foundation of religious belief, the need for scientific certainty compels evolutionists to their strong attachments to conventional theory.

Consequently, to challenge the theory of evolution is to be branded a "creationist." Because the debate has been presented by the media as an either/or issue, with evolution and creation the only two sides of the debate, most believe this is all there is to it—though in fact, nothing could be further from the truth.

When the "creationist" label doesn't conveniently fit the alternative theory in question, the accusation of "pseudoscience" is leveled against the offending alternative historian. However, with increased public awareness and access to new discoveries, the tired ramblings of accepted dogma will continue to be challenged by stimulating, open dialog among those wishing to discuss the highly plausible alternate theories.

Myth or History?

An increasing amount of evidence during the past decade has suggested a history of humankind extending far beyond the accepted textbook timelines. The idea of anatomically correct humans (*Homo sapiens*) in deep antiquity—civilized, agriculturally based humans with an understanding of astronomy, geometry, architecture, and other more sophisticated sciences—existing so far back in time as to coexist with early hunter-gatherers and other primates is not easy for orthodox historians to accept. To say that the broad acceptance of this idea would have a powerful impact on the scientific certainty of human evolution is a grand understatement. Indeed, its effect on evolutionary theory would be earthshaking—not to mention the effect it could have on some organized religions.

For anyone seeking to cut through the confusion as to what to believe about human evolution, I recommend reading *Forbidden Archeology* by Cremo and Thompson; *Shattering the Myths of Darwinism* by Richard Milton; and *Evolution, Creationism and other Modern Myths* by Vine Deloria Jr. These three books are scholarly works that put human evolution in its rightful place: as a theory in serious need of reconsideration.

Alternative historians have paved the way toward a new understanding of human origins that incorporates the early and current research of orthodox anthropology, paleontology, and archaeology with other scientific methods (e.g., archaeoastronomy, engineering, mathematics). Even the written and oral traditions, myths, and legends of traditional peoples throughout the world are being openly researched and analyzed for further insights. Fifty years ago, many of these methods were not considered acceptable (let alone standard) methodologies for approaching the study of human origins. Today they are proving to be of tremendous assistance in reevaluating early discoveries and aiding in the interpretation of new ones.

A famous case in point illustrates the potential validity of historical records previously regarded as "pure imagination." Over a hundred years ago, a seven-year-old boy named Heinrich Schliemann, enamored by pictures of the mythological city of Troy, determined that one day he would find the lost city. In 1873, Schliemann discovered the site of Homer's Ilium right in the location where it was said to have been, a discovery that moved Troy from the realm of myth to that of historical reality.

Apollonius of Rhodes wrote the famous *Argonauta*, which tells a story about the Greek hero Jason, who made his legendary voyage in search of a "golden fleece" some three thousand five hundred years ago. The story has long been thought to be but one of many Greek myths. However, excavations in some of the areas mentioned in the story have confirmed that the myth was indeed based on real people and real places. Myths and legends, when researched methodically and extensively, have also revealed hidden meanings associated with astronomical and geological events.

Our true history may be just beginning to unfold. With the advent of satellite imaging, NASA has recently discovered lost civilizations in Cambodia, South America, and India. Man-made megalithic structures have also been found off the coasts of Japan and Malta. A recent discovery off the coast of Cuba reveals what appears to be a complex of temples and other structures resembling Mayan architecture. Because of their two-thousand-foot depth, these ruins are believed by some researchers to have sunk around fifty thousand years ago! Are these the remains of some of the world's most ancient civilizations?

One would think that archaeologists would be doing cartwheels through the hallowed halls of academia when informed of so many new and exciting discoveries—but such is not the case. Most of the research on these and other mysterious discoveries is being conducted by independent scientists, journalists, and other curious individuals intent on solving unanswered questions.

If and when some of these new discoveries prove accurate through current methods of dating technology, this will be further confirmation that human beings were building sophisticated cities and temples fifty thousand to sixty thousand years ago.

And where there is civilization, there is agriculture.

"Stone Age" Technology

If we accept the theories of human and cultural evolution, our species was not evolved enough to practice agriculture until around ten thousand years ago, and there could have been no large-scale agriculture until five thousand years ago with the advent of the Sumerian culture, often dubbed the "first great civilization" or the "cradle of civilization."

But recent discoveries of other sites yielding evidence of ancient civilizations contemporaneous with Sumerian—or even earlier—have altered the picture.

For example, the highly advanced cities of the Indus-Sarasvati civilization of ancient India are likely to have preceded the Sumerians and measure an extraordinary three hundred thousand square miles—many times larger than the Sumerian ruins! (Even Egypt's fifteen-thousand-square-mile area pales in comparison.) Other sites of pre-Sumerian civilizations may exist near the pre-Incan site of the Sachsyuaman fortress, above Cuzco, Peru. No one knows who these megalithic builders were or how they worked, but they possessed a technology that allowed them to cut and fit four-hundred-ton stones into complex, megalithic puzzles. Attempts to fix the date of another ancient site, Tiawanaku, have yielded varying results, ranging from one thousand to twenty thousand years ago. The ruin's upward displacement, however, suggest that it must be at least many thousands of years old.

At the rate new discoveries are being made, there soon will be many more findings predating Sumerian, perhaps by thousands or even tens of thousands of years. When and where, then, did civilization really begin?

In trying to answer this question, we must remember that archaeology, paleontology, and anthropology still operate within guidelines designed to fit the scientific dogma of Darwinism, which still today comprises a Procrustes' bed to which all new evidence is forced to fit—even when the evidence itself may contradict it. Thus release of this information to the public may be delayed by years. And we have to understand that we have only begun to uncover the many secrets of our planet's history—and our own.

To orthodox historians, the idea of technologically advanced civilizations having existed in deep antiquity is generally regarded as unacceptable because (it is said) there is no proof in the form of technological artifacts. But this is often a tortuously slanted argument. For example, the detailed machining techniques used on some of the interior blocks of the Great Pyramid and other places in Egypt clearly exhibit highly technical knowledge—yet the actual machinery to produce these techniques has not yet been found, so even with evidence of the *use* of advanced technology in remote times, some historians still want to see the actual technological artifacts that *produced* this evidence.

This seems a fair enough request, if they would join the alternative historians and put their time, energy, and resources into looking for these missing artifacts. Indeed, it would seem to be a matter of scientific principle that they would do so. Yet something holds them back. Perhaps it is sheer intellectual inertia, or resistance to the difficulties involved in having to adapt any discoveries of ancient technology to the cultural evolution model. At any rate, a likely place to start would be around some of the newly discovered anomalous, man-made structures located under the sea. These submerged cities are likely to hold evidence for the true origins of agriculture as well.

One fact of the times strongly supports such a search: the proliferation and availability of modern scientific technologies. When the politically correct theories on human origin were first formed, a little over a 150 years ago, they were supported by a relatively small number of scientific fields of study using a limited range of technical methods. Today, with so many scientific disciplines, specialties, and technologies at our disposal, it is an especially apt time for reexamining the existing theories to see if they really are worth keeping intact or are in need of significant overhauling.

For example, even minimal research into the mathematical, astronomical, and engineering feats of the great pyramid of Cheops in Egypt, supposedly built a few thousand years ago, reveals an architectural masterpiece that required the stacking of one million stone blocks weighing two and a half tons (with some interior blocks weighing up to two hundred tons) to a great height with a mathematical precision unequaled anywhere in the world. Yet applying orthodox theory, one would have to believe that the people who built it were primitive men using a jury-rigged apparatus of ropes and logs!

Their purpose in building this great structure is believed to have been to create a tomb for a deceased pharaoh whose life was based in a polytheistic cult obsessed with superstitions concerning the afterlife. In this case, the evolution theory lacks even common sense—yet it is still promoted by orthodox historians. Not only is it irresponsible for professional scientists to promote such an unsubstantiated theory, it is also an insult to human intelligence. If certain scientific disciplines are to claim a monopoly on historical knowledge, then in all fairness, these disciplines should be able to demonstrate how and why their theories are valid.

Even with modern technology, it is unlikely we could reproduce this masterpiece with such mathematical precision. It is interesting that orthodox scholars so often make meticulous demands for proof of advanced technology in antiquity—yet in instances such as this one, their own theories either ignore the current evidence or explain it away, often with absurd theories.

Bones, art, megaliths, pyramids, and other anomalous structures from remote periods are among the clues found around the world pointing to human occupation lost in the mists of time. Some of these examples are so old that the dates given for them are tenuous at best. The attempt to fit ancient buildings into a time frame of the past five thousand years is futile when one realizes how clearly evident it is that many of these have been built and rebuilt *over previously abandoned structures*.

One could argue that the famous Sphinx of Egypt, even with an update of ten thousand years ago, does not exceed the orthodox timeline for the onset of agriculture. But common sense suggests that the civilization with the technology and technicians to build the Sphinx must have been already in place well before construction began. How long before? We do not know—but we do know with certainty that these people were not hunter-gatherers living in "Stone Age" conditions!

Egypt is only one of the mysterious ancient civilizations for whom the infancy of its art, writing, sculpture, and architecture has yet to be found. These ideas and artifices of civilization had to have had origins stretching back in time well before suddenly appearing, despite the fact that the evolutionary increments of development are lacking in archaeological strata.

In fact, the occurrence of knowledge being won, then lost, then rediscovered "for the first time" is far from uncommon even in our documented history. Columbus's discoveries of America and Galileo's pronouncement that the earth was round are two such examples. It is firmly established historical fact that Columbus was not the first to discover America, and the ancient Egyptians, Maya, and Chinese all knew that the earth was round long before Galileo's time.

Our Agricultural Origins: The Orthodox View

While metallurgy, language, and writing each played a role, agriculture is regarded as perhaps the most influential factor in forming civilization after primate man stood erect and walked (supposedly) out of the plains of Africa. Let's take a brief look at the orthodox view of the origin of agriculture and review it from some alternative perspectives. The following timeline incorporates modifications by historians in order to accommodate recent discoveries that deviate from the original theory.

- 100,000 years ago: Modern humans appear and migrate out of Africa.
- 60,000 years ago: Humans increase migrations, build simple boats and begin sea travel.
- 40,000 years ago: Humans arrive in Australia. Some hunter-gatherers begin to protofarm. Cave art appears.
- 30,000 years ago: Humans arrive in the Pacific Islands.
- 13,000 years ago: Humans walk across the land bridge (Beringia) from Eurasia to America and consume local fauna to extinction, often called the "Pleistocene overkill."
- 12,000 to 11,000 years ago: The Neolithic revolution begins.
- 10,000 years ago (now pushed back another 10,000 years): Signs of plant and animal domestication appear in the fertile river valleys of modern-day Iraq, Iran, and Turkey. The ice age ends.
- 5,500 years ago: Architecture, language development, writing, metallurgy, science, and religion appear.

According to this general outline, starting roughly ten thousand years ago with the glacial ice melting and flooding much of the lowlands, hordes of people headed to higher ground in search of food and shelter. In so doing they had to acclimate themselves to less space and were forced to practice agriculture full-time in order to sustain their growing populations.

As farming increased, so did population density and with it, the need for more farming, ultimately leading to permanent settlements with communities working together to produce enough food to sustain them through cold winters. While they were reluctant to give up their nomadic lifestyles, converting to agriculture from the hunter-gatherer lifestyle gave these people a sense of security that helped to regulate their lives, eventually enabling them to develop the resources to create civilizations.

Meanwhile, other peoples continued to migrate, consuming and eventually causing mass extinctions of much of the fauna in many locations. As their populations continued to increase, they too were forced to settle and farm.

There are eight areas recognized as the world's original agricultural regions: China, Papua New Guinea, South America, Middle Asia, Ethiopia, the Near East, the Mediterranean, and India.

Uncertainties in the Theory

This outlines the generally accepted theory; however, additions to this theory are ongoing—and not all historians accept the theory. Viewpoints on any number of issues vary among scholars.

Although this outline begins one hundred thousand years ago, conservative estimates are that it took hominids some four million years to evolve into modern humans. During most of that time, our ancestral "cousins" were dependent on wild plants and animals for food. Out of such an ancestry, why did some of us, modern *Homo sapiens,* later become farmers?

Some experts suggest that certain qualities inherent in human behavior were conducive to domestication, namely *sedantism, proto-domestication* (recognition of species predisposed to domestication), and *wealth accumulation.* The *deliberate planting of stored seed stock* is also an action ascribed to our species and not typically found in lower primates.

Finally, *high population density* could be a factor that encourages agricultural development. Yet in spite of numerous attempts to produce a model using all these factors to show how agriculture started, these ideas have proven inconsistent and have left experts in disagreement.

For example, to name population density as a cause for the invention of agriculture raises more questions than it supplies answers. Early peoples would have had other options for dealing with their situation. We wonder, why our early ancestors did not kill newborn females, as some modern hunter-gatherers do? Why did they not simply procure greater amounts of abundant wild foods to accommodate their population increase? How do we explain that most protoagricultural hunter-gatherer groups and many farming communities are sparsely populated?

Some historians cite the contrasting lifestyles in Central America, the Yangtze basin, coastal Scandinavia, and the archaic American Southwest to illustrate the inconsistency of the population-density idea. Specifically in America, domestication occurred long *after* a major climatic change but well *before* any significant change in population growth. Available evidence also suggests that an increasing population size only complicates social structure, rather than promoting more agriculture. Yet in spite of these holes in the population-increase hypothesis, some orthodox historians still claim population density is one factor that caused early hunter-gatherers to first begin farming.

The protodomestication hypothesis postulates two types of hunter-gatherers: the *common* hunter-gatherers, whose life has changed little; and the *protofarmer* hunter-gatherers, who managed their plants, developed more complex agricultural practices, and eventually became full-fledged farmers. This idea conveniently supports the cultural evolution theory, with its scenario of Paleolithic protofarmers harvesting large quantities of wild grasses as staple foods.

At present, though, sedantism, protodomestication, wealth accumulation, and population density are all generally recognized as being natural *influences on* rather than *causes of* our agricultural origins.

Migration and *colonization* are prevalent in the historical and ethnohistorical records, but this type of evidence is presently unpopular in archaeology. Where rapid changes in material culture, burial customs, and settlement systems coincide with the evidence of exogenous domesticated flora and fauna, archaeologists need to reconsider worldwide prehistoric migrations. A recognized example of this exists in southern Scandinavia, where it is evident that agriculture spread through colonization leading to indigenous adoption and other types of innovation. Some anthropologists suggest that something beyond a natural or biological influence must have motivated early hunter-gatherers to turn to farming, especially in areas where resources were already abundant.

The fact remains that we do not know if agriculture led to the origin of civilization or if the process toward civilization was already well underway by settled hunter-gatherers when agriculture began. Updates, revisions, and contrary evidence are all needed to eventually arrive at some definitive answers.

There are many "whys" yet to be answered. Because of this, the field is wide open for other theories.

The Reemergence of Agriculture: Alternative Theories

Experts are uncertain about what actually happened to humans before and during the hypothesized ice age. The many old bones and stone artifacts have held some interesting surprises concerning this period. In an attempt to reconcile some of the perplexing evidence found in strata layers, alternative historians have developed two very important theories that are rapidly gaining acceptance by many historians. These theories are known as *catastrophism* and *cultural diffusionism*.

Catastrophism

The theory of *catastrophism* suggests that several global catastrophes occurred at different periods in the remote past, forming geological features of the earth suddenly rather than gradually, through the evolutionary process.

Many historians acknowledge that several catastrophic events occurred around 3,200 years ago, though some suggest that these were not on a global scale. However, these events clearly affected many areas of the world. What caused them is still a point of contention among some experts. Some point to the likelihood of a comet or other celestial body falling to earth and resulting in volcanic disruption with accompanying tidal waves. Geographic evidence supports this idea.

Current research also indicates that similar catastrophic events occurred about 11,500 years ago and earlier, but on a worldwide scale. For example, most scientists accept that a cometary impact was quite possibly what caused the demise of the dinosaurs millions of years ago. If a small comet or large asteroid shower pelted the earth during the past fifty thousand years, such an event could easily have set off a chain reaction of storms, floods, or any number of other destructive natural phenomena. More than two hundred myths and legends from around the world attest to these types of natural disasters. Many climate adjustments occurred from seventeen thousand to five thousand years ago. The earth became extremely cold around twelve thousand years ago and sea levels rose by 325 feet. Any surviving coastal civilizations would naturally have moved to higher ground.

It stands to reason that before crops can be harvested, agricultural tools have to be developed. The grinding of grains also requires at least a rudimentary stone technology. Most evidence for agricultural technology occurs during the upper Paleolithic periods, but in the case of the Levant and other instances, such tool development extends as far back as the middle Paleolithic period. Indeed, evidence of early agriculture has been found dating to 26,000 BC (Solomon Islands); 16,000 to 20,000 BC (Indonesia); around 16,000 BC (Thailand); and 15,000 to 16,000 BC (Egypt). This evidence usually takes the form of tools accompanied by plant parts or residues.

However, around the world many examples of tools required for gathering and processing cereals having been found that predate the beginnings of domestication. There are likely many more examples remaining to be discovered, but ruins of civilization earlier than these dates would be covered in thick layers of sediment or submerged thousands of feet beneath the sea. Reflecting upon these dates, it seems apparent that natural disasters brought a severe halt to agriculture, later to be resumed in conjunction with each flourishing civilization.

The upper Paleolithic period is more richly evidenced with human remnants, as compared to the later lower and middle Paleolithic periods, where only the most durable items (such as stone tools) can be found. Earlier examples of stone tools exist as well; however, most of them are unrecognizable as to their actual function. Plant matter decomposes over time under the influences of natural forces and is therefore lacking in the two earlier Paleolithic phases.

In 1901, a mammoth elephant was found in Siberia, frozen upright with food still in its mouth. Further examination revealed buttercups and other spring plants in its stomach. This could have happened only if the climate had dramatically shifted in a very short time.

It would take some very astute humans to survive the aftermath of the sort of cataclysmic events that have occurred numerous times during the earth's long history. These disruptions permanently destroyed some species and often left harsh and brutal environments. Any human survivors would have had to carry the burden of responsibility for reestablishing civilization. Caves conceivably became shelter for these enduring survivors, who left some of their sophisticated artwork, unusual artifacts and precious seeds as proof of their tenancy. Some of these cave dwellers, unable to reestablish their agricultural practices due to severe weather, would have been forced to revert to a hunter-gatherer-scavenger lifestyle. Other better-prepared survivors may have set sail to foreign lands with whatever tools of civilization they were able to save.

Legends of primitive peoples who survived the cataclysm tell about welcoming the "culture-bearers" who arrived by sea or descended from high mountain peaks. According to written and oral traditions, many primitive peoples were relieved and grateful to have the leadership and direction from these multiracial people from afar.

In many of these instances, the "culture-bearers" came in peace, taught agriculture, and helped organize civilization. The indigenous peoples were so enamored by the extraordinary scientific abilities of these strangers that they not surprisingly revered them as "gods." (Unfortunately, we also have stories of the European colonial conquests for at least the past five hundred years where the "culture-bearers" came only to rob, rape, murder, and dominate the lives of indigenous peoples to the point of cultural destruction, including the loss of health and traditional knowledge.)

Eventually, the civilized survivors of an ancient world would again share the planet with surviving hunter-gatherers and hominids of various types. Those who had reverted to a hunter-gatherer lifestyle after several generations may have suffered a kind of amnesia, having lost the urge to re-create civilization. However, many of these nomadic people preserved stories of how their ancestors once lived in great cities with monumental buildings plated in gold and silver, before the world was destroyed by fire and water, in a time when the days were warm and sunny, where grazing livestock and flowing fields of golden grain provided nourishment.

The ancient civilizations of Sumer and Egypt represent just two of the most recent examples of such fallen civilizations rebuilt by ancient survivors of far older civilizations that have yet to be discovered.

Catastrophism, along with its increasing amount of documented evidence, sheds light on many of the questions previously unanswered in the historical records. It is a theory well supported by scientific discoveries, as well as both oral and written traditions, that helps to explain the many unusual artifacts unearthed from the past that simply don't fit the orthodox timelines or cultural model. It also gives credence to the idea that agricultural practices existed in our remote past.

Cultural Diffusionism

The theory of cultural diffusionism describes the cross-cultural exchange between primitive and advanced civilizations before, during, and after what is termed the "agricultural revolution."

Recent findings in Egyptian mummies of cocaine and tobacco, both believed to have originated in the New World, mark the exchange of goods between the "old" and "new" worlds during the times of the Pharaohs. This is one of the few publicly announced discoveries that show ancient peoples were communicating and trading across vast distances. I have personally examined numerous stelae, stone statues, and carvings throughout South and Central America and Asia depicting Africans, bearded Semitics, and Asians, all of which had to be thousands of years old.

Sweet potatoes have been found in Southeast Asia as well as Africa; to this day we are not certain of their origin. Amaranth, a grain used extensively throughout South America, is the same domesticated species used by some of the most remote Tibetan tribes, who have used the grain long before any outsiders came to visit. Peanuts have a long history in both Peru and China; cacao exists in Mexico and India . . . the list goes on. All of these common intercontinental crops are documented to have existed well before the 1500s.

An abundance of historical literature expresses world travel and trade in ancient times. In addition to artifacts and agricultural products, strong evidence for diffusionism exists in many social and cultural practices, linguistics, and genetic markers.

One of the most popular legends of culture-bearers comes from the Sumerian culture from around 3500 BC. Numerous cuneiform tablets have been excavated from what is now modern-day Iraq. These tablets reveal a detailed account of culture-bearers introducing agriculture and civilization to the Sumerians. This early example of colonization became popular among lay people through the *Earth Chronicles* of Zecharia Sitchin. However, scholars of Sumerian history criticize Sitchin's work because of the author's premise that these Sumerian culture-bearers came from another planet.

Whether one reads the scholarly interpretations of the Sumerian legends by Sitchin, Kramer, Jacobsen, O'Brien, or others, the stories carry the same theme of colonizers from *somewhere else*—whether they are postulated as having come from outer space or a sunken continent or as being evolved hunter-gatherers is beside the point. What is significant is the fact that they came bearing the already established gifts of agriculture and civilization.

The supporting evidence for some of these stories indicates that they have more substance than mere exaggerated myths. The "culture-bearers from elsewhere" subject is repeated with slight variations in legends from the Maya, Inca, Babylonians, Egyptians, Chinese, Indians, and other ancient cultures.

In tracing these legends, with their themes of floods and transplanted agriculture, we find that some of the stories could be relatively recent, while others may stretch back into Paleolithic times or further. Some of these legendary events could reasonably have occurred as far back as forty thousand to fifty thousand years ago.

After surviving the devastating effects of ice, floods, and other environmental extremes, many ancient civilized peoples, through their tenacious will to continue, became heroes or gods, the culture-bearers of the past.

According to legends, men and women of cultural and racial diversity and various statures arrived from the four corners of the earth, descending from mountaintops or arriving by sea to bring the seeds of civilization. They taught the primitive peoples agriculture and created laws. They taught biodiversity so people could work in harmony with the land, rather then merely living off it. They abolished cannibalism and human sacrifice. Grain was a new food for many; for others it was the reintroduction of a food that had been missing for generations. Today, grain universally symbolizes the most sacred food of our ancestors and is used as a tribute to those who brought us from the darkness of primitivism to the light of civilization.

If legendary timelines are accurate, then orthodox timelines need to be reevaluated to acknowledge that man was an agriculturalist for more than just the past ten thousand years of his two-hundred-thousand-year hunter-gatherer existence. Orthodox theories have recently begun to incorporate the idea that some early Paleolithic peoples were protofarmers before the currently defined timeline, as discarding the abundance of this new evidence would make rational scientific thinking appear hypocritical. However, modifying existing beliefs to conform to the evidence without really changing them significantly or genuinely entertaining other possibilities is unfortunately the norm.

In other words, in order to address the issue of agriculture in civilization existing before the accepted ten-thousand- to twelve-thousand-year period, it is fairly easy to keep with conventional theories by saying something like this:

At the beginning of the upper Paleolithic period, around forty thousand years ago, there were some primitive peoples in various parts of the world who were managing animals and plants to such an extent that we can consider them the earliest of agriculturists (protoagriculturists) . . .

As opposed to saying something like this:

Based on all the existing evidence, including research from other countries and historical traditions, from fifty thousand years ago until ten thousand years ago, we have evidence of extraordinary cave artworks, delicate medical operations (cranial surgeries and amputations), astronomical notations, ceramic artifacts, textile and basketry weaving, grinding stones, and writing. All of these are earmarks of civilization, once thought impossible before ten thousand years ago.

This latter approach would leave historians faced with having to explain who on earth these people could have been; how they evolved, or if they evolved at all; where they came from; and why they developed all these striking earmarks of civilization when the majority of the ancient world's population of hunter-gatherers never even came close to establishing civilizations until quite recently? And even then, they did so only because of the influence of already-established civilizations— why not as a process of natural evolution?

In the past ten years, an extraordinary amount of evidence has surfaced that points to cultural diffusion having been practiced in remote times, helping to introduce new foods between civilizations throughout the world. If a group of people specialized in a certain food, herb, or spice, it was often traded or sold to another culture, sometimes thousands of miles away, thus increasing the range and variety of available foods for these people.

Archaeological discoveries of ancient stone statues and carvings thousands of years old revealing many different racial types have been found in areas thought to be isolated from the outside world. Myths and legends exist in almost all traditional cultures regarding the origin of various foods brought from afar in times long past. How long this has been going on no one knows for certain, but it has been going on longer than the ten thousand years of our accepted history of civilized agricultural peoples.

In just the past five years, we have been forced to reevaluate our beliefs about the simple-minded primitive Neanderthals and other early hominids. Although there are no indications of large civilizations and agricultural practice among them, they apparently were not the stereotypical club-bearing cavemen portrayed in our history books. New findings of Neanderthal and Cro-Magnon man reveal advancement well beyond what was originally thought. Both had larger brains than *Homo sapiens* and equal time to evolve, yet both died off and neither ever reached the level of sophistication of modern *Homo sapiens*.

The overall pattern revealed by current discoveries shows civilized human activities extending continually further back into prehistory. Yet with some exceptions, most of these discoveries are still somehow "managed" by keeping them well within the confines of the cultural evolution paradigm. Writing at about the time of the founding of the United States, the eighteenth-century philosopher Jean-Jacques Rousseau wryly observed:

> The falsification of history has done more to mislead humans than any other single thing known to mankind.

More than two centuries later, Rousseau's words ring truer than ever.

An Unfinished Puzzle

Agricultural history has been based largely on the study of seeds and bones that remain in strata for thousands of years without breaking down. It is perfectly natural to assume, based on a scanty fossil record, that our Paleo ancestors consumed large quantities of meat along with the gathering of wild plants. After all, that is what we find with some modern hunter-gatherers, although most include higher quantities of carbohydrates in their diets.

Because there is little evidence in the way of preserved plant matter dating from earlier than twelve thousand years ago, it is often assumed that before that time, all plants consumed by our forbearers were wild roots, leaves, fruits, and wild grasses. After all, the assumption goes, human beings had not yet evolved to the point of agricultural necessity, having existed up to that point in varying states of primitiveness.

The human affair with agriculture and the currently accepted theory of its origin can be likened to a large puzzle: a few of the pieces fit nicely into place—and others are forced into the remaining empty spots, whether or not they actually fit!

The puzzle is far from complete. At this juncture, there is no proof that all humans on planet earth were primitive hunter-gatherers-scavengers before ten thousand or even twenty thousand years ago, and there is plenty of evidence that evolved agricultural peoples existed long before ten thousand years ago.

Today we as "civilized" societies represent the majority of the earth's people, with a minority consisting of nomadic hunter-gatherers still existing in the more remote parts of the world. It is plausible that at different times in prehistory, this trend may have been reversed, with civilized agricultural peoples being the remote minority.

The idea that our present civilization represents the ultimate in evolutionary achievement is a cultural bias that limits our future and ignores some of the evidence from prehistory. Perhaps the rise and fall of great civilizations is an event pattern that has occurred numerous times in prehistory. Before dismissing this idea as mere speculation, consider how often the accepted theories of human and cultural evolution have had to be updated to fit ongoing discoveries. We must remember to consider all the evidence and keep an open mind when confronted with new discoveries.

Some prominent historians believe that as hunter-gatherers, we had plenty of free time to do whatever we wanted, and that it was the heavy toil of agriculture that began our downfall. Some of these same historians also believe that agriculture brought with it all sorts of problems and had an overall corrupting effect on the happy lives of the formerly free-living primitives. But such beliefs are based partly on the observation of modern agricultural practices and some early "slash and burn" practices—not of the biodiverse methods practiced by the ancient peoples of the world. Allowing for the results of sudden earth changes, agriculture was not so much a cause of peoples' demise as some would believe.

When we listen to the ancient sagas and allow their accounts to help provide a coherent context for our scientific strata evidence, we find an increasingly persuasive picture in which ancient civilizations equal to and in some ways more advanced than ours have played a very real part. The constituents of advanced civilizations quite possibly shared this planet with a variety of primates and primitive humans for many tens of thousands of years in cycles of the receding and the reemergence of agriculture.

39
Traditional Ancestral Diets

When considering traditional ancestral diets as a model from which we can draw to improve our own food choices for better health, we must understand that these diets vary considerably according to a host of factors, including soil conditions, cultural habits, changing weather, availability of resources, and others. Despite these smaller variations, we can place traditional diets broadly into one of two categories depending on whether the people who practiced them were *hunter-gatherers*[1] or *agriculturalists*.

Conventional historians assert that the earliest traditional human diets were those of the hunter-gatherers; however, this established theory is now being questioned by a host of alternative historians. Explorers, anthropologists, and other scientists have offered compelling evidence of long-lost agriculturalist civilizations that before their disappearance had reached levels of development equal to or more advanced than our own.

The theory for advanced agricultural civilizations in prehistory parallels challenges to the mainstream theory of cultural evolution, which proclaims a slow evolutionary process from primates to primitive humans who used stone tools and fire, culminating in the first civilizations between 5500 BC and 3500 BC. While this "cultural evolution" orthodoxy has its supporting evidence, its theory is limited by the hypothesis that civilization began about this time and that all prehistoric humans lived as hunter-gathers until about ten thousand years ago, when they began to discover agriculture. The alternative point of view suggests that *both* agricultural and nonagricultural peoples may have coexisted for thousands or even tens of thousands of years—long before the accepted (and more conservative) estimated timeline for the advent of agriculture.

As one explores publications with conventional and alternative perspectives on ancient history, it becomes difficult to avoid the profound realization that we modern humans have been around for a long time and have experienced numerous cycles of catastrophic destruction. Through sheer tenacity and the will to survive, we have repeatedly emerged from the ashes of destruction to rebuild civilization.

Today, many historians blame our agricultural ancestors for the downfall of several civilizations, when the true causes were more likely drought, floods, fire, or any other number of natural phenomena. *Homo sapiens* have lived through ice-age conditions and numerous other periods of setback, somehow surviving them along with primitive humans and a variety of other primates.

Many of the primitive humans of Paleolithic times did not participate in cultural advancement beyond their basic living needs and have survived outside the boundaries of civilization for countless generations. Estranged from urban living, some of these groups of prehistoric hunter-gatherers learned to make and use stone tools and have continued to do so for hundreds of thousands of years. Sometimes their slow-paced development came to an abrupt halt when they were conquered by other hunter-gatherers or by agricultural peoples.

Today in some parts of the world, indigenous tribes of hunter-gatherers continue to exist in much the same way as those of antiquity. At the same time, colonizers from powerful nations continue to seek new lands and peoples to conquer. Things haven't changed that much for the hunter-gatherers, and the "Stone Age" of the past, in some ways, is alive and well today.

Apart from our two categories of traditional peoples, past and present, we can define a third category of humans: one that is growing at a phenomenal pace and may be destined to replace the other two traditional groups altogether. This third category represents an extreme departure from our two natural ancestral dietary traditions, moving to one based on artificial foods. The people in this group use an "imitation diet," which we'll touch upon near the end of this chapter. For now, let's get back to our two ancestral groups and their diets.

Clues from the Past

It is important to keep in mind that anthropological and archaeological conclusions are very often based on hypotheses and conjectures derived only from evidence that conforms to—or is *made* to conform to—preexisting paradigms. Through this exclusive evidence, history is then reconstructed and often presented to the public as though it were fact.

By reexamining this evidence and combining it with other reliable sources, we are able to create alternate theories and arrive at different conclusions from those we have been given. Let's consider the primary means of obtaining supportive evidence, see how it is used to formulate commonly accepted beliefs about Paleolithic dietary history, and realize how these conclusions are not the only interpretations possible.

There are four basic means of obtaining evidence when trying to understand our ancestors' traditional diets; other methods are usually extensions or variations of these four.

1. The analyses of stone tools, animal bones, and charred seeds found in prehistoric sites, mostly in or around lake settlements, hearths, fire pits, and caves.
2. Examinations of a few prehistoric human and other primate specimens, mostly incomplete fragments of skulls and skeletons.
3. Examinations of the world's prehistoric cave and rock art, depicting hunting scenes. This method also includes other art forms, such as pottery and textiles.
4. Cultural comparisons between ancient hunter-gatherers and modern hunter-gatherers. These also include comparative analyses of bones, teeth, and genetics of preagricultural and agricultural peoples to speculate and generalize about their health characteristics as compared to one another.

Each of these examples of evidence, regardless of the context in which they are found, is conveniently placed in the context of a single established theory: the cultural evolution theory. However, all four data collection methods have resulted in additional, anomalous evidence that does not fit the accepted paradigms; such anomalous evidence is often simply discarded.

For example, anthropologists have found human bones and stone tools in North America dating back thousands of years before what they consider the earliest human occupation of this region. Also, many examples of very ancient stone tools have been found throughout the world that show craftsmanship superior to more recent examples. This suggests that stone toolmaking did not always evolve gradually or consistently, as is usually suggested. Agricultural tools, too, have been found in early strata, dating well before the accepted timeline for agricultural origins.

Historical dating is based on the assumption of uniformity, a gradual and consistent depositing of strata over millions of years. This idea of uniformitarianism does not fully consider the evidence for the many global catastrophes that have occurred throughout history, sometimes with effects so devastating that virtually all remnants of civilizations were obliterated. Human relics, bones, tropical plants, dinosaur bones, and any number of other remains have been found mixed in strata dating back millions of years, when each theoretically should have been found in its own particular stratum, far removed from all others. This sort of evidence appears in several parts of the world and clearly proves that nature does not always behave in a consistent, regulated manner.

Nevertheless, for convenience and consistency's sake, I will use the standard dating sequences of human remains and other historical artifacts for purposes of discussion throughout this section.

Lack of plant evidence in strata at some Paleolithic sites seems to indicate that hunter-gathers consumed mostly meat, with few fruits or vegetables, because animal bones were often found in abundance around prehistoric hearths, while plant remains rarely show up in very early strata. However, plants have a much higher decomposition rate than bones or stone tools, and this is the reason we don't find evidence of plant consumption in ancient strata. Pollen samples are often used to obtain scientific data on prehistoric plant matter, but results can vary considerably.

While animal bones and carbonized wild grass seeds found in pre-historic lake settlements seem to indicate that meat and wild seeds were part of the hunter-gatherers' diet, we should not assume that no or few plant foods were consumed just because few flora samples show up in prehistoric strata. Some obvious exceptions to diets including plant consumption would be ice-age sites, where people similar to modern-day Inuit lived and whose environment lacked a climate suitable for plant growth. But while evidence from ice-age settlements is plentiful, these sites do not represent the only lifestyle of early humans, who had to endure changing global conditions over hundreds of thousands of years. Some historians are now suggesting even the *regular* inclusion of cereal grains, both wild and domestic, by prehistoric hunter-gatherers.

For example, we find evidence today of early agricultural tools in several areas of the Near East where groups of robust peoples we call the Natufians once lived.

Of particular interest is the presence of sickle blades, sickle handles, and even some intact sickles. The blades often have a sheen or gloss, which is taken to indicate that they had been used to harvest cereals, either wild or tame. Grinding and pounding equipment, both stationary and moveable, was also abundant. All the equipment for cultivating cereal grains is present in the Natufians' industries, but there is no indication that either plants or animals were domesticated. The Natufian people lived in an area in which wild wheat and barley are abundant today and presumably were abundant at that time.[2]

The Natufians are a good example of grain consumers whose skeletal remains reveal robust health. In fact, most indigenous hunter-gatherers living today include a large quantity of plants in their diets. The assumption that agriculture and the domestication of cereal grains began for the first time in the Neolithic period is tenuous.

While we can no longer deny the regular use of wild grasses by some early hunter-gatherers, we must also understand these early peoples may have had uses for wild grasses other than as food. Examples of charred

wild grasses have been found in Paleolithic sites and are often interpreted (in attempts to support the evolution of cultivated plants theory)
as primitive examples of preagricultural food sources from which later
evolved cultivated cereals. While in some cases this is possible, as a few
Paleo feces have revealed the remains of grass seeds, it is more likely that
this evidence represents the early use of grasses for fuel, baskets, bedding, or any of a range of other purposes commonly found today among
the world's nonagricultural indigenous peoples.

First Farmers, Later Hunter-Gatherers

In the dense Brazilian rainforest archaeologists are shocked to find a
one-thousand-year-old, fifteen-square-mile network of towns and villages that were connected by a system of broad, parallel highways. The
reason researchers were shocked is that the pre-Columbian rain forests
have long been thought to have always been a wild ecosystem unaltered
by humans and occupied by various hunter-gatherer tribes.

The indigenous Xinguano and Kuikuro tribes now living there were
unaware of the accomplishments of their "ancestors" until this discovery. Following are some highlights from news articles:

> Ancestors of the Kuikuro people in the Amazon basin had a "com-
> plex and sophisticated" civilization with a population of many thou-
> sands during the period before 1492. These people were not the small
> mobile bands or simple dispersed populations that some earlier stud-
> ies had suggested. . . . The people demonstrated sophisticated levels
> of engineering, planning . . . in carving out of the tropical rainforest
> a system of interconnected towns making up a widespread culture
> based on farming. . . . The people also altered the natural forest,
> planting and maintaining orchards and agricultural fields.[3]

In reference to the ancient settlement that included raised cause-
ways, canals, and other structures, the article states, "They are organized in ways that suggests a sophisticated knowledge of mathematics,
astronomy, and other sciences."[4]

Current aerial photographs indicate that the entire Amazon forest may have been engineered with settlement mounds, irrigation canals, agriculture, and roads at some time in the distant past. These new findings are literally shattering the "pristine myth" that the Americas, before being "discovered" by Columbus, were an untouched Eden occupied by primitive hunter-gatherers.

It is not known when this massive engineering project took place, but it could have occurred numerous times over thousands of years, each time ending with the lush forest completely engulfing the long-abandoned areas. Excavations at many neighboring South and Central American pyramids reveal a repeating history of building and rebuilding by subsequent settlers.

These discoveries also question the origins of what appear to be wild food plants in the Amazon forest. Perhaps many medicinal herbs and food plants gathered by resident tribes today are but free-running examples of what were once cultivated crops of ancient agriculturists. Dates for other recently discovered agricultural sites in Peru and Bolivia are being pushed back nearly five thousand years as long-standing theories are being challenged.

In the desert of the Supe Valley, near the coast of Peru, lie the remains of Caral, a city that flourished nearly five thousand years ago. Findings reveal a peaceful city of pyramids and homes founded on farming and trade. Spanning thirty-five square miles, Caral all but destroys the theory that civilization was the result of warfare. While discussing ancient agriculture in South America in his book *The Living Fields,* Jack Harlan refers to the views of several other researchers:

> Levi-Strauss (1950) and Lathrap (1968), among others, have suggested that most, if not all, hunter-gatherers in South America are "dropouts" from farming.[5]

In Graham Hancock's seminal work *Fingerprints of the Gods* we find another example of "lost agriculture" in Egypt. On pages 412–13, he refers to Hoffman's *Egypt Before the Pharaohs* and Wendorff's and Schild's *Prehistory of the Nile* when discussing mysteries of "Paleolithic agricultural revolution." Grinding stones and sickle blades used in the preparation of plant foods were found in the Nile Valley and dated to around 13,000 BC.

While this may not be so unusual in and of itself, what makes it interesting is that fishing declined in the area at this time and barley suddenly appeared—just before the first settlements were established. Moreover, hunter-gatherers replaced grinding stones and sickles with stone tools about 2,500 years later. Based on the evidence, Hancock suggests that agricultural practices were established around 13,000 BC in Egypt, but the great Nile floods of 11,000 BC led to the abandonment of agriculture and caused a prolonged relapse to a more primitive lifestyle.[6]

How many other ancient civilizations lost their agrarian-based cultures to an adaptive hunter-gatherer lifestyle? Such may have been the case with the ancient precivilizations of Egypt, China, Mexico, Indus Valley, Sumeria, and others that later reemerged as what now appear to be our "earliest examples" of civilizations.

Sites of large urban developments from antiquity have been found in various areas of inland and coastal regions. Ancient urban peoples clearly used their resources and knowledge of agriculture in harmony with nature to effectively support their growing populations. Some of these cities were comparable with modern cities in size and population, complete with sophisticated waste management systems, drainage, running water, and irrigation canals. The Giza plateau in Egypt contains an elaborate maze of underground tunnels carved out of solid limestone bedrock with precise right-angle turns that stretch for miles. Modern research in this area suggests that these tunnels represent an elaborate irrigation system used to transport water from local rivers to what were once neighboring cities and their agricultural centers. Other records available from these civilizations reveal lifestyles embedded in the advanced sciences of agriculture, astronomy, architecture, and engineering.

These qualities do not appear to have been an evolutionary process; in most cases throughout the world, they rather appear to have been a legacy left by previous civilizations. These and other findings help to prove the capabilities of ancient humans, dispel the "all preagricultural peoples were primitives" theory, and strongly support the notion of culturally advanced people with sophisticated abilities living in prehistory.

Time and again, when discoveries do not support an orthodox theory because that theory would crumble if the controversial evidence were made known, those discoveries have been kept from public awareness. The fact of such a state of "withheld evidence" is undisputable.

Why has so much evidence not supporting accepted theories of human history been dismissed? Raising this question would of course be unnecessary if all the puzzle pieces of history already fit nicely into place—but they don't. Ideally, the world's recognized anthropologists, archaeologists, and historians would assemble, discuss all the evidence available, decide how the information pertains to all possible theories, and present their findings to the public. Until that day, dissatisfied newcomers will need to investigate sites, dredge through archives, run tests, publish their own findings, and speak out to gain credibility for an alternative theory.

When we start to include all the rejected pieces of this extraordinary puzzle, it becomes crystal clear that there is a great deal more to human history and prehistory than conventional theory would have us believe. These rejected pieces are the very information that could help solve life's greatest mysteries. Until all the cards relative to the traditional lifestyles of ancient peoples are placed on the table, we are left with no choice but to seriously entertain the idea of planet-wide coexistence between hunter-gatherers and agricultural peoples in prehistoric times.

Stature and Health among Traditional Peoples

Some anthropologists claim our hunter-gatherer ancestors were taller than the agricultural types—and therefore healthier. The idea of greater height as a barometer of better health is typical of the Eurocentric point of view stemming from early anthropological research. Just as typically, when examined in a global context, both presently and in the fossil record, it is misleading and incorrect. I have personally witnessed robust health among both types of traditional peoples from different parts of the world of varying heights and builds.

Oxygen, carbon dioxide, and radiation levels, among other environmental conditions, vary immensely throughout our past, all likely affecting the conditions of flora and fauna, including hominids. Fossil evidence from Paleolithic times generally shows most flora and fauna to be quite large. Using the "man is an evolved animal" theory, is it so unusual to find larger hominid fossils during Paleolithic times as well? Paleolithic flora specimens appear gigantic as compared to their counterparts, even in the Neolithic period. Fauna specimens of the Pleistocene period, including those of the wooly mammoth, giant sloth, saber-toothed tiger, and giant bear, are much larger than many of the mammals that followed.

Today, many free-ranging, domesticated ruminants are smaller than their wild counterparts, yet they are not less healthy simply because they are smaller and domesticated. Can we unequivocally say that prehistoric megafauna and flora of a particular era were healthier simply because they were larger than the specimens of a later age? Not really. What we can surmise is that many plants, animals, hominids, and humans from a particular time in prehistory differed from many of those that followed, and that each adapted as much as possible and were suitable to the environment of their day.

Just because the cranial capacities of Cro-Magnon and Neanderthal were larger than that of today's human being doesn't mean they were smarter than we are. To assume this would be the equivalent of saying, "All generally tall Germanic peoples are smarter than generally shorter Japanese people."

Many tall traditional peoples have robust health, but so do many short traditional peoples, some averaging less than five feet in height. The agricultural highland Peruvians, for example, are short in stature and healthy, according to the studies and research of Weston A. Price.[7]

Early Western explorers of South America and Mexico were often carried over treacherous mountain terrain for miles on the backs of sub-five-foot-tall Peruvians and Mexicans. These same tiny agricultural people of the Peruvian highlands could run for thirty miles or more, starting at nine thousand feet above sea level, where the air is extremely thin, to coastal regions, and then return the same day with fish they had caught or traded for their ruler's dinner—hardly examples of weak, unhealthy people.

To accurately study the history of stature and health in our ancestors, we would have to include the giant skeletons from the many fossils found throughout the world. In the mid-1800s and up through the early 1900s, many human skeletons ranging in height from seven to eighteen feet were found in North America and around the world. These fossils were excavated from mounds, caves, and many different levels of strata. Some dated back to the Jurassic period, more than 185 million years ago. Newspaper reports, along with many reputable witnesses, attest to the truth of the discoveries—yet none of these unusual fossils have ever been entered into the fossil record.

Some of these skeletons were found with axes and stone tools. Some specimens had even gone through the process of mummification. Were these giants healthier *Homo sapiens* than average-sized *Homo sapiens,* or were they a different species altogether!

Generalizations on health and stature between ancient agricultural peoples and hunter-gatherers based on fossil evidence can be misleading. For one thing, it is not clear how many ancient agriculturists had reverted to the hunter-gatherer lifestyle in prehistoric times, nor do we know how many cycles of agriculture and civilization there may have been in our complex history as *Homo sapiens.*

The possibility of such a reversion process, demonstrated by the modern examples of the Amazonian tribes mentioned earlier—whom scientists once thought had a long history as hunter-gatherers, only to find that their ancestors were agriculturists who developed sophisticated city states—could very well be one of many examples. The Amazon discoveries may be the first examples of what could be a worldwide phenomenon. These findings, in addition to the myths and legends told by many ancient hunter-gatherers and agriculturists, could help to explain the sudden emergence of agriculture in some parts of the world. They would also help to explain the discoveries of domesticated cereals and other crops found in archaeological sites with no wild progenitors and no signs of previous agricultural experimentation.

Does diet play a role in physical stature? Certainly. People who consume dairy products, for example, tend to be taller than nondairy eaters. However, this does not mean that dairy consumers are healthier than those who consume little to no dairy products. Today, people in Western countries are becoming taller but generally eat inferior foods, compared to those of traditional people. Increased stature today is often caused by foods laden with growth hormones and other hormonal stimulants, the result actually being a decline in health correlating with increased height! While diet may affect stature, peoples' heights and hat sizes have little to do with robust health, high intelligence, and longevity.

Defining Traditional Diets

If the theories of human and cultural evolution are reasonably valid, we can accept the idea that our diet should consist of foods our ancestors gathered, hunted, and fished. But what do we really know about these ancestral diets? And how do we know what we know?

With little evidence from our prehistoric ancestors other than some telltale signs from bones and stone tools, much of the available information about traditional diets has been gleaned from studies of various present-day indigenous peoples, who continue to live primarily as their ancestors lived.

However, some of today's indigenous peoples, through the influence of other cultures over time, have added new food sources to their diets, creating a modified version of what their ancestors ate. The introduction of new culinary tastes and experiences by outside cultural influences has been a common practice throughout history and likely prehistory as well. Sometimes new foods have improved the health of the people. At other times, the change has contributed to their demise. Traditional peoples who have incorporated large quantities of modern refined flour, sugar, and processed foods into their diets have experienced a sharp decline in health during the last two centuries.

There are many different opinions on what constituted a preagricultural diet; most of them can easily find scientific evidence to back their theories.

For example, it has been said that our Paleolithic ancestors did not consume dairy products. According to evolutionary theory, it is assumed that dairy products are not incorporated until the onset of agriculture and animal husbandry during the Neolithic period. But we are not at all certain that this is the case. A UPI *Science News* report challenges one such widely accepted notion about the onset of dairy consumption:

> . . . traces of milk some 6,000 years old in Britain, the earliest direct evidence known of human dairy activities . . . "first direct evidence milk was consumed by humans in the early Neolithic, or Stone Age."[8]

Although still fitting the accepted timeline for animal domestication, this report places the use of milk at a far earlier date than previously thought for Britain. People began herding animals earlier than six thousand years ago in the Near East, but the idea of primitive herders being the only humans who had connections with animals—other than hunted prey and the domesticated dog—is an assumption based on a lack of evidence from anything earlier than about twelve thousand years ago. Perhaps the use of animal's milk, like grain domestication, extends much further back into prehistory than the incomplete facts and assumed theory suggest.

With more evidence supporting the existence of Paleolithic agriculture, it is reasonable to assume that animal domestication occurred at an earlier time as well. Could the extensive harvesting of wild grasses by some Paleolithic hunter-gatherers, as noted by researchers and scientists, have been for the purpose of feeding their domesticated livestock? This is highly plausible in that our fossil record for early animal domestication in the Near East includes bones from both wild and domestic sheep and goats. The morphological similarity of modern and ancient sheep and goat bones is so close that even under close examination they are often indistinguishable from each other.

As with the hypothetical "Agricultural Revolution" and the origin of grain domestication, perhaps it is also unwise and far too early in the game to confine animal domestication to an imaginary time period.

Ancestral Nutritional Problems

Due to at least one hundred thousand years of extreme climatic fluctuation, from the late Pleistocene up through the Holocene, about twelve thousand years ago, it is difficult to accurately compare the health of hunter-gatherers and agriculturists in antiquity. Both groups throughout history have experienced periods of abundance, scarcity, and famine, depending on the prevailing climate, geography, and resources.

For example, the early Egyptians, like other past civilizations, faced times of war, famine, drought, and other environmental problems throughout many generations since prehistory. For thousands of years, these people enjoyed a wholesome, varied diet abundant in both plant and animal products. Because of these facts, we cannot simply state, as some have done, that some human fossils revealing signs of ill health resulted from a diet high in grain and low in protein and fat. The analyses of a few or even a hundred mummies or other fossils of ancient peoples from around the world at various times of history is hardly enough to conclude—again, as some have claimed—that all ancient Egyptians or other agriculturists suffered from ill health for the past ten thousand years or more, as compared to Paleolithic hunter-gatherers.

Some historians suggest that because hunter-gatherers were mobile and thought to consist of groups smaller than one hundred, they were less susceptible to the diseases and health problems faced by agricultural civilizations. Small, moving groups tend not to pollute their water supply or attract rodents and insects, all strong contributors of disease in civilization. While this may be true to some degree, it is also known that hunter-gatherers at times endure famine and an insufficient supply of animal protein. When this "meat hunger" occurs, what little amount of meat is available typically becomes rationed. The males who hunt down the food are given priority, while women and children have to subsist on whatever amount remains uneaten, if any remains at all. This lack of protein has been known to last anywhere from several days to weeks for those less fortunate tribe members. Some hunter-gatherers today show signs of malnutrition from protein deficiency.

The notion that "small and mobile is better" is placed into a more

realistic perspective when we consider the knowledge of early agriculturalists. Like those of hunter-gatherers, the sophisticated civilizations
of early agriculturists also had natural medicines to help combat disease.
Both groups had a working knowledge of the medicinal qualities of the
plants and animals in their environment, knowledge that was passed
down through the generations. Herbology, traditional Chinese and
ayurvedic medicines, and numerous other healing systems are contemporary examples of such wisdom that have been passed down through
many generations.

Use of the natural antiviral, antibacterial qualities of herbs and
spices by early agriculturists is also suggested by archaeological records.
The domestication of cats in 9500 BP may have been an effort to control rodents in settled communities. Evidence is accumulating that
points to severe health problems among some groups of ancient hunter-
gatherers during various periods throughout history, not to mention
the taboo subject of cannibalism. These new discoveries are challenging
previously held beliefs, making it unreasonable to assume that hunter-
gatherers possessed superior health over agricultural peoples.

In the present day, the health of some modern agriculturists practicing traditional farming methods far exceeds that of some modern
hunter-gatherers; in other cases, the opposite is true. There is no reason
to suppose the same would not hold true with our ancestors as well.
There are studies showing that some ancient agricultural peoples had
remarkable bone densities and extraordinary life spans.

In other words, civilization is not necessarily a disease-inducing way
of living. Our ancient agricultural ancestors developed ways of handling
the many negatives of a largely populated, less mobile lifestyle, just as
nomadic hunter-gatherers have found ways to cope with their cyclical
environmental changes.

It is quite easy to gather scientific evidence for either the hunter-
gatherers or agriculturalists in order to fit a particular dietary agenda,
such as a low-carbohydrate or low-fat perspective. If we wanted to down-
play the diets of the hunter-gatherers, we could emphasize the long history of cannibalism practiced routinely among some groups until only
recently, as documented by anthropologist Marvin Harris and others.

Many hunter-gatherers have suffered (and still do today) from long-standing parasitic infections. Hunter-gatherers often feed in an area until it is depleted. Their lives can be marked by internal strife, short life expectancy, population control by infanticide, incest, rape, and violence from tribe to tribe. On the other hand, the lifestyles of some agricultural peoples have had their shortcomings as well, with dental caries, arthritis, the practice of genocide, epidemics, and numerous other problems. In fact, the two groups share so many characteristics in common that if we were to swap problems between the two groups, we might very well find that eventually they would both end up with the same problems they had before, albeit with slight variations.

Based on the evidence, what we can safely conclude is that physical and mental health problems occur in both groups of people when nutritional balance is adversely affected by external influences. Comparing the modern diets of both groups is impractical and misleading, because many hunter-gatherers today still maintain a natural diet largely similar to their ancestors' diets, whereas most modern agricultural people in developed areas maintain a diet based on artificial foods. And while it is helpful to understand the functions and behaviors of isolated nutrients in foods, the approach of modern nutritional science is severely lacking in the nutritional common sense and wisdom of our ancestors—both groups of them.

In essence, researchers have not found a specific meat- or plant-based Paleolithic diet that represents an overall example that we could reasonably call "our ancestral diet." Food choices vary considerably within both groups. Staples of insects and monkey brains, for examples, are daily fare for the hunting and gathering Mentawai tribe of Sumatra, while the agricultural Incan descendants living in the highlands of Peru find their sources of nutrition in cuy (a domesticated guinea pig) and cultivated quinoa.

Dr. Weston A. Price has a very balanced perspective on traditional peoples and their diets, pointing out the numerous health benefits of living a natural lifestyle through his studies of traditional peoples throughout the world. Although the diets of the groups of people he studied varied considerably due to climate, environment, and geographic location, Dr. Price was able to show how natural, unrefined foods contribute to robust health. He concluded that it is not a matter of whether a people practice agriculture; rather, it is a question of what essential foods constitute a healthy diet. Among people with ample amounts of nutrient-dense foods, he found better overall health, as contrasted with those lacking in sufficient amounts of these foods.[9]

In the past, as today, people throughout the world lived in widely varying conditions and circumstances. Today some people live in poverty and suffer from numerous nutritional deficiencies while others live afflu-ent lives and still suffer from nutritional deficiencies. The most impor-tant difference between agricultural people of the past and people of the present is that the overwhelming majority of people of the present suffer from "environmental amnesia" and have lost their intimate connection with their natural surroundings, while many people of the past, whether rich or poor, maintained harmony with nature through their food and agricultural practices.

Diet Evolution

From the evolutionary perspective, man's earliest primate ancestors ate a diet of fruits, nuts, leaves, roots, and a small percentage of meat, not unlike modern-day chimpanzees and apes. These primate "ancestors" were said to have evolved to the point of being able to use stone tools about 2.5 million years ago. Stone tool usage represented the beginning of technology and led to an increase of meat and fat consumption in the form of small, easy-to-pursue animals. Large quantities of animal bones found at some archaeological sites, along with stone tools from this period confirmed regular consumption of prehistoric game animals.

This period of increased meat consumption coincided with an increase in brain size and is considered an important side effect of consuming nutrient-dense food in the form of animal fat and protein. However, the increase in brain size could also have been caused by the need to utilize the brain more in order to hunt prey. Increased brain size gave hominids a new branch among the primates on the ancestral tree 1.8 million to 500,000 years ago. Then, the hominid *Homo erectus* appeared with a fully functional brain that gave him the capacity to hunt big game.

While other hominid species appeared throughout these long periods, it was not until about two hundred thousand years ago that modern humans made their appearance. This period also coincided with the first evidence of cooking. By cooking their food, modern humans increased the available energy content of plant foods, especially complex carbohydrates (wild grasses, tubers, and roots), which, in combination with big game animals, supposedly contributed to another leap in the evolution of brain function.

After about 190,000 years of continuous hunting, fishing, gathering, scavenging, and cooking, modern humans began to farm. Hunter-gatherers presumably had hunted the megafauna to extinction in some parts of the world. Lack of available prey then led to the need to farm the land.

Many hominid species in the evolutionary tree are not mentioned, and some of the dates vary among historians; what you have just read is a simple outline of a widely accepted—though unproven—theory of diet evolution.

The Neanderthals

Although evolutionists do not believe humans evolved from chimpanzees or apes, they do believe that humans and chimps have a common ancestry. Characteristics associated with being human include loss of thick body hair, bipedal movement, tool- and weapon-making, use of fire, creation of clothing, and language development. Each is thought to have evolved along with our ancestors. Evolution, rather than representing a ladder leading upward in a straight line, is better understood as a tree with many hominid branches that include *Homo erectus* and *Homo sapiens*. All hominids, relatively, are "cousins" that somehow, through millions of years of mutations, eventually culminated in modern humans.

However, DNA analysis of Russian Neanderthal remains dating back twenty-nine thousand years reveals "that modern humans are not related to Neanderthals,"[10] disproving conventional scientific opinion. Instead, this research indicates, Neanderthals represent a completely different species of hominid. Additional tests on Neanderthal remains found in a cave in Germany show the same results. Both studies imply that Neanderthals "don't have the diversity to encompass a modern human gene pool."[11]

Another theory suggests that Neanderthals didn't have the technological means to survive the increasingly harsh winters of the ice age. One has to wonder about this theory, when evidence for Neanderthal intelligence has been well documented. They buried their dead in specific astronomical directions, showed signs of artistic creativity, knew how to make fires, lived in caves, and ate a diet consisting exclusively of meat. The same theory suggests that modern hairless *Homo sapiens* had what it took to survive because they could make throwing spears, fishing nets, and fur clothing. It is difficult to believe that Neanderthals, with their developed brains, could not have figured out these basic survival skill as well. Still, however, the experts continue to debate the role of Neanderthals in their social and genetic relations to modern humans.

Guess Who's Coming to Dinner?

What really caused the demise of the Neanderthals, wiping them from the fossil record around thirty thousand years ago? Human bones found at some Neanderthal sites strongly indicate the regular practice of cannibalism. This should not surprise us, since our human history right up into recent times includes numerous examples of cannibalism.

Anthropologist Marvin Harris writes about the history of cannibalism. In *Good to Eat* Harris states:

> When first contacted by Europeans, the peoples of New Guinea, northern Australia and most of the islands of Melanesia, such as the Solomon Islands, the New Hebrides and New Caledonia, practiced some degree of warfare cannibalism.[12]

Later on, while discussing other issues related to diet and lifestyle, Harris makes a point to say that not all Polynesian islanders practiced cannibalism.

All three of the Polynesian groups that practiced warfare cannibalism also lacked the highly productive agriculture and fisheries which characterized the politically centralized Polynesian islands.

A few agricultural peoples also practiced cannibalism, but cannibalism tended to predominate among peoples lacking centralized governments and the accompanying agricultural systems.

It is interesting to note that in the tribal lore of modern tribes who practiced cannibalism, there is a common belief that consuming another person, be it conquered warrior, relative, or other, endows the consumer with the powers or energies of the person consumed. The consumption of a powerful opponent, then, means more power and energy for the consumer. While this may sound barbaric or disgusting to our sensibilities, many primitive and civilized peoples perceived nature and food of any kind as energy.

There are a few recorded examples of cannibalism among agricultural peoples as well. One of these describes the Aztecs, who first sacrificed their victims to the gods before consuming them, with only the upper classes and priests allowed to partake of the ghastly feast.

While the reasons for consuming human flesh may differ between meat-hungry tribes and civilized cannibals, the basic shared belief of obtaining the strength and power of a competing rival may very well be the reason for the demise of the Neanderthals and other "robust and powerful" hominids in the past. With the onset of the ice age and competition for food between "modern humans" and Neanderthals, including the history of cannibalism among both, perhaps desperate times led to desperate acts. Perhaps humans outnumbered Neanderthals, or maybe early hunter-gatherers considered a powerful Neanderthal a prize meal, if they could capture one.

In light of new discoveries in anthropology and archaeology, it is increasingly difficult to define the character of early human and other hominid species. Some evidence confirms the barbaric and primitive qualities that previously defined prehistoric cave men. Other evidence reveals a fully conscious and intelligent species, not unlike modern humans at their best.

A basic problem with the orthodox view of ancestral Paleolithic diets is that it is based on a series of assumed progressions from nonhuman primates that eventually culminate with modern humans, yet an actual link between these primates and humans cannot be shown to exist. This is also the case with *Homo erectus* and Neanderthal: there is no genetic link that proves modern humans actually evolved from any hominid species. Without such a link, diets of other species need not be a basis for human dietary practices, modern or ancient.

Even though some of these hominids used fire and stone tools and competed with modern humans in hunting, the simple truth is that ancient humans (hunter-gatherers and agriculturalists) are the only true ancestral examples we have with which to accurately assess human dietary history. It is difficult to say whether or not diet had any influence in making us human; however, we can definitely say that it played a major role in the establishment of civilization and human development. And diet may very well be the most distinguishing factor between our hunter-gatherer and agricultural ancestors.

The Hunter-Gatherers

Some historians think that prehistoric humans were parasites of the land because they would diminish both plant and animal resources before moving on to their next habitat. However, new discoveries are being made almost daily that shed further light on the lives of prehistoric peoples, including Neanderthals, revealing extraordinary abilities as exhibited in their astronomy, art, pottery, and textiles. Evidence of mummification indicates knowledge of preservation and elaborate burial rituals.

Up until recently, we have associated all these activities with civilization, not with primitive hunter-gatherers. Is it possible to have all these earmarks of civilization and no agriculture? Why did these prehistoric hunter-gatherers take so long to cultivate plants and domesticate animals? Some experts of cultural evolution now say that hunter-gatherers have, to some extent, been using agricultural techniques all along.

If what these new findings suggest is true, then we have numerous examples of prehistoric hunter-gatherers that were advanced in some areas that even many modern hunter-gatherers have yet to reach. For modern hunter-gatherers, little has changed and their lifestyle appears much the same as that of their ancient ancestors. It seems as though evolution has ceased for them, and that their culture remains confined to the simple tools and materials necessary to survive the elements.

The fact that examples still exist in parts of the world is remarkable, considering the extremely long time spans attributed to the evolutionary process and the intrusions into their territories by civilizations throughout history. How much longer hunter-gatherers will be able to continue living as they do remains to be seen. Will they disappear, like Neanderthal and Cro-Magnon? Both of these prehistoric peoples were supposedly more robust than agricultural peoples and they both had hunter-gatherer lifestyles and diets. How did the comparatively frail human with little body hair, survivor of an ice age and the crowning achievement of hominid evolution, come to outlive the other *Homo* specimens?

The answer we have been taught to accept is based on the limited view that human culture developed in a mechanical way through the use of stone tools and other material basics. Moreover, adherents of the cultural evolution theory inaccurately assume that current hunter-gatherers represent the only living examples of what humans were like before ten thousand years ago!

The hunter-gatherers have never lost their original primal instincts for survival. Today there are people from this group who know of agriculture but prefer to maintain their nomadic lifestyles. Tens of thousands of years of hunting would naturally hone one's skills, especially when confronted with predators competing for food. Lacking the speed or agility of the lion, for example, the knowledge of what, when, and where a lion hunts is something these ancestors would have learned at an early age.

Having such close ties to the environment also allows the hunter-gatherer to observe animals' relationships to plants and develop various uses for those plants through continuous sampling. This, in turn, leads to the development of natural medicines.

Knowledge of plants and animals is a commonly recognized skill of hunter-gatherers; it is this close relationship with nature that modern-day hunter-gatherers share with their ancient ancestors. Nature has been and remains their teacher.

The Paleolithic Diet Riddle

The following statements are some of the most commonly expressed opinions on traditional preagricultural diets by experts in the fields of paleontology and anthropology:

- Early Paleolithic man had a diet much like other forest-dwelling primates. This would be similar to what chimpanzees eat today and includes mostly fruits, some other plants, and small amounts of insects and rodents.
- The diet of the early hunter-gatherers consisted of about 80 percent gathered foods, including shellfish, eggs, plants, and about 20 percent meat.
- Man was a gatherer-scavenger; his diet consisted of mostly wild roots and other plants, occasionally supplemented by small amounts of scavenged animal flesh left by predatory animals or taken from them when possible.
- Early man's original diet was based on fish, seafood, and other marine life until he was forced inland from coastal regions by rising sea levels, where he learned how to hunt game.
- The diet of early man was mostly meat, up to 80 percent or more, derived from hunting game.

If we were to create a multiple-choice question asking which of the above was the diet of our Paleolithic ancestors, the answer would have to be "all of the above"!

The reason for such diversity in opinions on early ancestral diets is that evidence has been found to support them all. Naturally, as more evidence accumulates the theories are revised and updated, but current evidence shows there are a variety of regional diets for the early and modern hunter-gatherers. Based on this evidence, some of these early diets were healthy and supplied more than adequate nutrition for people, while other diets did not. Obviously, lush, tropical, coastal environs could provide a healthy diet of abundant plant foods with moderate amounts of animal products, whereas arctic dwellers would derive most of their nutrition from mammals and seafood and with less plant foods.

Those who toe the party line of cultural evolution persist in the belief that hunter-gatherers and agricultural civilizations did not exist side by side in prehistory. They also often glamorize hunter-gatherers as being taller and with superior health as a result of their nomadic diet, as compared to the much "later" agricultural peoples.

Aside from the fact that some of the evidence used to compare these two categories of peoples is from the remains of nonhuman primates, there is still no consensus on a particular diet for our hunter-gatherer ancestors, nor is there likely to be one. Not only that, it is simply untrue that health declined with the introduction of agriculture. Agriculture and animal domestication alone had nothing to do with the decline of health in humans. There are numerous examples where agriculture improved the health of people by introducing a wider variety of nutritional resources and reliable sources of protein foods.

How long humans have been in a state of declining health cannot be accurately determined through the study of fossil evidence alone. Many as yet unknown factors continue to haunt our past. What can be determined are the observable results of the past two hundred years of environmental destruction from chemical agriculture and processed foods on the health of humanity.

It is true that some anthropologists have supported the claims of "preagriculture health superiority," but it is just as true that not all anthropologists and experts in the field agree with each other. Harvard anthropologist Ofer Bar-Yosef writes:

Natufian skeletons of the Levant represent robust and healthy individuals.[13]

From this same source, we have:

A number of seminar participants (Keeley and Bar-Yosef, among others) did suggest that the most extreme forms of population pressure leading to skeletal pathologies would be unlikely to be related to domestication. . . .[14]

Several diet gurus have suggested that grain domestication was the deciding factor in the decline of health after hunter-gatherers "transitioned" to agriculture, and therefore, that grains (carbohydrates) are best reduced or eliminated completely for optimum health. This idea is often rationalized by claims that our hunter-gatherer ancestors did not eat grain and were healthier because of it.

This is patently untrue: it is now well known among anthropologists and archaeologists that many early preagricultural peoples harvested large stands of wild grains, and it is believed that these grasses served as a regular staple in prehistoric hunter-gatherer diets. Today we know that these wild grains are suitable only for grazing animals; the domesticated versions are the ones with high nutritional content and when properly prepared, are an important source of human nutrition. Nevertheless, it is still believed that these large stands of harvested wild grains played a substantial part in many Paleolithic diets, particularly those of the Near East.

It has also been proved that when sustainable agriculture is practiced, including biodiversity along with other ecologically sound methods of animal husbandry, the people thrive. These were the original methods of agriculture, some of which are still practiced today by the Quiché Maya and the Incan descendents in the highlands of Peru and elsewhere among modern-day, natural agriculturists. Biodiversity in agriculture and animal husbandry can provide additional varieties of nutritious foods that actually improve health.

Ancient Ecoagriculture

The understanding of cosmic cycles was a common theme among many ancient peoples, as were biodiversity and other methods of sustainable agriculture. Because of this, the food produced and consumed by these people living in harmony with nature would have been of a much higher quality (and thus nutritionally superior) to the highly processed food of mono-agriculture systems today.

Our urban populations are nourished mainly on imitation foods devoid of health-promoting properties. We call this "progress" and rationalize it by the needs of a rapidly expanding population, yet the "progressive" methods used in chemical agribusiness to improve on nature are shortsighted and have led to severe degradation of the planet's natural resources. Civilizations of antiquity used everything that was natural, in stark contrast to today's world, where we create toxic plastics, Sheetrock, and synthetic clothing materials, thereby creating disharmony within and between our environment and ourselves.

The great civilizations of antiquity were agricultural and pastoral. Most of these civilizations used a wide variety of foods for daily consumption when environmental conditions were stable. The most common dietary links to all of the great civilizations of the world were found in their basic choices of foods and how they were used. All grew grain and an abundance of plant foods and raised various animals with which to prepare their meals.

Archaeological evidence suggests that ancient peoples knew the importance of biodiversity and the nutritional balance of proteins, fats, and carbohydrates. Ethnobotanist Edgar Anderson explained that there are ample instances from South and Central America that show that both ancient and modern agricultural peoples had individual gardens, which included vegetables, herbs, a bee yard, a fruit orchard, a dump heap, a compost heap, and a few domestic animals for food. Plants were isolated from each other by intervening vegetation so that pests and diseases could not spread from plant to plant, and everything was conserved. Even mature plants were buried between the rows when their usefulness was over.[15]

Evidence for worldwide trade of foods and other goods among ancient civilizations is also increasing. These trade routes increased the varieties of foods and affected more than only agricultural peoples: many newly introduced foods adapted to semiwild states in forests and jungles and are now regularly consumed by modern-day hunter-gatherers. One striking example may be the many varieties of medicinal plants, fruits, and other foods found in the Amazon jungle. Current evidence strongly suggests that this vast jungle was once engineered and occupied by agriculturists. One wonders how many of the useful plants and animals currently found there were introduced thousands of years ago by early agriculturists.

The Mayan peasants in the Chiapas region of Mexico are often considered "unproductive" by large agricultural companies because they produce only about two tons of corn per acre, but the other foods produced through natural farming methods on that same acre can amount to as much as twenty tons. It has also been calculated that their farm incomes would be reduced by a factor of three if they didn't use biodiverse methods of farming.

In Thailand, a home garden can contain up to 230 species of plants. African home gardens often include fifty species of trees with edible leaves, and while Nigerian home gardens comprise only 2 percent of total Nigerian farmland, not too long ago these individual home gardens produced almost half of the agricultural output of Nigeria by using the same natural methods as the Thais and other traditional cultures.

Many ancient agriculturists not only concerned themselves with ecology, they also developed brilliant uses of what today would be considered useless land for farming. China, Peru, and Mexico made use of steep, rocky hillsides through a method of farming called *terraced agriculture*. Mountain streams were diverted to irrigate layer upon layer of terraces, sometimes extending thousands of feet above sea level. These terraces produced (and still do today) large quantities and varieties of grains, beans, and vegetables. The Aztecs of Mexico created floating gardens in the swampy areas of Lake Texcoco by piling rich earth from the lake bottom onto rafts made of weeds. These raft gardens would eventually be anchored to the lake bottom by the roots of the plants and trees planted on them. Large quantities of food were produced on these island gardens, all without chemicals or harm to the environment.

While the ecological crises of today that are associated with farming are caused primarily by the environmentally devastating use of monoculture and other unsound farming methods from industrial agribusiness, many of the ecological problems of the past were caused largely by environmental factors.

Granted, there is ample evidence for agricultural devastation in ancient history. One example is the slash-and-burn method practiced by some agriculturists and hunter-gatherers. Environmental destruction caused by human need for sustenance was not uncommon with both groups of people in varying degrees. However, these methods were not the only ones used by these groups in the past or the present. Using our modern, environmentally destructive agricultural methods as a basis for comparison for all ancient hunter-gatherers or agriculturists is extremely inaccurate and does not take into account the sustainable methods of growing food practiced by many of our ancient agricultural ancestors, who were able to nourish large urban populations of hundreds of thousands of people with natural, whole foods.

The fact that the ancients cooperated successfully with nature while possessing advanced technology is cause for deep reflection. Defining life through the science of nature in large urban civilizations, an accomplishment unknown to twenty-first-century *Homo sapiens,* does not mean conflict will not arise from external influences or even internal strife. But think how today, with less effective methods, we live with the problems of hazardous wastes, poor food distribution for current population needs, and the threat of global warming.

Many traditional peoples throughout the world still practice the old ways of agriculture and their land has long been producing and thriving. Unlike the denaturing processes that we use on our modern food products, ancient food technology included natural processing methods of pressing, grinding, fermenting, salting, smoking, and other storage methods still used today in many parts of the world by traditional peoples.

The ancients chose, grew, and harvested their foods according to nature's cycles. They adapted to tastes through natural preparation methods according to the needs of their environment. They wisely planned their waste management, drainage canals, and food production—right down to what ended up on the table. Food was a very important part of their daily lives. It played an important role in all scientific and religious beliefs and was treated with reverence and respect. For our own health and that of future generations, it is imperative that we integrate similar methods of cultivation on a global scale.

Who Do We Think We Are?

The term *modern humans* is often used by historians to describe our ancient *Homo sapiens* ancestors who appeared on the evolutionary scene around two hundred thousand years ago. This is a generally accepted timeframe for when humans resembling those of today began their long, gradual path toward civilization.

However, it is often suggested that primitive hominids were well on their evolutionary path to becoming modern humans as far back as five hundred thousand years ago. The theory that nonhuman hominids evolved through mutations into *Homo sapiens* is based on scanty fossil records and is steeped in controversy. What is indisputable is that nonhuman hominids did coexist with the earliest humans and their alleged relatives, *Homo erectus,* Neanderthal, and Cro-Magnon.

As mentioned above, two cultural groups of modern humans are recognized as having existed within the past two hundred thousand years. The first group, who according to most anthropologists are the first and only cultural examples of Paleolithic humans, are hunter-gatherers. The second group represents agricultural and pastoral peoples, who supplement their cultivated foods with hunted and gathered foods from the wild.

These two groups of people represent the only nonape, nonmonkey specimens of hominids alive today, with the exception of the elusive giant hominids, about which we know little, who live in the deep forests of the Pacific Northwest, inaccessible mountain regions, and a few other remote parts of the world.

Hunter-gatherers and agriculturists, while anatomically alike, differ in their cultures and dietary traditions. Agriculturists are thought to have evolved from hunter-gatherers about ten thousand years ago when the domestication of plants and animals are thought to have first begun. Recent discoveries suggest that this "guesstimated" evolutionary timeline is way off the mark and that agricultural peoples have existed along with hunter-gatherers for a much longer period than the ten thousand years allotted. A print of a shoe sole has been found in Triassic rock in Nevada dating from 213 to 248 *million* years ago. Another example reveals *human* footprints—not those of an ape or missing link—preserved alongside those of a dinosaur.[16] These examples have yet to be challenged effectively by any Paleoscientist or anthropologist.

What are we to make of this unusual evidence? Is it too much of a stretch to suggest that these particular anomalies were isolated occurrences made by a time traveler from the future? Or could these tracks be from highly evolved humans who coexisted with cave men and dinosaurs? What if the methods used to date these tracks are highly inaccurate, and the tracks are actually from a more recent period, say, ten thousand to fifteen thousand years ago?

The possibilities for explanation are endless—yet there are too many other examples like these to ignore them all, and addressing these anomalies by denial or by discrediting the individuals who bring them to our attention does little to further our understanding. For numerous examples of evidence pertaining to human existence in prehistory I strongly suggest reading *Forbidden Archeology* and *The Hidden History of the Human Race* by Cremo and Thompson.[17]

Did a few small bands of hunter-gatherers from different parts of the world evolve beyond all other hominids and convert to farming a mere ten thousand years ago? A hypothesis held by the orthodox view is that agriculture was established by small bands of hunter-gathers who had depleted their regional food supplies. These people then introduced it to others, and it spread. Meanwhile, in about seven other parts of the world, similar situations occurred.

Many historians hold to the "small bands of hunter-gatherers" part of this theory, but they also believe there would have been ample supplies of game and other resources in the regions where agriculture began when it did, and therefore suggest that there would not necessarily have been a need for agriculture. But why, with all those resources available, would they have then turned to farming?

A theory based on evidence from Scandinavia suggests that there was colonization by other people. It is suggested that these colonists were other bands of hunter-gatherers who might have been advanced in their own protoagricultural experience and experiments. These groups could have practiced some seed planting or basic harvesting techniques. It is assumed that the spread of agriculture occurred with an increase in the populations of the original agricultural groups. Once agriculture was established, we learn, it led to increased fertility, which in turn created an increase in population and greater dependency on agriculture.

Were the majority of Paleolithic peoples so well supplied with edible flora and fauna that they didn't need to convert to agriculture ten thousand years ago? Or is it possible that the road to agriculture was not a slow, gradual evolutionary process instigated by a few groups of imaginative hunter-gatherers after all? The genesis of agriculture is still highly disputed by many historians.

Education as a Factor of Civilization

As an animal, man is the most plastic, the most adaptable and the most educable of all living creatures. Indeed, the single trait that alone is sufficient to distinguish man from all other creatures is the quality of educability—it is the species character of *Homo sapiens,* according to British-American anthropologist Ashley Montague.

The differences between human and other primate intelligence are that humans possess discernment, vision, and determination when faced with life's challenges. These qualities enable us to creatively work out problems by using our brains beyond the basic level of primate instinct. Using fire and creating clothing are two basic examples of human ingenuity that apes and chimpanzees have not achieved.

Based on current research, the earliest humans and Neanderthals shared these fully developed brain qualities, as did Cro-Magnon, though until recently they were considered illiterate primitives with still much to learn. For some unknown reason, Neanderthal and Cro-Magnon would not survive long enough to utilize their brain capacity to the extent of modern humans.

We are told that *Homo sapiens* evolved "because they had reasons to evolve." These reasons are generally presented as a series of accidents, happenstance, mutations, and various other ways of describing how we developed from primitive to civilized people. Were language, writing, agriculture, metallurgy, and all the other earmarks of civilization really accidental discoveries? Or were they sudden brainstorms by evolving and insightful cave men and women?

For that matter, if the world was populated with primitive cave people with fully developed brains, why is it that only a small percentage of them evolved to the point of agricultural awareness in only a few places in the world? Why didn't the rest of the world's populations evolve as well?

The fact is that many groups of hunter-gatherers never evolved at all beyond their original states, and this was not due to being isolated from those who had so evolved. One would think that after a good five hundred thousand years (or at least two hundred thousand years) of hunting, gathering, and scavenging, *all* modern humans would have finally evolved from simple stone tool usage to a more settled agricultural lifestyle, especially if we are to believe that nutrition played a role in this development and that agricultural awareness and civilization in general was a process of evolution.

Research has shown that both apes and chimpanzees can learn how to paint pictures and communicate with sign language; these are two things they wouldn't do in their natural habitat, yet clearly they do have the necessary intelligence to learn these things. If prehistoric hunter-gatherers had all the necessary intelligence to evolve to the point of modern civilization, why did it take almost two hundred thousand years for them to do so?

There are several theories that suggest answers to this question. One is that there was no reason to evolve from a leisurely life of hunting and gathering with abundant available resources. Another reason is that early humans evolved in stages and developed only what was necessary for daily living. For example, stone tools were essential for hunting and butchering animals. Eventually pottery was needed to hold and transport water, so someone somehow came up with the idea of pottery and the use of ceramics . . . and so forth, right up through the invention of smelting copper and iron.

Let's go back to the apes and chimps for a moment. If they had the intellectual capacity to learn how to paint pictures and communicate with sign language for millions of years, why didn't they eventually evolve to do it naturally? The answer "no need to" would certainly make sense, because they have no need to do so now, either. But let's see where this reasoning leads. Given that humans have had the intellectual capacity to evolve at a rapid rate, create civilizations, and practice agriculture for half a million years yet didn't, can we use the same reasoning to say that we had no need to create civilizations while we still existed in small, communal bands of hunter-gatherers? And if this is true, then why did a few select groups of people throughout the world "evolve" to create agriculture and civilizations, while most did not evolve at all, relatively speaking?

Nutritional differences, hunting practices, reproduction and population pressures, settlements, the use of stone tools, environmental changes, social pressures . . . some historians say these are responsible for the advancement of civilization. These factors are doubtless critical aspects that are associated with and contribute to civilization—but what actually motivated certain humans to literally leap forward while others remained as they were? We have already discussed the issue of ample wild food resources in areas where agriculture began, so there doesn't seem to be a need to learn how to domesticate crops and animals or develop civilizations. In the development of civilization, however, *education* is intertwined within the social fabric of human relationships.

Illiteracy is a common problem in our modern world. We are faced with the unfortunate situation where some children do not have educational resources. Other children and adults are often faced with educational challenges for different reasons. And while proper nutrition plays a major role in brain and nervous system health, many uneducated children and adults simply lack the guidance from qualified teachers to lift them from their ignorance to a point where they can read and write. It is likely that most humans, were they raised without teachers and education, would remain illiterate their whole lives. There are many unfortunate examples of people living this way throughout the world.

In other words, humans from an early age need teachers, experienced educators who often become role models, leaders, and guides in order for civilization to progress. Some people are easy to teach, while others represent more of a challenge and require extra time and patience. Our traditional sources (oral, written, and legendary) of history and prehistory suggest that many of our primitive ancestors were taught the basics of agriculture and civilization by experienced teachers. Perhaps this was an experiment, similar to modern educators teaching chimpanzees how to paint and communicate today.

Even though many prehistoric hunter-gatherers did not advance to the point of civilization, it doesn't mean they didn't continue to learn from each other and whomever and whatever they encountered in life. For them, much of their education and learning experience came from the absorption and assimilation of the natural world through the direction of a shaman, medicine man, or other spiritual teacher. This form of leadership is common among modern bands of hunter-gatherers and may have been part of many Paleolithic groups as well. However, sophisticated agricultural practices and other earmarks of civilization are not a part of their education. This would tend to validate the evidence of our traditional sources, which suggest that civilization and agriculture were handed down from qualified teachers to selected peoples.

On the other hand, paleoanthropologists and archaeologists are persistent in hanging on to the human and cultural evolutionary model when explaining the beginnings of preagricultural peoples. Orthodox scientists disregard the oral traditions of many modern hunter-gatherers that claim origins from ancient, agriculturally based civilizations destroyed by cataclysmic events.

Bertrand Russell could easily have been describing the tenacious hold of the "cultural evolution" idea and studious disregard of such ancient oral traditions when he wrote:

> The fact that an opinion has been widely held is not evidence whatever that it is not utterly absurd.

Similar stories of this type of ancient heritage can be found around the world today among all types of traditional peoples. Gradually more kernels of truth are emerging from these legendary stories as new discoveries are being made, corroborating the idea that the great civilizations of the past were fully formed and show little signs of an evolutionary process from the onset.

We know that they left either oral or written traditions that describe their lives. We don't know how ancient civilizations originated, and so we blindly accept the conventional theories as answers. The decomposition of natural materials, which was all our agricultural ancestors had, may be part of the reason why we find so few traces of their history before 10,000 years ago. Furthermore, if conventional scientific paradigms fail to acknowledge the evidence for the advanced civilizations that existed tens of thousands of years ago, how can scientists claim to know what occurred *millions* of years ago in Precambrian and Cambrian times? The truth is that we really do not know with any certainty.

Unlike with hunter-gatherers, who are mainly content with a lifestyle similar to that of their ancestors, the agricultural lifestyle and diet have changed considerably within the last few hundred years. Most urban and rural humans are now so far removed from the precepts of their ancestral heritage, it appears the stage has been set for an ultimate showdown between man and nature. Greed, arrogance, and strife have become the distinguishing characteristics of twenty-first-century *Homo sapiens*. Refined foods with their artificial additives contribute to unprecedented health problems, and forced growing methods have adversely affected agricultural conditions and ecological balance throughout the planet.

Meanwhile, we ourselves have become addicted to constant entertainment and other distractions that suppress creativity and spiritual awareness. While we may have prevailed through our intelligence as the majority in developing certain technologies, most us have become oblivious to rational thought.

How do we reverse this destructive "cultural" trend? Could we adopt a hunter-gatherer diet and lifestyle and live a life devoid of technology and distraction? No, we have come too far for that. And it wouldn't work anyway, as this lifestyle could not support our current population. We would very quickly decimate our food supply. Furthermore, the hunter-gatherer lifestyle is not conducive to progress and intellectual advancement, as has been shown by more than two hundred thousand years of continuous repetition around a stone tool technology.

While agricultural technology has not been properly focused, this is not to say that science and technology haven't helped us better understand the elemental nutrients in food. Rather, it is that every attempt to improve real, natural food has been unsuccessful. Today's nutritional science lacks traditional wisdom and fails to acknowledge the importance of food *quality*. Its agenda is geared to support large food corporations that have little interest in health.

With profit-only goals, these corporations buy science in order to support the kind of technology that creates artificial and highly processed foods, emptied of the ingredients essential to sustain our species. Homogenization, pasteurization, growth hormones, steroids, synthetic vitamins, preservatives, and genetic modifications are some of the facets of modern technology that have failed to improve the food our agricultural ancestors brought to the table.

In every instance where modern Western culture-bearers have introduced their food, which indigenous peoples know as "white man's food," the people's health has declined. By contrast, when our ancient ancestral culture-bearers introduced new foods and farming methods to other cultures throughout the world, the recipients thrived. To this day, the peoples who use traditional foods and natural agricultural practices do well. It stands to reason that these simple, basic ancestral foods of traditional agriculturists must be the proper nutrition for civilized mankind as well.

One would think that with all our scientific knowledge, we would have improved on the more than ten thousand years of traditional dietary practices—but we haven't. Perhaps this is because traditional foods cannot be improved.

Ancient China and India are two examples of traditional cultures with a very sophisticated understanding and long history of food as nourishment and food as medicine. In many ways, their holistic food science is far superior to our modern, left-brain methods of nutrition analysis. Modern nutritional science has done little to solve the problems of malnutrition and obesity, either in the "developed" nations or "third world" populations. What it has done is to contribute greatly to the hundreds of extreme and absurd dietary fads so prevalent today, which in turn have done little more than create greater confusion and ill health.

One can imagine future residents of planet Earth, twenty thousand or more years from now, uncovering traces of artificial buildings and other examples of today's civilizations—perhaps an intact package of preservative-laden pastry. What will they think? Will they recognize a connection with this evidence and the demise of civilization?

The Interconnection of Science and Religion

All was not peace and love with the ancients. Indeed, human history as we know it was not exempt from periods of violence and warfare. However, some sort of paradisiacal "golden age" is mentioned in nearly every ancient culture. Architecture of past civilizations reflected nature's designs and used materials from the surrounding landscapes. Ancient peoples were aware that the frequencies of energy in nature flowed in constant, recurring cycles. Ancient civilization itself synchronized with the natural world to the extent that religion was their science—and science their religion.

Our ancestors equated nature with the divine in all they did and had a deep understanding of the interconnectedness of physical and spiritual worlds. This unique unification between science and religion extended throughout the ancient world and distinguished the great civilizations of the past from those of the present. While ancient beliefs are often confused and misrepresented by orthodox views as "ritualistic cults," ancient peoples had a working concept of the soul and its purpose in the universe. Some of their ideas, though altered over time to fit the changing religious and political climate, were filtered down to us as days of fasting and other "holy days."

What conclusions can we say we have reached through research pertaining to our hunter-gatherer and agricultural ancestors and their dietary traditions? Try as they may, researchers cannot define either group as having consistent qualities within their respective cultures.

Let's summarize what we do know about some of their known cultural qualities and see what new ideas we have gained.

1. Ancestral Lineage

Long-accepted beliefs about prehistoric humans are changing, as both groups turn out to be more advanced than previously depicted. New discoveries challenge the dating for agricultural origins and show there is little evidence to support the theory of cultural evolution from hunter-gatherers to agriculturists.

2. Art, Religion, and Ritual

The myths and legends of both groups of peoples reveal the great depth and broad scope of understanding of nature that extends well beyond the basic survival concepts of primitive culture. Rituals, once interpreted as primitive rites of passage, idol worship, and religious superstition, are now coming to be regarded as exercises based on profound wisdom.

While peaceful, spiritual lifestyles may have predominated at some time, regular instances of cannibalism, incest, and other practices unacceptable to some modern civilizations occurred among both hunter-gatherers and agriculturists.

Links between different ancient cultures and tribes are being discovered that reveal cross-cultural communication over vast distances. These cross-cultural links are supported by archaeological evidence and further confirmed by universal legends of culture-bearers and global catastrophes. New discoveries are shedding light on these issues, again causing us to reevaluate past interpretations about cultural evolution.

3. Diet and Health

Neither hunter-gatherers nor agriculturists can be pigeonholed into a specific dietary category. Diets vary among both modern and ancient groups, with a wide range of foods depending on environment and lifestyle.

Both groups have experienced examples of reverting to the other as a result of environmental changes: drought, famine, floods, and depletion of resources have resulted in agriculturists reverting to hunter-gatherer lifestyles and vice versa. Both groups include examples where their diets are nutritionally sound and healthy, and other examples where their diets have been inadequate, leading to deficiencies and health problems.

Many of the positive health aspects both groups have experienced have been due to their close interaction with and exposure to nature. This type of lifestyle, along with high quality foods, enhances endurance, immunity, and overall strength.

Today we have disrespectfully distanced ourselves from the natural world—to our own detriment. We are well aware of the repercussions of living against nature, which include rampant disease; environmental devastation; and a pervasive sense of psychological, emotional, and spiritual alienation that lead to a host of societal ills, including profoundly criminal and self-destructive behaviors.

Perhaps this is why some few individuals and enclaves of people have chosen lives of celibacy and meditation in isolated environments, where they can reconnect with the knowledge of the ancients, the source of wisdom.

To know that our ancient ancestors were so highly evolved, both scientifically and spiritually, is an inspiration for many of us—and hopefully one that will motivate us to seek our species' continuance in a more sublime expression than our present path would suggest.

Here we are, against evolutionary odds, living at a fraction of the cultural potential expressed by the wisdom of civilizations past. It would seem that we are treading a delicate balance. If we begin to fill in some of the missing pieces of our heritage with what we know to be true, we can undoubtedly rebuild our planet's ecosystem, ensure our longevity, and fulfill our cultural destiny.

In the next two chapters, to demonstrate bringing these tools of scientific and historical perspective to bear on diet, we'll look at two examples of specific foods—chocolate and grains—both from a conventional perspective and from an alternative perspective based on current evidence.

40
Cacao
The Essence of Chocolate

One of the most popular foods in the world, chocolate is also one of the most versatile. It can find its way into (and have its way with!) delicate cakes, creamy puddings, mousse, cookies, candies, beverages. . . . When used for sauces or as a seasoning mixed with spices and herbs, it can even transform a savory meal into an exotic culinary experience.

Few foods on the planet have as much appeal as chocolate. It can dominate sweet desserts or entire meals while still maintaining its peculiar character and distinctly recognizable taste. Like fine wine, varieties of chocolate can be measured by flavor, taste, and other more subtle qualities, all of which determine the distinctions between the chocolate used in those chocolate bars found in your local convenience store versus chocolates from fine chocolate makers, especially those who use ecologically grown, harvested, and processed varieties.

Anatomy of a Pod

Theobroma cacao is the name of the tree that produces the podlike fruit from which cacao seeds are derived. The slender tree averages about twenty feet in height and thrives in humid, tropical forests beneath the shade and shelter of other taller trees that make up the forest canopy. Cacao trees take about seven years to mature and can live up to fifty years, bearing fifty to sixty football-size pods per year. These pods, when mature, can become red, purple, yellow, orange, or green.

Unlike most fruits that grow and ripen at the end of branches, cacao pods grow directly out of the main branches and from the trunk and bark of the tree. Each pod contains twenty to forty almond-size beans (seeds) embedded in a soft white pulp. The pulp has a sweet citrus flavor with a pear-like texture and has long been a traditional food for hunter-gatherers residing in the steamy forests of Mesoamerica. The creamy pulp is essential for the fermentation of cacao beans, an important stage of transformation on the way to actually becoming chocolate.

The Transformation

Cacao is the name given to the seeds before they are processed; once processed, they become *chocolate*. Here is a somewhat simplified version of the first stages of chocolate making:

First the ripened cacao pods are split open and the pulp and beans scooped out. The mixture is then spread on mats to ferment for four to six days in a shady area; the fermenting beans are turned occasionally by raking. The degree of fermentation is crucial to good chocolate and must be carefully observed and timed. The fermenting pulp eventually turns to liquid and drains away as the temperature rises, leaving the seeds with little residue of pulp.

During this time, the seeds begin to germinate, but high temperature and acidity levels prevent them from reaching full germination. The seeds are then sun-dried for another five to seven days, then cleaned and roasted for about forty minutes at 100 to 200 degrees to enhance flavor. The paper-thin skin surrounding the beans is then removed, leaving what is called the "cocoa nib." This is unprocessed, dark, unsweetened chocolate.

From here just about anything goes: milk, sugar, nuts, spices, and numerous other ingredients can be added to make both familiar and not-so-familiar delicacies.

The origins of this unique and exacting processing method for chocolate are lost in time. Wherever it came from, we can be sure the people responsible for it knew a great deal about science and food processing.

A Little Chocolate Science

Chocolate contains more than four hundred known pharmacological chemicals. There is still much to learn about this food, but three important chemicals whose interesting effects we have studied are *phenylethylamine, anadamide,* and *theobromine.*

Phenylethylamine is an amphetamine-like substance that selectively elevates those brain chemicals associated with pleasure. It is known to raise blood pressure and increase the activity of neurotransmitters.

Anadamide is a compound found naturally in the brain, seminal plasma, and ovarian fluids. It is similar to THC (tetrahydrocannabinol, the active ingredient in *cannabis*) in that it activates cannabinoid receptors (parts of a cellular system that regulate some reproductive fluids) and is responsible for creating enhanced feelings of well-being.

Theobromine is a mild stimulant with similar effects to caffeine but only about one-tenth its potency. Its diverse actions include: myocardial stimulant, diuretic, smooth muscle relaxant, and dilator of coronary arteries. Cacao also contains a small amount of caffeine, along with strong alkaloids similar to those found in coffee and tea.

Cocoa butter, the fat contained in cacao, consists of approximately 35 percent oleic acid, 35 percent stearic acid, 25 percent palmitic acid, and 5 percent other. It is the third-highest source of saturated fat, after coconut oil and palm oil. Overall, the cacao bean is about 30 percent fat, with an additional 14 percent carbohydrate and 9 percent protein. Cocoa butter liquefies at just above body temperature; since it is mostly stearic and palmitic acid, it does not raise cholesterol. It is also a stable fat, meaning it doesn't go rancid quickly. In fact, the fat content of cacao is one of its healthiest qualities. Cocoa butter is a valuable fat with multiple uses; the finest-quality chocolate has high quantities of it in the finished product.

Ancient History

No one really knows how our fascination with cacao began, nor do we know the true origins of this remarkable food. However, some evidence does exist to reveal clues that could one day help to solve the mystery of the origin of chocolate.

Archaeological evidence points to the Olmecs as the first people to use cacao. The word *cacao* itself was given to us by the Mayan peoples who once populated much of South and Central America. Historically, they are believed to be the people who came after the Olmecs in these regions. While Mesoamerican hunter-gatherer tribes may have harvested cacao pods to extract the creamy, custardlike flesh that surrounds the actual cacao seeds, the elaborate processing of cacao seeds began with the agrarian lifestyle of the Olmec civilization.

In many ways, the Olmecs are as much a mystery as is cacao. The word *Olmec* means "rubber people," reflecting the fact that evidence for early Olmec civilization was found in areas where trees that produce the essence of rubber were found. These enigmatic people are known for their elaborate stonework, consisting of colossal multiton stone heads (some over six feet in height and almost as wide) carved from hard basalt that was somehow brought to the Yucatán and surrounding areas of Mesoamerica from great distances. Some of these heads have helmets and stern faces, resembling warriors of some lost civilization, while others have faces with serene expressions, as if in a state of meditation.

The Olmecs are also known for their building of megalithic temples, sophisticated irrigation and drainage technology, crystal lenses, and much more. They are said to be the earliest civilization of the Americas. Their influence stretches throughout the Yucatán peninsula and into the remote jungles of Guatemala. Archaeologists are continuously finding new Olmec sites and uncovering information that helps broaden our understanding of these intriguing people of the past who were responsible for introducing the world to chocolate.

A recent title of *Proto-Mayans* has been given to the Olmecs because it is believed that they preceded the Maya and may have even intermixed with them to form future branches of the Mayan race. Conservative timelines for the Olmecs place them at around 1500 BC at the earliest; more realistic timelines place them in Mesoamerica by at least 3000 BC. Where they came from is anyone's guess, but they appear to have arrived fully organized and structured with civilization and agriculture.

There is no indication of any evolutionary process, from primitive hunter-gatherer to technologically advanced civilization, among the Olmecs. In fact, much of the archaeological evidence indicates a controversial mixture of racial types. Stone sculptures have been excavated that clearly reveal the various racial types of African, Mongoloid, Semitic, and Caucasian peoples. This strange cultural mix strongly points to cross-cultural diffusion at some remote period in history, and to the likely possibility of early settlement in the Americas by several racial types having traveled together.

An argument against this point of view pertaining specifically to cacao has to do with the unique growing environment cacao needs to thrive. Since the plant needs the hot and humid conditions of a rain forest, the argument against the diffusionists' point of view is that the product must be unique to the rain forest of the Americas. The fact that the plant is not found anywhere else is also cited. However, this argument does not take into consideration the possibility that similar environments may have existed in the distant past and long disappeared in a cataclysm, as indicated by numerous oral and written traditions—or that cacao could have been genetically designed by the Olmecs or some other advanced peoples. After all, it is a rather unique crop with strange attributes.

Sophisticated Food Science

Why this emphasis on the Olmecs? And what does it all have to do with chocolate?

What is so interesting is the extraordinary and detailed processing of cacao seeds from the *Theobroma cacao* tree to the finished chocolate, beginning with the Olmecs who handed it down to the Maya, Aztecs and everyone else who followed them. Such elaborate processing is not something one learns through trial and error.

Transforming the bitter and essentially inedible seeds of the cacao pod into chocolate was a well-thought-out process comprised of complex and detailed phases, and would have required a sophisticated understanding of each stage of the process. Furthermore, where would one get the idea to take such a bitter, inedible seed to make it into something edible, let alone something of such great importance? Some knowledge of biochemistry would have been necessary to undertake putting cacao seeds through such a process, and whoever first did so would have known beforehand what the outcome would be.

The chemical interactions that take place during the fermentation stage of cacao processing and the combination of shade and intense sunlight used to induce these and other chemical reactions reveals a comprehensive understanding of food science. It is a bit more complex than the hunter-gatherer, who observes an animal's interaction with particular plants and from there begins to imitate that behavior. Nor does it sit comfortably with the idea that someone at some time in the past witnessed a rotting cacao pod fermenting in the shade, by chance had a brainstorm, and spontaneously deduced the remaining details and steps needed to derive chocolate from the seeds.

For what purpose would one want to put so much energy into processing cacao seeds? It's important to realize that to the Maya and Aztecs, cacao seeds were worth more than gold. Moreover, they, like the Olmecs before them, knew all too well the physical and psychological effects of chocolate. Chocolate was also fermented to make alcoholic beverages and they most certainly combined it with various mind-altering plants and fungi.

Like other advanced civilizations of antiquity, the Olmecs had a sophisticated understanding of food science, including breeding, cultivation, and processing. The complex food science involved in turning cacao seeds into chocolate was something the Olmecs knew about when they arrived in the Americas. For that matter, they may have even brought the cacao plant with them from their original homeland—now lost to the sea from one of the cataclysmic events that took place sometime within the past 11,500 years.

Cacao is one of many food plants of the world with unknown origins. What appear to be wild cacao trees can be found throughout the jungles of Mesoamerica—yet whether these are wild or simply cultivated plants that have run wild is anyone's guess.

Ritualistic Uses of Chocolate

Historically, cacao was handed down from the Olmecs to the Maya and from the Maya to the Aztecs. At some point in this lineage, the Olmecs seem either to have disappeared or to have been integrated into or evolved into the early Mayan cultures. Artifacts from some early Mayan archaeological sites closely resemble Olmec art. It is from these early Mayan periods, as well as later ones, that traces of cacao have been found in excavated pottery, sometimes in tombs or areas where evidence suggests the practice of ritual human sacrifice. There is ample evidence to show that cacao was used as part of some of these rituals, especially those where enemy captives were sacrificed to appease the gods.

How cacao was used in ritual sacrifice is more clearly ascertained through evidence left by the later Aztecs of Mexico. It is important to understand the context in which this occurred. In *The True History of Chocolate,* Sophie and Michael Coe explain that the Aztecs did not practice human sacrifice for reasons of blood lust, cruelty, or an obsession with death. Rather, it was practiced because of an overshadowing fear that the world as they knew it might end, with everything in it perishing. This fear had its roots in myths and legends left by their ancestors.

In fact, this fear of a worldwide catastrophe where few humans survive to repopulate the earth appears in legends among hundreds of traditional cultures around the world. It appears to be based on actual experience passed on in the form of oral and written traditions by survivors among previous generations.

Though there is clearly a historical basis for the idea that human sacrifice was practiced by these cultures, much of the information we have pertaining to human sacrifice among the Aztecs is now recognized as embellished fact, in many instances highly exaggerated examples originally concocted by apologists who lived during the Spanish conquest.

The killing of most of Mexico's indigenous peoples in 1521 by the Spanish conquistadors and their religious zealots, along with the beating into submission of those few who remained, is a sad story indeed.

It is because of these barbarous acts that the conquerors were compelled to alter historical facts by destroying all but a few written records and proclaiming the Maya and Aztecs to be primitive, inhumane people—when in fact both were highly civilized peoples with extremely organized, productive, and thriving civilizations. In many ways, their polytheistic cultures were actually far more advanced than that of their conquerors, especially in their understanding and implementation of architecture, agriculture, and medicine.

Sacrifice was but one context of the many for the ritualistic use of chocolate among traditional Mayan and Aztec peoples. It also played an important role in weddings, royal feasts, and other special days throughout the year. Moreover, when it was served during these occasions, it was not consumed indulgently, without meaning or purpose.

Cacao seeds were also a source of monetary exchange for both the Maya and the Aztecs; it was their currency for purchase and trade among themselves and with other peoples. That it was a food specifically and exclusively for the ruling elite, including lords, long-distant merchants, and warriors, is supported by numerous sources, but according to some researchers, the evidence supporting this idea is still inconclusive. Some believe there is also evidence to support a long history of public consumption as well.

Cacao was available to commoners if they were assigned status as soldiers in the Aztec army. This may have been for practical purposes, as chocolate can act as an appetite suppressant and with large armies to feed, cacao would certainly help supply energy to the soldiers while also helping to curb their appetites.

Food of the Gods—and Goddesses

Cacao is mentioned several times in the Popol Vuh (Book of Counsel), a sacred book of the Quiché Maya of the Guatemalan highlands. One particularly interesting mention has to do with the gods having created humans in their final form after several previous attempts that ended in failure. In order to do this, the gods had to find the right foods with which to form human bodies. The foods were found in what was called the Mountain of Sustenance, and although several foods are mentioned in the legend, two very important ones were maize and cacao.

The Aztecs have a similar story that includes a mountain and the god Quetzalcoatl, who instructed ants to bring seeds to the surface that were hidden in a mountain. To both the Mayan and Aztec peoples, cacao was known as a "food of the gods" and was consumed primarily as a beverage, of which there were many variations.

Numerous ingredients were added to chocolate beverages, which were for the most part served unheated, although there is evidence that the Maya consumed both heated and unheated versions. Some of the added ingredients included chili powder, vanilla, maize, honey, and flowers. Each addition had a specific purpose and effect, but the ultimate and most widely cherished part of these beverages was the foam that would appear floating on the top of the drinking vessel. This bubbling foam was created by pouring from one vessel, in a standing position, into a receiving vessel at ground level.

Women served cacao to men of high rank or royal status. Whether or not it was forbidden to elite women of a thousand or more years ago is hard to say. If it was—women of that time doubtless being as resourceful as they have always been—one would suspect that traditional Mayan and Aztec women somehow managed to get their share of chocolate too.

There are three recognized varieties of cacao used to make chocolate today, although each of these varieties have adapted to various environments since first discovered, causing them to take on unique characteristics of the environment in which they are grown.

Criollo "native" cacao is considered the finest available and was the variety introduced to the Spanish when they first set foot in Mesoamerica. While it is the finest, it is also the most difficult to cultivate. *Forestero* is of lower quality but is hardier and more prolific than criollo. The third variety of cacao, *trinitario,* is a cross between the first two types.

Although Cortéz brought cacao seeds to the Emperor of Spain in 1502, it wasn't until 1585 that chocolate officially arrived from the "New World" (Vera Cruz) on the shores of Seville, Spain, where it continued in its status as a food for the elite upper classes. However, it wasn't long before it became available to the public as well.

Once available to the masses, this unique food quickly spread its influence throughout the world. No longer limited to the humid forests of Mesoamerica, and although stripped of its original spiritual and ritual history, chocolate has now become the focus of new exotic and erotic rituals in its unique position as a global food phenomena. Moreover, while still a food of the gods, with its overwhelming appeal to women, it could easily and deservedly be called food of the goddesses.

Chocolate and Sex

Is chocolate a healthy food—or is it perhaps one of those very special foods where it really doesn't matter whether it's healthy or not?

It certainly has some healthy ingredients, particularly cocoa butter. It contains stimulants and it contains sedatives. Much like coffee, it begins with a bitter flavor but can be altered to suit one's taste. According to traditional Chinese medicine, its bitter nature makes it resonate in the heart and small intestine. It has a dry and cold effect on the body when consumed as dark chocolate, and a damp and cool effect when consumed as milk chocolate.

It has long been recognized as a substitute for sex—yet for the true chocolate lover, sex may serve as a substitute for chocolate! Given our brief discussion of some of chocolate's ingredients, it is easy to see how it could influence sex on a biochemical level.

With specific components that can induce feelings of well-being while at the same time cooling the fire of sexual passion, it can induce a mental state of sexual delirium. Chocolate has less of an influence on the physical aspects of sex, as far as stimulating sexual fire goes, but it does have a strong influence on the more mental or psychological aspects of sex in the form of sexual fantasies, especially those where aggressive physical stimulation is used for sexual enhancement. While physical stimulation may be reduced under the influence of chocolate, chocolate may serve to enhance more subtle psychological aspects of sex having to do with emotional sensitivity.

Two Sides to Chocolate

The great and powerful Aztec ruler Montezuma believed it to be an aphrodisiac; an old Aztec legend speaks of it in a less positive light.

The legend speaks of Motecuhzoma, an earlier great Aztec emperor who, curious about the legends and origins of his people, decided to dispatch a group of sorcerers to seek out the legendary Aztec homeland called Aztlan. After a long journey, the party eventually arrived at Aztlan, which was situated on an island in the middle of a lake. Upon meeting the islanders, the sorcerers told them they had gifts for the goddess Coatlicue (Serpent Skirt). The goddess lived on top of a hill; the sorcerers were instructed to follow a guide up the hill to meet the goddess.

The old guide climbed the hill with ease but the sorcerers found they could barely walk up the steep incline. The spry old man asked the group of Aztecs what they ate in their land that would make them so heavy and fatigued. They told the elder guide they ate foods that grew there and that they drank chocolate. The elder then told them that this would make it difficult for them to reach the place of their ancestors.

When they finally reached the goddess, they presented her with their gifts. When she asked what chocolate was, they told her it was drunk and sometimes eaten. She told them that this was why they could not climb the hill: they had become old and weak, burdened by the chocolate.

There are many more details to the story, but this will suffice for getting the point across!

Thus the ancient stories present two sides to this mysterious food. One side portrays chocolate as an important and essential gift of the gods; the other, as expressed by the goddess Coatlicue, portrays it as a weakening and debilitating food.

Perhaps chocolate carries the potential for both extremes and, like other specialized foods, deserves to be understood for all that it truly is.

A Demanding and Sensitive Food

The cacao tree is subject to a multitude of diseases. Those known to attack it include fungus, pod rot, and extraneous growths. It is extremely sensitive to exposure, and low temperatures kill the seeds. Cacao is difficult to grow and requires both year-round moisture and regular irrigation to thrive. Overall, cacao is a very needy and demanding plant, and if it doesn't get these needs fulfilled it will die. These properties are all entrained in the final product—and therefore, in the eater of that product.

The sensual allure of chocolate is something few people can resist. It's as if this mysterious food has the ability to influence the senses in ways that no other food can. It can create deep feelings of satisfaction that can lead to expressions of self-importance and confidence. It can impart feelings of relaxation, euphoria, and sexual playfulness. It can even be a substitute for sex by sedating one's inner fire and replacing it with a sultry yet superficial demeanor.

Chocolate can stimulate and energize the body and mind. It can influence our thoughts by leading us down well-trodden paths of psychological awareness, while at the same time challenging us to open doors of perception we never knew existed, sometimes revealing thoughts and expressions of blatant truths and confusing deceptions that somehow meld into each other with convincing acumen.

Chocolate seems to have it all when it comes to being a favorite treat. It is the food of choice many people lean on in times of stress. When life doesn't seem to be going right, when anxiety has peaked, when the passion is gone, when there is no one who will listen, understand or believe, there is always chocolate to comfort us and ease the pain. While there are endless reasons—or excuses—for indulging in chocolate, for many the simple fact that it exists is reason enough.

41
The Gift of Grain and Flowering Plants

Grain is the first agricultural crop of the civilized world. One might even say that cereal grains and pseudocereals (the term for nongrass grains, such as quinoa, amaranth, and teff) hold the genetic blueprint for civilization.

Satisfying and versatile, grain has become the staple for making porridge, noodles, and bread. When accompanied by traditionally grown sources of proteins and fats and fresh vegetables, unrefined grain provides an excellent source of complex carbohydrates to nourish and support the functions of the brain and nervous system. This nutrient-packed, highly versatile food is easily stored and has served as the foundation of creative thought and spiritual harmony for countless generations.

Ancient peoples revered grain as a gift from the gods and have associated it with teachings of peace and unity. Modern science has offered many theories about the origins of cereals, legumes, and other cultivated plants, but none are conclusive, and the mysteries surrounding the world's major food crops remain unsolved.

Flowering plants first appear between 130 million and 150 million years ago and have since multiplied to become the more than two hundred thousand species known today.

Modern plant species consist of two basic groups, wild and domestic. The domestic varieties supposedly evolved about ten thousand years ago, through human intervention. More than seven major agricultural regions have been discovered that are thought to have been the original domains of ancient hunter-gatherers, who would eventually speed up the evolutionary process of wild grasses, transforming them into domestic cereals.

A Hypothetical Scenario

According to orthodox theory, domesticated cereal and bread grains were descended from wild emmer, einkorn, and barley. Harvesting and threshing these wild grasses is nearly impossible because when mature, they quickly drop ripened seeds that persistently retain their hulls—a characteristic that make the grasses impractical to harvest.

Neolithic hunter-gatherers, so goes the popular theory, therefore selected individual, mutated grass seeds—the largest ones that might have held fast to the ripened grain heads rather than dropping off—and replanted them in seedbeds. Through selection, cultivation, and natural interfertility over hundreds—some say thousands—of years, the mutated seeds eventually produced the modern grains typified by nonshattering rachises (the lower section of the seed that attaches to the stalk) and a hull that separates easily in threshing. Such seed crops became known as "free-threshing" or "naked" grains, a highly nutritious, easily harvested food crop suitable for human consumption.

And so, after thousands of years of foraging and gathering plants, planting mutant seeds in prepared seedbeds and waiting for generations until the seeds finally produced the results they were looking for, our Neolithic ancestors successfully created modern grains from wild grasses.

This hypothesis, while interesting, leaves many unanswered questions.

Assumptions, Missing Links, and Mutant Grains

First, close analyses of wild grasses and modern cereal grains reveal that, while some similarities exist in some cases, there are numerous domestic grains without wild progenitors, or at least without any that have yet been found. When progenitors are known, the related specimens may bear little to no resemblance in morphology.

Furthermore, within a species, both wild grasses and cultivated grains can have variances in their chromosome sets, numbering two, four, six, or more. These variances result in marked morphological differences, suggesting the possibility that genetic tampering between the wild grasses and cultivated grains could have occurred at some point in the remote past.

Admittedly, the origins of emmer and bread wheat are unknown, but it is theorized that these grains were produced from accidental hybridization between a species of tetraploids (four sets of chromosomes) and a weed that supplied the missing chromosomes needed to produce these domestics. Unfortunately, we do not know what this specific weed was. And with einkorn wheat, little is known about the mystery weed or even the actual process that supposedly turned wild or weed wheat into the diploid (two sets of chromosomes) domestic einkorn.

It is further assumed that a later hybrid of einkorn and a weedy grass became emmer wheat and that from there, probably through hybridization with other weeds, tetraploid wheat combined to produce spelt. This explanation seems confusing to some and rational to others; either way, it becomes questionable when we realize that these "missing link" transitional weeds have yet to be found.

There have been numerous modern experiments with cultivation, breeding, and genetics that have linked wild grasses to domestics. However, the idea that accidental hybridization along with hunter-gatherer experimentation could have created modern cereal grains more than ten thousand years ago is pure hypothesis and anything but a scientific certainty.

Research shows that in 17,000 BC, people were collecting wild emmer on the shores of Galilee in Israel. The assumption that it was used as food comes from the idea that these carbonized wild emmer wheat seeds must have been preagricultural and therefore the progenitors of what would eventually become domestic emmer, an important food source in the region. However, it is uncertain exactly what these carbonized seeds were actually used for.

Carbonized seeds of wild einkorn wheat dating to 10,000 BC have also been found in northern Syria. This einkorn was thought to be wild because the seeds are thinner in appearance than some fuller domesticated versions. However, the wild and domesticated aspects of carbonized grass seeds are often indistinguishable from each other, and not all thinner or smaller grass seeds are wild. Furthermore, when wild and domestic carbonized seeds can be distinguished from each other, age is not necessarily a factor, as both have been found together at ancient sites.

Without having the actual wild progenitors of these ancient carbonized seeds and instead having to go with the assumption that currently existing wild species of grasses are the offspring of the elusive (i.e., non-existent) progenitors, even though some are genetically related, makes it difficult to determine anything with any accuracy.

The wild einkorn grass that grows today in the Fertile Crescent has been and still is used for ruminant grazing, weaving, bedding, and fuel. Therefore, evidence of carbonized grass seeds at archaeological sites does not necessarily mean that early peoples consumed these wild grains. The suspected wild progenitors of emmer and wild einkorn are examples of living grains that are not normally consumed by humans or any other primate, and for that matter may simply be surviving examples of what might once have been domestic species. (See chapter 37, The Origins of Agriculture.)

Emmer, einkorn, and barley cereals are highly concentrated nutritional sources as compared to wild grasses, which offer little to no nutritional value to humans because we cannot effectively digest them. Ruminants thrive on wild grasses; when they consume domestic cereals, they tend to develop numerous health problems. This is especially true for cattle: while they may grow fatter and faster on domestic grain, cattle thrive more healthfully on their natural diet of wild grasses.

Another example of blurred history surrounds the origins of rice.

Not too long ago, rice was thought to have a history dating back about 1,500 years. With a recent discovery in China, this estimate has now been pushed back to 11,000 years BP. There are about 150,000 varieties of rice, yet the difficulty of determining wild species is complicated by thousands of years of crossbreeding among these varieties.

Thus, we are faced with creating hypothetical progenitors for the first domesticated rice.

And then there is the case of oats. Cultivated oats are diploids, while most of the ubiquitous wild oats found throughout the Mediterranean are a series of related polyploids. To some botanists, this strongly suggests that the cultivated crop must have given rise to the wild diploid species and not the other way around (ironically providing a new and literal meaning to the phrase, "Sowing their wild oats"!).

It is unlikely that our Neolithic forebears would select mutated forms of wild grass seeds over regular seeds simply because of size or adherence to the stalk at maturity. Most mutations in the plant and animal world are inferior to their parents. Are mutated grass seeds an exception? And if so, why are there no examples to be found of these Neolithic experiments that show the evolutionary steps through this selection process between wild grasses and domesticated cereals? Even the grains with wild predecessors are only related to each other genetically, and it is still not clear how one may have become the other.

Three Gifts

Even as the fruitless search for wild progenitors of domesticated grains continues, other food crops continue to have similarly paradoxical origins.

Squash and pumpkins, for example, vary considerably in size, yet the flesh of the domestic varieties have a pleasant, sweet taste. Wild species of squash, though, tend to be small and extremely bitter—not something one would normally consume. It is generally believed that wild gourds were originally used as ceremonial rattles. This is a reasonable assumption, since many Native American tribes use gourds for rattles today and have done so for thousands of years. Later, gourds began to serve as storage containers and supposedly evolved over succeeding generations as edible vegetables in the form of squash and pumpkins.

Not surprisingly, this evolutionary process is thought to have occurred in the same way as did cereal grains: by hunter-gatherers planting wild gourd seeds in separate seedbeds until they somehow transformed into sweet, soft-fleshed squash and pumpkins.

Cucurbita, the squash and pumpkin family of plants, originates in the Americas. How it transformed from a gourd to an edible vegetable is still a mystery to plant scientists; however, indigenous folk wisdom supplies an intriguing scenario.

Remember the Native American legend that describes three sisters, each bearing a gift of food in her hand, who descended from the Pleiades constellation and gave a trio of foods to the people to supplement their hunting lifestyle: squash, beans, and corn?

There is clearly nothing arbitrary about this triad: it is a unique combination of foods with surprisingly symbiotic traits. Squash, beans, and corn improve and support each other's growth while sustaining the earth.

Furthermore, this "sacred trio" also provides an exceptionally strong nutritional symbiosis: corn (maize) is deficient in tryptophan, isoleucine, and lysine—all of which are supplied in abundance by squash and beans.

Legends such as that of the three sisters are preserved through oral tradition over many generations; the range of possibilities for their interpretation is naturally challenging. In this case, for example, perhaps the three culture-bearers were not visitors from the Pleiades, but colonists from some exotic land. Perhaps the Pleiades constellation was simply visible in the sky at the time of the arrival of these gift-bearing strangers. Or maybe the strangers were indeed from the Pleiades!

The point is that while the literal verity of many of these legends remains elusive, the words of the traditions continue unchanged. And if the Native Americans' ancestors (or any other traditional culture with similar legends) knew how to genetically alter wild plants into their most sacred food crops, this knowledge certainly would have been part of their legacy as well. However, like so many other traditional peoples around the world, Native Americans also have a legend of mysterious, gift-bearing strangers *who already possess* the knowledge of plant domestication.

Mysterious Maize

Let's consider for a moment another of this remarkable trio of nutritional gifts: maize.

Agronomists recognize maize as an evolutionary anomaly. According to *The Cambridge World History of Food,* by Kiple and Ornelas, the oldest known remains of the (supposed) wild ancestor of maize are pollen grains that were found on an archaeologist's drill core during excavations for a new building in Mexico City. The remains were said to be dated at about seventy thousand years old, long before there were humans in that region.

It is thought that these pollen grains may be from an ancient ancestor of maize, but this is not considered conclusive, as there are as of yet no known specific ancestors to maize. Teosinte, a wild weed, is believed by some agronomists to be the ancestor of maize, yet other plant specialists suggest it is more likely to be the other way around: maize is the ancestor of teosinte. There is no such thing as wild maize, although there are garden escapees growing in seemingly wild habitats.

So what is this sevnty-thousand-year-old Mexican maize pollen sample? No one knows for sure, but if we are to maintain the cultural evolution theory and established timelines associated with it, we must assume that there were no sophisticated agriculturists around at that time, let alone humans. How about human hunter-gatherers experimenting with wild grasses? No, this region is considered the "new world!"

The earliest maize remains found in Mexico consist of tiny ears and were first thought to be the progenitor of the large domestic types. However, it is now known that this ancient tiny grain is but another early species of domestic maize. This is not unlike the examples of the thin wheat grains spoken of above that were excavated at sites in the Fertile Crescent and dated at 10,000 BC. Because the wheat is thinner or smaller does not mean it is wild, especially when grains of differing types (both wild and domestic) can vary in size and shape.

Maize, commonly known as *corn* in the Americas, contains the largest seed heads (one or two ears per plant) of all grains, each set in rows (always with even numbers) and covered in husks that prevent self-reproduction. Reproduction is assisted by maize's loose flowers that allow for free-flying pollen, whereby the promiscuous female organs openly receive wandering spores.

Wild plants have been used by traditional peoples throughout history and still are today. The leaves and seeds of many wild plants are often used as food consumed in numerous ways, and as ingredients in herbal remedies, poultices, and other medicines. However, some grains (amaranth, quinoa, teff) and their wild relatives are important staple foods for many throughout the world. These grains have unusual patterns of domestication that differ considerably from their wild grass counterparts. They are so varied in speciation that it is unclear where the line of domestic varieties and those of wild varieties begins.

Amaranth and Teff: More Gifts of the Gods

The idea of preselection of larger seeds by primitive ancestors also becomes questionable when considering the long history of cultivated tiny grains. Amaranth, a traditional grain (sometimes referred to as a pseudocereal) of Mexico, Peru, China, Africa, India, and remote parts of Tibet, has a seed head that contains up to fifty thousand seeds as tiny as poppy seeds. How one particular species of amaranth ended up in so many places in antiquity is an unsolved mystery. Since it is not reported to exist as a wild weed species, this globe-trotting species of amaranth is believed to have originated from genetic mutations selected by its "domesticators."

The close botanical cousin of quinoa, "pale" or "blond" amaranth, with its superior flavor, pops better and germinates faster than other types of amaranth. Most wild species of amaranth offer highly nutritious and tasty leaves and a single wild plant can yield thousands of seeds. On the other hand, a single plant of domestic blond amaranth can yield hundreds of thousands of seeds. One plant can plant one acre and one acre of seed production can plant twenty thousand acres.

Amaranth has nearly complete amino acids, with protein that is 90 percent digestible (higher than that in milk) and is used more efficiently by the body. There is more calcium (3.5 ounces) in a comparable amount of amaranth than in a glass of milk; it is high in niacin, lysine, and iron and contains no gluten.

The Greeks called amaranth "everlasting" or "immortal" because of the durability of its seed. Everywhere it is found, it is said to have metaphysical traits of feeding the soul as well as the body. Like other cereals, amaranth is regarded as a revered gift of the gods by all who use it as a dietary staple. In Mexico, it served as the basis of elaborate ceremonies by the Aztecs until it was almost eradicated by Cortéz as part of his final conquest. Amaranth was a ritual plant of the Pueblo Indians; the Hopi believed it was a gift from their beloved otherworldly friends, the Kachinas.

Who were these domesticators of amaranth that spread this remarkable food throughout the world long before recorded history?

Another extraordinary grain is the life-saving teff, a traditional grain of Ethiopia. The world's tiniest grain, teff is so small that five grains can fit on the head of a pin. These exceptionally small grains are cultivated by the Ethiopians, in whose diet they have played a major role from time immemorial; teff has long been recognized by Ethiopian peoples as yet another "gift from the gods."

The tiny teff seedlings are quite fragile and delicate when young, and must be cared for until fully grown. When mature and ready to harvest, the seed head forms a beautiful but tiny heart-shaped display. Ethiopians believe this is the plant's response to the tender loving care given to it while it is young and in need, a belief which is probably the origin of another name for teff, "lovegrass."

Teff is both a highly nutritious food and a low-risk, drought-resistant crop, this latter being an especially important factor in the erratic and unpredictable environment of Ethiopia. Teff provides about two-thirds of Ethiopians' nutrition. While attempts have been made, science has not been able to improve on the qualities of this life-sustaining food of Africa's traditional peoples.

A Fragile Theory

It is becoming increasingly difficult to accept the orthodox theory suggesting that our Neolithic ancestors somehow genetically altered the chromosomes of wild grasses, bred them for adaptability, increased their nutritional profile, and made them dependent on human cultivation to thrive. This would have been a tremendous scientific endeavor, and one that has not since been repeated with any benefit to our species. With the ending of the ice age and plenty of game available, how desperate were our Neolithic ancestors to spend so much time and effort attempting to alter wild grasses?

In his book *Everything You Know Is Wrong,* researcher Lloyd Pye suggests that our ancestors would have had to look at wild grass and imagine what it could, should and would become over generations. Were they even capable of this level of thinking? Such an enterprise would have required specific and highly specialized scientific knowledge along with generations of time for the effort to succeed.

If we concede that civilization was *not* a slow, gradual process and that it coincided with the appearance of large-scale agriculture in only a few select areas of the world, then it is hard to deny that the knowledge for agriculture and grain cultivation must have already been present from the outset. As further proof of this conclusion, we are still growing and consuming the same basic grain crops of our ancestors, albeit in inferior versions.

The Case of Genetically Modified Organisms

It is scary to contemplate how modern, genetically altered grains could replace something that has nourished and supported the health of the human species for well over ten thousand years.

However, some ask, is ten thousand years too short a time for humans to physiologically adapt to grain as a food? After all, we supposedly thrived for a few hundred thousand years without it. . . .

But this question presupposes "facts" that no longer stand up to scrutiny. In fact, the Neolithic period may not have been the first time grain was cultivated, harvested, and consumed as a principle food. It had to have come from somewhere. The lack of evidence for an evolutionary process, combined with consistent widespread legends of culture-bearers as its originators, along with the sudden emergence of agriculture in a few select regions, all suggest that the cultivation and dietary use of grains could very plausibly have arrived from someone who already knew it well as a defining characteristic of his or her own culture.

Through the introduction of cereal grains, human beings were changed—intellectually, culturally, and physiologically—into what and who we are today. Can the modern human species adapt to artificial foods as a primary source of sustenance? Sure it can—and humanity can change again, perhaps at a much faster pace than our Neolithic ancestors did . . . though not necessarily with the same salutary results.

Much of Europe has recently refused to accept the genetically modified cereals and other plants offered by many multinational corporations—organizations that are in fact modern culture-bearers with sordid histories of environmental devastation. Perhaps Europeans remember their own role in bringing "white man's food" to primitive cultures, or perhaps they are wisely distrustful of promises made by profit-driven companies. Either way, they know that GMOs are not the answer to the world's food shortages, and so should everyone else.

We might want to ask ourselves, Who is responsible for the most recent adaptation of the human species to artificial foods? And do they have humanity's best interests in mind?

After answering that rather easy question, we might then ask ourselves, Who was responsible for human adaptation to agriculture in Neolithic times—and did *they* have humanity's best interests in mind?

The nutritional package designed by the culture-bearers of ancient times was in so many ways extraordinarily well designed for human development. If the means of obtaining and reproducing this package of nutritious, life-sustaining foods through sustainable methods of agriculture is reestablished on a global scale, we all stand to benefit.

42
Dangerous Brains
The "Lo-Carb" Fad and Diet Extremism in the Twenty-first Century

Proponents of a high-protein, low-carbohydrate diet use the following general outline of human evolution and reasoning to support their claims:

2.5 million years ago: Primitive humans begin to use stone tools and hunt small animals.

Claim: Until this time, our earliest primate ancestors consumed a diet much like modern chimpanzees. As a direct result of the increased nutrient-dense protein foods—that is, small animals—our ancestral hominids' brains begin to increase in size.

1.8 million to 500,000 years ago: *Homo habilis* and *Homo erectus* evolve into *Homo sapiens*.

Claim: These three species have larger, more fully functional brains than their hominid ancestors and have the capacity to figure out how to hunt big game.

200,000 to 100,000 years ago: Neanderthal appears and is accompanied by modern humans. They cohabit the planet and eventually Neanderthal dies off. Fire and cooking are discovered.

Claim: For the next 190,000 years, humans continue as hunter-gatherers.

10,000 years ago: Modern humans begin farming out of necessity.

Claim: Through the advent of agriculture, man begins to cultivate grain, thus increasing his carbohydrate consumption. This mere ten-thousand-year period is insufficient time for modern humans to physiologically adapt to a high-carbohydrate diet from grains—and as a result, the health of *Homo sapiens* begins to decline.

Conclusion: The best diet for humans is that of our Paleolithic ancestors—the diet on which we have evolved over the long term. This is proven by the fact that our Paleolithic ancestors were healthier than our more recent agricultural ancestors.

This is a nice, neat conclusion—but it doesn't stand up well to close inspection, and its supporting claims are riddled with contradictions and inconsistencies.

For example, throughout these long stretches of time, various human species have evolved and disappeared. The "established dates" of the chronology given above are spurious: such efforts at fixing dates for evolutionary epochs vary widely, according to what and whom you read and when the material was published.

Experts vary so in their opinions and conclusions because information is constantly being updated and revised through new discoveries. There are numerous inconsistencies in fossil records. The result of this shifting picture is that all the foregoing conclusions and inferences remain little but unproven theories.

Indeed, upon close examination, they raise more questions than answers.

How are we "not physiologically evolved to handle a carbohydrate-centered diet" if our earliest ancestors, during their ape and chimpanzee stages, consumed such foods almost exclusively in the form of fruits and other plants for who knows how long?

If we are going to subscribe to the theory of cultural evolution, we are accepting the fact that our ancestors had to adapt to eating larger quantities of meat and fat long *after* already having established a physiology designed to handle large quantities of carbohydrates as a primary source of food! There is no reason to believe that large portions of these carbohydrate foods did not stay with evolving hominids all the way through the evolutionary process and right up to the present, as is evidenced in many modern hunter-gatherers.

Is it likely or even possible that once our so-called earliest ancestors got the taste for meat and fat, mostly in the form of small animals, they then simply gave up all the carbohydrates they had been consuming for untold generations?

There would be only one reason for any hominid to give up large quantities of a given type of food after having eaten it for hundreds of thousands of years, and resort instead to the exhausting and dangerous task of hunting big game: if the environment stopped producing it.

Why would the environment stop producing an abundance of plant foods? This might occur during long periods of consistently freezing weather. Ice ages undoubtedly had a major impact on diet and health and represented long interruptions in our ancestors' patterns of living. Arctic-type climatic conditions would have resulted in low carbon dioxide levels, thus contributing to less and smaller plant growth.

This scenario certainly would have encouraged phases of greater animal food consumption, leading many early hominids to hunt full-time. Temperate climate phases, on the other hand, would have brought an increase in plant and other easily gathered foods, similar to those in modern-day hunter-gatherers' diets.

Why did it take so long to create stone tools and go for the big game?

From 2.5 million years ago to 1.7 million years ago, our ancestors were still scavenging and eating small animals. Ancestral hominids finally reached the point where they could now use their larger brains to hunt big game. . . .

Or so says the theory. However, current findings have caused some paleoanthropologists to lean toward the scavenger theory for Paleolithic humans as a means of obtaining their unpredictable sources of animal foods.

It is well known that most plant matter is scarce in the archaeological record because it decomposes without a trace, unlike bones and pottery. If a variety of carbohydrates were available from the earliest times whenever the climate was suitable, it then stands to reason that they would have been available and consumed in large quantities continuously throughout the evolutionary process. It is always risky to compare modern hunter-gatherers to those of Paleolithic, Mesolithic, and Neolithic times because many of the food sources from those earlier periods are no longer available, and those that are have gone through various changes over the eras.

Does the big-game diet fare any better in our nutritional history of brain advancement?

Concerning the increased consumption of meat and fat from small, easily obtained animals and its correlation to the increase in our ancestors' brain size, this is a reasonable assessment, because nutrient-dense foods do nourish the brain.

However, what about the time it took the brain to develop? Did human ancestors just sit around for nearly a million years, drooling and fantasizing about the large prey so abundantly available in their environment while consuming small animals and fruits, until they finally figured out how to put their large brain to some use so they could hunt the big game? Is that a reasonable scenario?

So much for the attribution of brain development to nutrient-dense protein foods in the form of small animals. These foods may have contributed to brain *size,* but they obviously didn't help much to promote brain *function.*

It is true that most varieties of game contain omega-3 fatty acids, zinc, L-carnitine, B_{12} and other vital nutrients utilized by the human body for strength and immunity. But remember, we are assuming that our ancestors' larger brains gave them the capacity to hunt, and that the consumption of larger quantities of nutrient-dense animal foods likely played a role in further brain development. At least this is what conventional theory holds. But was it this increase in animal food that caused the human brain the develop?

Questioning Human Evolution

Scientists who go about teaching that evolution is a fact of life are great con men and the story they are telling may be the greatest hoax ever.

Dr. T. N. Tahmisian, Atomic Energy Commission

The second stage of advancement is said to have occurred around 1.7 million to 500,000 years ago when our hominid ancestors gathered their stone tools and took the risk of hunting big game.

This begs the question: did they do this to supplement their existing diet of plants and small animals, or did they give all that up for the big stuff? It is still too early to tell how these slowly evolving big-game hunters are doing with their fully evolved brains as compared to their small-game-hunter ancestors, who took what seem to have been forever to get it together to hunt big game.

With the theory of slow, gradual ascension from apes to modern humans entrenched in our textbooks, it is no wonder that the image of the lumbering Paleolithic brute is so well established in people's minds, even though most paleoanthropologists today are doing their best to change this conditioning. This is likely to remain a difficult challenge as long as the theory responsible for this image has not changed.

At this point, we have a hypothetical historical situation in which our earliest ancestors consume mostly fruits, insects, and (occasionally) small animals as a regular diet, much as apes and chimps do today. Then, according to theory, 2.2 to 2.5 million years ago a special line of hominids evolves. These new hominids have to learn to spot predators hiding in the tall grasses of the savanna in Africa. Since they no longer live in trees, they begin standing upright in order to see over the tall savanna grasses, and are the first species to become truly bipedal. . . .

But hang on. Have you ever actually seen the tall grasses of the savanna? Even standing on someone's shoulders and looking out over these tall grasses, one would be hard pressed to spot a low-crouching, well-camouflaged lion. Anyone giving this idea even a little common-sense thought can see the absurdity of it.

And why didn't any of the other monkeys, apes and chimps evolve beyond their original status? Were they so frightened by crouching predators (and are they still today) that they were able to ignore evolution and refuse to venture from the safety of the trees (and still do so today)?

The theory of human evolution is described in part as a primitive species going through processes of gradual change, through which this species eventually evolves into a more efficient and thus more advanced species. We start with nonhuman hominid ancestors whose diet consists of fruits, other plant parts, insects, and a greater quantity of small, hunted animals, which may eventually contribute to an increased brain size. Loss of body hair for ease in perspiring and other morphological changes also take place at some point. These hominids evolve further and develop skills to hunt large game, which results in increased meat consumption.

But isn't this heavy game consumption really an example of adaptation to a food that was foreign, at least in large quantities, and apart from small animals? At this point our hairless hominids are really eating the same diet they have been eating for millions of years, with the addition of greater quantities of large game.

Meat-Eating Newcomers

Neanderthal and anatomically modern humans eventually appear out of the same evolutionary branch as *Homo habilis* and *erectus*. The appearance of both groups comes to fruition about two hundred thousand years ago (some say one hundred thousand). As noted in the outline above, fire is discovered for cooking at about this time; indeed, the advent of cooked food may have been an additional influence on larger brain development.

Modern man and Neanderthal continue the patterns of big game hunting for around one hundred thousand more years. Neanderthals are robust and mighty hunters with fully developed brains; yet, whether by some trick of fate or simple ingenuity, it is we smaller-brained modern humans who survive and the Neanderthal who die out.

Now, I enjoy a nice barbecue with friends and family on occasion. Still, one cannot deny that over the past several decades, we have been bombarded with scientific studies showing the dangerous, cancer-causing effects of grilled and charred foods, especially meats. I cannot help wondering how researchers can claim that our Paleolithic ancestors were so much healthier than later farmers. Isn't this pretty much exactly how our big-game, Paleo-hunter ancestors were cooking *all* their meat? After all, they had not yet learned to manufacture cooking pots. Their food preparation had to be similar to modern grilling—if anything, only more intensely so, owing to their food being in direct contact with flame.

Direct flame is well known to cause high levels of free radicals in the blood of subjects consuming charred food. Most of the evidence found relating to food in prehistoric kitchen middens and other Paleo sites has been from charred remains. If this charred food represents the largest part of our ancestor's diet, then antioxidant foods, such as fresh vegetables, could not have helped much to counter the effects of the toxic free radicals.

Either all the modern studies of the cancer-causing effects of char-broiled meats are way off the mark—or the "healthy eating habits" of our Paleo ancestors have been grossly misinterpreted.

Or perhaps both conclusions are circumstantial and dependent on other influences.

The two-hundred-thousand-year-old discovery of fire use by early *Homo sapiens* fit nicely into the cultural evolution model—until one considers a recent find in the northern Dead Sea Valley.[1] This new information places fire use at 790,000 years ago—more than *three-quarters of a million* years in our past—thus throwing the evolutionary timeline wildly off kilter.

At a campfire site near an ancient lake in what is now Israel, researchers found evidence of meat consumption, including bones that had been broken to extract the marrow. Who these hominids were is unknown, but it is suggested they may have been a transitional form of *Homo erectus,* the precursor to *Homo sapiens* (modern humans).

Does this report mean that cultural development could have occurred 590,000 years sooner than we thought? If so, we could be facing a significant modification in our cultural evolution theory. Or do scientists need to recalculate the arrival of *Homo sapiens*? At any rate, the effort to reconcile this new timeline for fire use with the accepted orthodox timeline boggles the mind.

There's more. Orthodox theory implies that we are "just surviving" for 120,000 years, often threatened by a harsh environment and forced to hunt large game. Recall that Neanderthal are robust, great hunters who possess larger brains than we have today, as are Cro-Magnon, our relatives. Yet both go extinct. As I mentioned earlier, this apparent contradiction may be partly explained by the evidence of the worldwide practice of cannibalism, a taboo subject with the low-carbohydrate-diet enthusiasts. Perhaps the physical taming of fire has little to do with taming the spiritual fire, which while hard to quantify is equally necessary for civilization.

If we consider only the smaller-brained *Homo sapiens* and evaluate our progress for the past 200,000 (or is it 790,000?) years, we reach the mathematical conclusion that it takes us *at least 190,000 years* of hunting big game before we figure out that we can domesticate animals for food instead of chasing them down and competing with dangerous predators.

This means we are still foraging, hunting, gathering, scavenging, caving, and roaming right up until around ten thousand years ago.

So much for the thousands of years of including large game into our diet and the effect it supposedly had on the development of our brain.

Small Brains, Big Ideas

Suddenly, about ten thousand years ago, as if out of nowhere, *Homo sapiens* begins agriculture in several parts of the world at once. Whole grain is cultivated and added to already existing nutrient-dense protein food sources; human brain development leaps to unprecedented heights.

We continue hunting to supplement our domesticated plant and animal food sources. Furthermore, we move out of the caves, start making clothes from plant fibers, build monuments, and begin learning astronomy, geometry, and other sciences. With this new dietary addition of cereal grains, we become fully civilized in a very short time.

Yet before this time, when on hunter-gatherer diets, *Homo sapiens* progresses very little—even over the course of hundreds of thousands of years.

Perhaps grain and plant cultivation combined with animal husbandry is cause enough for this giant step in human progress and brain development. Could this extraordinary development have been the first and only such dramatic shift in humanity that occurred since our sojourn out of Africa? Stone tool development, hunting, the discovery of fire, some ritualistic burials, and cave artwork are explained easily enough through orthodox theory. Many of these developments are said to have occurred within the past forty thousand years. However, *Homo sapiens'* leap to agriculture and civilization is not as easily explained.

For almost two hundred thousand years, our ancestry makes few basic changes, but ten thousand years ago we suddenly make extraordinary changes with the advent of agriculture, which carries us to the present era, in which we have already been to the moon and are well on our way to visiting the rest of the solar system.

Is it true that our relatively large-brained human predecessors could not have thought of smelting copper or other metals? Did they not have sufficient desire and that one inventive mind among them to build a flying glider, even out of simple wood-and-tar materials? And is it true they did not build any cities for 190,000-plus years?

Is the story of prehistoric humankind nothing but a grim struggle for survival?

The expert might respond, "Well, we haven't found any evidence to indicate anything other than what orthodox theory suggests." My response is, "That's not true. Keep looking—because what we do know at this time is limited to the knowledge of a few ancient historians and a couple of hundred years of excavations and scientific research. More information is being discovered almost daily."

Voltaire once wrote, "History is the lie commonly agreed upon." Personally, I have not given up on our ancestors, the ones who gave us the knowledge to go beyond the basic need to survive and to explore our universe. Rather than being forced into agriculture about ten thousand years ago, as some historians hypothesize, many early *Homo sapiens* most likely began the practice of agriculture many thousands of years earlier, and were only much later forced to live in caves and subsist on mostly game, fish, and other wild animals because of extreme climatic changes until the ice age had receded.

The Carbohydrate Question

Some adherents of low-carbohydrate diets suggest we should eat like our Paleolithic ancestors. But what exactly does that mean? Which ones should we be eating like—the ones who ate more plant foods or the ones who ate more animal foods, the humans or the other hominids? Our Paleolithic ancestors' diets varied as greatly as do those of today's traditional hunter-gatherers around the world.

Most of today's low-carbohydrate diets lean toward the high-protein group and some suggest little to no carbohydrates; others permit tubers, fruits, and honey. For Paleo-diet advocates, grains are usually discouraged, especially wheat, barley, and other gluten-containing grains. There are numerous problems with this extremist thinking. There is no doubt that protein and fats are necessary for proper metabolic balance and general good health, but so are highly nourishing carbohydrates in the form of cereal grains.

Paleo-diet advocates often cite the Egyptians as an example of why one should not eat grains. Some Egyptians statues have bloated faces and waistlines, and fossil evidence of some Egyptians reveals low bone density. These and other problems are often cited as caused by a high-carb (grain) diet.

While this is true to some degree, any Egyptologist knows that in its long history, this extraordinary culture experienced widely varying periods of abundance and scarcity. The Nile, their primary source of water, was susceptible to extreme flooding at times; drought was also experienced periodically, sometimes lasting for generations. During times of abundance, Egypt's culture thrived, with a wide variety of health-sustaining foods. Cattle, vegetables, grain, fowl, and many other foods were essential components of their diet. In difficult eras, the culture suffered and had to make due with stores of grain and other foods that could be preserved.

Archaeologists have found an essentially similar pattern of extremes in every ancient civilization. To state that all Egyptians throughout history were weaker and less healthy than Paleo hunter-gatherers because of a diet high in grain is absurdly simplistic and ignores a host of important factors in Egyptian history. And Paleo hunter-gatherers in other areas were not exempt from such extreme changes, either (as is evidenced, for example, in periods where cannibalism was prominent).

However, the negative attitude toward carbohydrate consumption has little to do with whole grain consumption; it is rather based on the imbalances caused by highly refined and denatured products derived from poor-quality, refined grain products. We should face this problem not by eliminating carbohydrates, which are necessary for good health, but by replacing our modern, refined versions with *naturally grown complex* carbohydrates, such as those that have been consumed in cereal grains by traditional agriculturalists around the world for at least twenty-three thousand years.

The Age of Designer Diets

A balanced diet consisting of a wide variety of quality fruit, vegetables, grains, legumes, nuts, seeds, and animal protein supplies the widest spectrum of nutrients, well beyond what any modern fad diet can claim. The most extraordinary thing about this is that hardly anyone in the modern world has experienced this type of traditional diet for at least two generations! Instead, we have been overwhelmingly consuming a diet of highly refined carbohydrate foods accompanied by processed, commercially grown animal protein, toxic trans fats, and loads of pharmaceuticals. Any close evaluation of these modern food sources reveals the truth about why health is on the decline and obesity is on the rise—as well as why there are so many extreme dietary trends.

We are living in the age of designer diets. There are diets for every ill and every belief. I have yet to meet one person on a designer diet who, before commencing that new diet, had eaten a high-quality, balanced diet of traditional foods.

It is to some extent natural that such designer diets would appeal to us: we seek release and relief from the debilitating effects of processed foods that we have been manufacturing and consuming over the past century. Sometimes the appeal of a particular designer diet lies in the fact that we are trying to escape from (or to compensate for the effects of) some other designer diet that didn't fulfill our desire for weight loss, more vitality, or some other health goal.

Much of the food consumed by most people today consists of processed, denatured foods, laden with preservatives and many other non-essential substances that do little to support health and much to detract from it. More and more people are realizing this, so they naturally seek ways to remedy the problem and reestablish their health.

Enter designer diets: lots of them, and all different too—yet all of them offer similar promises. Those that stress natural, unprocessed, and preservative-free foods help us to gain insight on the importance of quality in our diet. These are the only ones worth considering, if we truly want to be sure what we are eating is healthy. However, even among these more naturally oriented approaches to diet, the balance of nutrients remains a very important consideration.

The first category of people seeking designer diets are those needing to escape from nutrient-deficient foods for whatever reasons, health, weight loss, and so forth. The second category of people seeking designer diets are those who have already tried at least one new, restrictive diet and failed.

Those of this second group try another designer diet, sometimes continuing the new diet for years, or perhaps only months. All eventually find the need to eat things not on the diet—some often, others only occasionally. This is natural: designer diets tend to restrict the very foods with which we are most familiar, and in eliminating them from our diets, we often feel deprived.

Another reason for distractions from a diet is a lack of energy due to a lack of balanced nutrition; increased use of stimulants is a common response, but sometimes these stimulants (coffee, tea, tobacco, etc.) can come to comprise a larger percentage of our diet than healthy foods. Actually, coffee, chocolate, and other stimulants are good barometers for determining how well one's diet is working: the more of them one consumes, the less effective the diet. The need for these foods, other than in moderation, is a strong message that suggests changes in one's diet are called for.

In general, modern *Homo sapiens* are unsatisfied nutritionally and, thus, metabolically. This is not the result of a simple-minded generalized notion of "carbohydrate overload." Nor is it caused by the consumption of traditional whole grains in the diet, often mistakenly classified by low-carb proponents as being in the category of "bad carbs."

High-quality whole grains are health-promoting when balanced with adequate amounts of protein, fats, and fresh vegetables. Organic, complex carbohydrates and processed, junk-food carbohydrates are as different from one another as a chicken is to an apple.

In fact, if there is any beneficial aspect at all of a low-carbohydrate diet, it is in the concomitant suggestion by many teachers to reduce or eliminate junk-food carbohydrates. Once such a shift is accomplished and protein and fat are increased, one's metabolism gets a jump-start from years of stagnation caused by excessive, poor-quality carbs. One is then energized, tends to lose weight, and experiences life differently, at least for a while. Thus, there may actually be a temporary benefit from following a low-carbohydrate diet—but beyond that temporary benefit, it is critically important to make a distinction between the qualities of different carbohydrates and to eat a variety of health-promoting foods, including grains.

The Fallacy of the "Single Cause"

All nutritionally related health problems invariably result from a combination of factors. For example, some think obesity is caused simply by excessive fat consumption, but it is the *quality* of fats and the *imbalance* between healthy fats, proteins, and carbohydrates that principally contribute to extreme weight retention. Refined carbohydrates also contribute to obesity, often even more than fats. All essential macronutrients play a role in every diet-related illness; it is never just one thing.

Try removing one category of nutrition from your diet; inevitably you will find yourself eating it again in some form or other. After more than thirty years in the natural health field, I have had the opportunity to hear many stories and witness many dietary tragedies.

Here is a common statement I hear from those trying to adhere to a low-carbohydrate diet: "When I *was* doing it I felt great!" This sort of wistful past-tense expression is typical with designer diets that depend on restrictions or limited choices. Deprivation of a variety of healthy foods makes these types of diets difficult to maintain.

Another statement I have frequently heard is, "I really enjoy the food, but I find myself cheating a lot." Again, depriving oneself of a variety of healthy foods eventually leads to compulsive overeating and other emotional problems.

Those with allergies to grain (wheat and gluten-containing products) should naturally avoid gluten-containing grains—*if* they do indeed produce an allergic reaction. I say "if" because there are people who are gluten-intolerant who can still eat high-quality grains traditionally prepared by fermentation, soaking, or sprouting. Also, for people experiencing this problem, it is important to consider that the problem itself was not caused by high-quality, traditionally prepared grain as part of a balanced, healthy diet. Gluten intolerance problems can be carried from generation to generation and are caused partly by refined-gluten-containing products, along with other immune-suppressing substances, especially drugs and chemicals of all kinds.

It is interesting to note how saturated fats of all types have been accused for years of causing a host of problems, from heart disease to cancer, yet today, traditional saturated fats are finally starting to be recognized as healthy and essential macronutrients. As it turns out, the problems once believed to be caused by these traditional fats were in fact caused by trans fats and refined polyunsaturated oils.

Protein, too, has been demonized in the past; now it appears to be carbohydrates' turn to take the stand and be accused of the majority of the Western world's health woes.

In order to prevent future problems, we must be careful not to make the same mistake we made with fats: that is, we need to avoid the simplistic error of classifying all carbohydrates in the same category. Certainly it is important to acknowledge the problem of gluten intolerance for some people, yet it is at least as important to consider the long history of grain consumption among healthy peoples eating a balanced traditional diet.

Dietary Common Sense

With quality carbohydrates, very few people have had "too much of a good thing." In other words, not many people have overdosed on unrefined, complex carbohydrates; most have their excessive carbohydrate experience by way of sugar and refined grain products.

However, there are still those scant few who believe they have developed problems from the excessive consumption of good-quality grains and legumes they had consumed for a number of years. While it may be true that grains were consumed in excess, grains cannot be accused of causing these people's difficulties. In my observation, these health problems typically develop from diets lacking an adequate balance of protein, fats, and other nutrients needed to balance complex carbohydrates.

There are many designer diets that promote high-quality, natural carbohydrates yet *discourage* the intake of high-quality fats and proteins, often favoring incomplete protein sources or "natural" junk foods, such as those derived from nontraditional soy products that have no health benefits. Consuming even high-quality carbohydrates, such as organic whole grains, without sufficient quality protein and fats can be an example of when too much of a good thing goes bad.

Indeed, this can happen all too easily with any nutritional source, be it carbs, proteins, or fats. *Unbalanced* high-natural-carbohydrate diets are no more beneficial to our health than unbalanced low-carbohydrate diets. When people eat a healthy diet with a variety of healthy foods in a balanced way, they have little need for designer diets.

This does not mean you will not need to adjust your diet on occasion to accommodate life's changes. However, when you have all the finest-quality tools at your disposal, you are more apt to successfully work out life's often complex health issues than if you have only a few good tools at your disposal and are unaware of what needed elements you're missing. With all the proper nutrients available and utilized, weight problems, energy loss, and similar concerns are easily remedied, and you become satisfied on many levels of your being.

In other words, it is easier to address diet-related problems by starting from a balanced traditional diet than it is to start with an extreme diet that will lead, sooner than later, to other extremes.

PART VI

A Call to Common Sense

43
The Golden Spiral of Traditional Foods

The figure on page 526 is a representation of dietary proportions roughly based on the well-known mathematical model called the Golden Rectangle or Golden Spiral, shown opposite.

This fascinating geometric model has been called by many other names in different parts of the world and different historical epochs. The spiral has often been termed the "universal master form," and has long been revered as a sacred symbol of life, death, and transformation. Found abundantly throughout nature in both the plant and animal realms, manifestations of the spiral with its logarithmic progressions have been represented in the arts and sciences of every culture, from the most primitive to the most advanced.

It is in the logarithmic spiral that we find a consistent thread of knowledge linking the beliefs and lifestyles of the great ancient civilizations through art, architecture, astronomy, engineering—and even agriculture, pastoralism, and food production.

Whether in India, China, the Middle East, the Far East, Africa, or North or South America, the study of traditional foods reveals a dietary pattern based on a remarkably consistent wisdom of sensibility, practicality, and proportion. On the surface, these traditions are characterized by obvious cultural diversity: thus one part of the world may include cereals of a particular species, while elsewhere another species takes precedence. The same holds true for vegetables, animal prod-

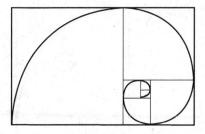

The Golden Spiral

ucts, beans, seeds, nuts, dairy products, etc. Yet there is an underlying consistency—one is tempted to say uniformity—in the basic proportions of foods and food groups each culture has used to feed its people.

There are, of course, broad differences based on climate and terrain. Coastal peoples naturally consumed more fish and seafood than inland peoples, who consumed more fowl and mammal products. Yet as fundamentally agricultural peoples, both groups consumed animal products on the whole in a roughly equivalent proportion to all other foods. While ruling classes often exercised the exclusive rights of the wealthy to adjust these proportions for their personal use, the general proportions were maintained among traditional peoples just as they are today.

Golden Ratio, Golden Age

It is my experience that a diet of traditionally grown foods, eaten in accordance with the principles of the golden spiral, holds the keys to health where so many other approaches fail. The culture-bearers of antiquity were able to create a golden age, a state that is possible only when all aspects of life are in harmony. I believe we can achieve optimal health, a clean environment, and new levels of cultural expression by consciously implementing these principles once again.

Careful investigation of the spiral nature of the traditional dietary pattern leads to a startlingly profound truth at its center: *light is the source of inspiration.* This is simply a poetic way of stating that the source of all is the powerful force of creation itself—what some refer to as God or by many other names.

1. Air
2. Water
3. Carbohydrates
4. Vegetables
5. Protein
6. Fats and Oils
7. Essential Supportive
   Supplements

The Logarithmic Spiral of Nourishment, based on the Golden Ratio

This omnipresent, omniscient force charges and generates the process and flow of energy through each stage of this spiral, supplying the raw materials for human sustenance and nourishment. These materials are comprised of macronutrients, vitamins, phytonutrients, carotenoids, and all other known and unknown ingredients inherent in our daily foods.

More than the sum of its ingredients, each individual food also carries specific energetic properties exclusive to its makeup and origin. These energetics have the ability to alter our health in profound ways.

The Spiral of Nourishment

Section 1: Air

When we are born, the first breath, a simple inhalation of air, is the beginning of an incredible journey in self-discovery that is individually unique.

Throughout our lives, air will serve as our most abundant resource for nourishment. Oxygen from the air will spark the fires of metabolism, helping to regulate all microcellular and macrocellular functions in the physical body. Although we experience individual variations in our respiratory quotients, the air we breathe will supply by far the greatest portion of nourishment as energy to support life.

The constant exchange of oxygen with carbon dioxide through the respiratory system plays an integral role in the body's ability to process all other forms of nutrients. Air is the one form of nourishment that is consumed constantly, whether you are awake or asleep.

Other forms of nutrition listed in the chart have a proportionally equivalent influence on oxygen's effectiveness—right down to the cellular level.

Section 2: Water

Water comprises more of our daily diet than we realize. Fruits and vegetables are mostly water. Grains, beans, soups, and boiled or steamed foods are prepared with water. About 75 percent of the human body is water. If we were to weigh all that we consume at the end of a day, water would comprise the second largest quantity after air.

It is important that pure water comprise the majority of liquids consumed daily in order to cool the body and cleanse the blood, cells and organs of toxins and wastes. Water is also essential for maintaining and regulating healthy bowel function and peristalsis.

While pure water is the ideal beverage and the one that hydrates our body cells most efficiently, our ancestors also consumed other liquids, including herbal teas, wine, beer, and water-based natural remedies.

Section 3: Carbohydrates

The ideal carbohydrates are those consumed by traditional peoples: whole grains, whole grain products (breads, pastas, etc.), pseudocereals (quinoa, amaranth, teff) and starchy vegetables (roots and tubers, including sweet potato, potato, yam, yucca, squashes, and others). In part because of their versatility, these foods should make up the largest portion of the diet.

This section also includes supplementary carbohydrates (all fruits and sweeteners). Some typical sweeteners are grain malts, honey, maple syrup, sugar cane, and the like. In traditional diets, supplementary carbohydrates were consumed in smaller quantities.

Among the carbohydrates and revered above all other foods are the "sacred gifts of the gods": the grains and pseudocereals. Ancient peoples believed these staples held the genetic memory of human origin and the spiritual essence of man and woman.

Section 4: Vegetables

Vegetables include all edible land and water plants. Roots, seeds, leaves, stalks, buds, and marine and freshwater algae are but some of the plant forms consumed around the world. Although many vegetables can be considered additional sources of carbohydrates, I have placed them in a separate section because of their dietary importance in the lives of our ancestors.

Vegetables contain a wide spectrum of nutrients and act as balancing agents when eaten in proper combination with other foods. For most people, vegetables are sorely lacking, exceptions being those instances where people practice certain ethnic traditions or dietary programs specifically based on ample quantities of fresh vegetables in wide variety.

Section 5: Protein

Progressing from greatest quantity to smallest, protein sources follow wild and domesticated plants as the next category in the spiral. This includes a broad range of traditional foods: eggs, wild game, fowl, waterfowl, cattle, lamb, goat, pig, organ meats, dairy products, shellfish, fish, beans, seeds, and nuts are some of the many types of protein consumed historically throughout the world.

Section 6: Fats and Oils

Fats and oils have a long history in dietary traditions, consumed either as a part of other foods or as foods in and of themselves. Olives, avocadoes, and nuts are whole-plant sources of fat; salmon, eggs, and beef are examples of animal sources. Some traditional, stand-alone fats include animal-derived butter, ghee, lard, and other animal fats; and the plant oils from olives, sesame seeds, palm kernels, and coconuts.

Section 7: Essential and Supportive Supplements

This section of the dietary spiral includes herbs, spices, salt, minerals, and natural medicinal foods such as bee pollen, specialized fungi, microalgae, and other whole-food-based supplements.

Supplements have several functions. They can enhance digestion, aid assimilation, improve flavor, raise or lower blood pressure, increase kidney or liver efficiency, and strengthen the immune system. Peppercorns and certain other spices possess antiviral, antibacterial, and antifungal properties.

Additional Considerations

The area of each section represents roughly the proportion that type of food occupied in our agricultural ancestors' daily diets; these proportions have held true for untold generations back through history and prehistory.

The nutrient category in each section of the chart is proportionally dependent on those of every other section for proper metabolic balance and health maintenance.

While the chart divides different foods into sections or categories, bear in mind that in the context of nature and tradition, this represents a single continuum: you will find most foods and food groups overlapping with the preceding or following categories. For example, "beans and nuts" embraces nutritional combinations of fats, proteins, and carbohydrates in varying amounts.

The sections are also designed for easy recognition of the food sources most commonly accepted as fitting in that section. For example, beans (legumes) are only about 25 percent protein, yet they are most commonly thought of as a protein source and have therefore been placed in the protein category. As another example, many cheeses are high in both protein and fat and could logically be ascribed to either category. Yet cheese, like beans, is more commonly thought of as a protein food, so it is grouped in that section. Leafy green plants, which also provide some protein, are grouped in their own section, as explained above.

Plant protein has an incomplete amino acid profile, while animal proteins contain all dietarily essential amino acids necessary for the body's growth and cell repair.

Plant oils have a different effect in the body than animal fats, and each type of oil or fat has its own unique effect as well. In fact, the body responds uniquely and distinctly to each different food.

44
Choosing a Healthy Diet

Just what is "healthy food"? Ideally speaking, *healthy food* can be defined as *natural foods:* plant foods that are grown either organically or biodynamically, and animals that are pastured and raised naturally. Natural foods that have been processed and prepared by traditional methods, including fermenting, marinating, drying, and so forth, also are healthy foods. Healthy food does *not* include foods that have been grown, raised, or processed through genetic experimentation, chemicals, preservatives, hormones and other unhealthy measures adopted by corporate agribusiness conglomerates. These methods of raising food, while able to sustain the human species to some degree, do not even warrant argument against natural methods of food production, because history, science, tradition, and common sense have already set the record straight on this issue.

Every now and then we find ourselves wondering about the wisdom and healthfulness of modern food production and their marketing spin, but most of the time the "science" goes unquestioned by an unwitting and obedient public. But we are right to wonder. Profit-driven production methods of the pseudoscience that backs their dubious achievements with spurious claims is commonplace in today's market—and the more we educate ourselves about these practices, the better off both we and our future generations will be.

The healthiest foods for all human beings are those that are raised and grown through natural methods and time-honored traditions.

One might argue that natural foods too are exposed to environmental toxins on a regular basis, or that organic guidelines can sometimes be considerably nonspecific, or that the water used in the growing process of naturally raised foods may contain toxins. In many places, this is true; unfortunately, that is the state of the planet, at this point. But adding additional chemicals, preservatives, growth hormones, and the rest just compounds the problem. Naturally grown foods in a semiunnatural environment are still superior to those grown in that same environment with all the added toxic ingredients. Therefore, for the best food capable of supporting health, as much as possible and as much as is realistic for you, consume organic and biodynamic foods.

Traditional Differences: The Real and the Make-Believe

One of the best criteria for determining whether or not a food is natural is to use a historical perspective; where or how a food shows up historically or in a traditional context helps to clarify the issue. The further back in history a food goes can determine and define how effective and useful the food has been, especially if the food is still in use today after thousands of years.

Even in this context, we will often find some natural processing methods involved with certain foods. Grains, for example, have been processed by soaking, fermentation, and grinding to make a wide variety of porridges, breads, and noodles for thousands of years throughout the world. This form of processing does not involve the use of chemical preservatives, however, and is perfectly natural and healthy. Another example of natural processing occurs with fermented foods. Pickling is a traditional and natural method of food processing that offers numerous health benefits.

Today, however, these and other traditional methods of food preparation are artificially mimicked in the commercial food industry, where inferior products manufactured with chemicals and preservatives are the norm.

Substituting the Substitutes

Well-known plant- and animal-derived commercial food products crowd the aisles and overstuff the shopping carts of today's consumers. Some of the most widely consumed groups of processed foods are cold cuts, hot dogs, and processed cheeses. While often containing the by-products of actual foods, these products essentially are highly processed food "substitutes."

The same also goes for the substitute foods some people call "modern natural foods." These "natural" versions of substitute foods are those products found in natural food stores that are designed to look and taste like substitute food products found in commercial grocery stores.

Items such as soy "tofu" hot dogs, fake bacon, soy sausage, and soy cheeses are food *products,* and not actually foods per se: highly processed products made from by-products of soybeans (mostly soy isolates) that offer little to no health benefits. Long used as filler for pet foods, these fake food ingredients, usually processed with chemical solvents and other unhealthy processing methods, are now used to create "natural" food substitutes that resemble the commercial food substitutes that have become so familiar to most of us who were raised in Western cultures.

One has to question why someone changing to a healthy diet would want to reproduce the nonfood items of his past with more "natural" versions of nonfood items to begin with. The original processed animal products do not offer the natural nutrition of real naturally raised animal foods, and the soy versions offer even fewer benefits and are not healthy substitutes for real food, no matter how we look at it.

In the case of the various new-fangled "meat" products, the use of nutritional science derived from traditionally consumed soy products (miso, tamari, etc.) is often used to support highly processed soy foods. This practice of nutritional indoctrination is deceptive and misleading, yet unfortunately it permeates both the commercial and natural food industries.

The same science is applied to substitute meat products. Processed beef parts with nitrates and preservatives in the form of, say, bologna is no substitute for air-dried, grass-fed beef, and the two cannot be qualitatively compared just because the bologna has animal parts in it.

Healthy, real food is just that; it cannot be substituted with imitations. So why would some of us want to include these and other food substitutes in our diets in place of real foods? If you're going to eat these kinds of foods and quality is important to you, it is far better and healthier to eat real sausages, real hot dogs, and other similar real meat foods made from real, grass-fed, naturally raised animals, free from chemicals and preservatives.

Who Is Choosing Your Food for You?

Familiarity, convenience, and indoctrination are three important reasons for choosing certain foods. Many of us have been raised on processed foods. Cold cuts, hot dogs, and other processed meat protein sources were and still are the mainstay of school lunches and weekend cookouts for many people.

These modern foods offer convenience, are easily preserved through chemicals and refrigeration; they don't require cooking and, most of all, they are designed and promoted by large companies whose sole purpose is profit, with little concern for public health—as evidenced in the quality of the majority of these products. What's more, many of us were and are raised on these processed foods, and they have become strongly familiar to us, both to our senses and to our biochemistry.

In many households, these processed animal products have replaced the traditional whole roast chicken, roast beef, lamb, duck, fresh fish, or other traditional healthy animal foods. In other households, these traditional animal foods are simply given less priority and consumed less frequently.

In the past few years, many health-conscious people have discovered the unhealthy qualities inherent in processed meat products and have stopped eating them. At the same time, though, many have also stopped eating traditional animal products, opting instead for the alternative diets and lifestyles offered by health food or natural food diets.

Knowing an advantageous opportunity when they see one, the soy industry recognized the need for plant-based protein sources in the rapidly growing trend of natural diet followers, and in the financial growth of the natural-products industry in general. The burgeoning variety of soy-based protein pseudofoods that resulted, along with a massive marketing effort including made-to-order scientific backup, quickly permeated the commercial and natural-foods marketplace.

The effort to influence the masses with their new soy-based meat substitutes is an ongoing campaign, but is now being joined by others. New meat substitutes made from fungi and other ingredients are being used to create still more artificial substitute foods, and these are all competing in the race to flood the marketplace with new products for public consumption . . . in other words, to take the place of real food.

So far, the greatest impact of these pseudofoods has been in the diets of health food enthusiasts—ironically, the very people whose original philosophies and ideals, along with their founding fathers' and mothers' commitment to quality, were centered on the importance of quality in growing, processing, and manufacturing of whole foods!

While the marketing of these new products may have misled many vegans, vegetarians and other health food enthusiasts into believing they had a greater variety of healthy protein sources with which to help balance their diets, the products also struck a familiar chord from the past. Followers of natural diets no longer had to pine for those processed meat products of their pasts: now they had substitutes! The new ersatz versions tasted just like the foods they'd left behind, plus they were low in fat and cholesterol and, let's face it, they were convenient, too. So convenient, in fact, that for many naturalists, these new substitute foods have come to comprise as much as 50 percent or 75 percent of their diets. Sometimes even more.

Unfortunately, this is not a good thing, and I say this with great respect for those who are attempting a true vegan or vegetarian diet based on whole foods, as well as from my own experience as a teacher and counselor of whole-foods nutrition. Some of the well-documented health problems resulting from this imitation-food phenomenon include: hypothyroidism and other hormonal problems, loss of hair, pallor of skin, loss of muscle tone, fatigue, digestive distress, and a host of other problems. According to some researchers, some of these problems may be irreversible, yet advocates of the soy protein myth and other fabricated "health" products are quick to quote numerous scientific articles touting the benefits of these imitation foods.

Who is behind these scientific articles? And what is their real agenda? One can also find numerous scientific reports touting the benefits of vegetable oils on cholesterol, heart disease, and other health problems—but scientific evidence can also be found that shows these same polyunsaturated vegetable oils *contribute* to these problems.

To anyone willing to take a close look at the science of nutrition, it becomes crystal clear that nutritional science, like so many types of "expertise" today, has a price. Not only that: just about every product on the market, be it natural or not, has two sets of conflicting nutritional data—one version to support it and another to debase it.

Convenience foods were designed to make life easier for modern civilization. We all can certainly use a little more convenience in our lives, but the commercial line of these pseudofood products have resulted in the unbalanced tradeoff of diminished health and vitality for convenience. And the natural versions of these convenience foods are no better than the original ones they were made to resemble.

This serves as a valuable lesson for all of us: nutritional science alone should never be used to make healthy dietary choices. Due to the influence of industry agendas, conflicting data is rampant in nutritional science. In fact, before even considering the "scientific evidence," it makes sense to first use common sense and look to tradition. Only then can one be free from the quagmire of confusion created by nutritional science.

It is common for modern nutritional science to have no basis in nutritional traditions; it is far less common for nutritional traditions to have no basis in nutritional science. Therefore, one should exercise caution when believing scientific reports on nutrition that lack a basis in traditional nutrition. Learn to make your own choices for yourself and your loved ones using tradition, common sense, and science.

The Whole Story

Two of the greatest barriers that often stand in the way of discovering our dietary needs can be found in deeply entrenched habits and beliefs about food and nutrition. Habits and beliefs about food, while different in meaning, are both linked with that invisible umbilicus that feeds and nourishes the ideas and concepts that created them in the first place: our appetite. Therefore, when choosing how and with what we will nourish ourselves, it is of utmost importance to constantly challenge our concepts and beliefs through other sources of information and traditions.

When using scientific information, we also need to seek both sides of the story. For example, current nutritional science states that tomatoes are a food exceptionally high in *lycopene,* a substance said to be highly beneficial to health. Because this information has come from what most people consider a reputable source of scientifically published papers, it is quickly assimilated as a new belief.

For many, this newfound data translates into a sound reason for eating lots of tomatoes: doing so ensures that they will get all those healthy benefits lycopene has to offer. But the very same science responsible for the isolation of lycopene in tomatoes has also isolated from the very same tomatoes other not-so-healthful, toxic alkaloid compounds that have been adversely linked to the very diseases lycopene may help to prevent!

Reviewing both sides of the available nutritional science, we come up with something like this: *tomatoes have a powerful substance that might help protect us from disease, but they also have other toxic substances that may contribute to disease.* Thus we have scientific data on a food that is both helpful and harmful—but only the helpful is emphasized for advertising purposes.

We could go on with detailed scientific reports supporting both sides of the story, but here is the point of the matter: when making food choices, it is best not to form an opinion based on one source of information alone, regardless of who or what it is.

I use tomato as an example because it is a food that has become common and widespread in just the last hundred years or so. While its history as a global food has been only recent, tomatoes and people have adapted to each other; tomatoes are now one of the most popular and commonly consumed foods. For many people throughout the world, these unusual fruits of the nightshade family are consumed in some form or other and recognized as highly suitable to a nutritious diet— and now, with the science of lycopene backing it, even more so.

But simply because we have discovered a food that seems to suit us or can be supported by scientific research does not mean it is something that should be eaten all the time, as has become a common habit for many people. The idea that, "If a food is good for you, then it is good to eat more of it," is not a wise dictate. *More* does not equate to *better,* regardless of the food in question.

The tomato is not the only food that carries potentially harmful components; so do many other healthy plant foods. For example, many plant foods contain toxic *lignans* that can serve as protective mechanisms for plants. This information doesn't mean one should consider tomatoes an unhealthy food, nor any other traditional food, for that matter. It simply means that we should be well informed about a food and its historical uses before we formulate a belief based on a single component that could lead to a regrettable habit of excess based on half-truths promoted for the sole purpose of profit.

These same one-sided nutritional science agendas can be found with other foods as well; coffee, chocolate, flax oil, and soy are just a few. The need to discover our personal dietary requirements is a matter that takes time, information, common sense, and some experimentation.

Eat Globally

Experimentation with food is not something to fear, nor is it something one should do with careless abandonment. The best way to begin experimentation is through traditional and ethnic cuisines. When approached in this manner, exploration of new foods can not only be an adventure, it can also be a most enjoyable and rewarding experience.

For example, ethnic cuisines often include spices and herbs— seasonings long known and proven to have health benefits among traditional peoples. Many people have had little experience with some of these properties and flavors. And people *within* many ethnic groups have experienced only their own foods and seasonings. It is important for all those living in our modern era to experiment with global foods, to find those with time-honored traditions of health and healing and to support the continuation of these foods through their original seeds and sustainable agricultural practices.

Global foods offer the most extensive choices for establishing a healthy diet. Experiencing other people's traditional foods can give us deep insight into ourselves and other people's cultural patterns, philosophies, cosmologies, and rituals, since food has always played a profoundly important role in the lifestyles of traditional cultures.

Truth or Dare

Not only can we experience newfound health benefits and new tastes when incorporating global cuisines in our diets, we also experience new *textures*. Some of these may be familiar, yet the familiarity could be in relation to a current unhealthy food habit. Replacing this unhealthy food with a newly discovered healthy food or foods having a similar texture can help satisfy the desire for that texture and open new doors to better health. Yes, even food textures can define how we make food choices!

Are you one of the many people who has the deep inner urge to crunch? A potato chip, corn chip, cracker . . . anything you can put in your mouth that crunches when you bite into it? Even worse, do you need to crunch so everyone in your immediate environment can see and hear it? Are you even aware you are doing it when you do it?

Once, while attending a precelebration dinner after one of my lectures, a young, rather vivacious young woman came up to me and began talking to me while crunching on crackers and dip, crumbs falling out of her mouth as she spoke. I tactfully maintained my composure as she interrupted a conversation between me and a close friend of mine. My friend, known for brazenly speaking his mind, stared at this cruncher in disbelief for a moment, then asked her how she thought anyone could understand a word she was saying with her mouth full, and how disgusting she was. He then walked away. (The young woman's response was injured incredulity: "What did I do?!")

This is an example of how powerful an influence food textures can have on developing habits and food choices. While speaking with one's mouth full is not proper etiquette, in this case it wasn't the full mouth so much as the fact she had to continue crunching in front of us and everyone else while trying to converse.

Rarely are our food habits formed by sensible and conscious choices; more often than not, they are formed through an individual's belief or through someone else's belief. This can come in the form of popular diet books, a health practitioner's charisma, or expert opinion, the identity found through the camaraderie of a group of like-minded people or other very common sources that we have all been influenced by, to some degree or other. These other influences, positive or negative, often include parents and relatives, peers and friends.

Whoever or whatever the influences on your dietary choices are, it's important to question how realistic they are *for you*.

One of the most powerful influences on our food choices today can be found among diet groups. Let's consider the example of group influence on our dietary choices.

Choosing the Natural Path

My experience with natural food diets has shown there are two primary reasons people have for choosing one of the many types available.

The first reason is public exposure of the intolerable and abusive treatment of factory-farmed animals, along with the chemical processing of these products and their resulting poor quality. One would be hard-pressed to argue in favor of the negative effects on one's health from consuming to much processed and refined foods laden with preservatives. However, these facts can also be misconstrued to mean that any and all farmed animal products are detrimental to health.

Many vegetarian crusaders, intent on the elimination of the atrocious practices involved in raising factory-farmed animals, are either blinded by their cause or simply unaware of traditional methods used to raise animals for food and of the important role naturally raised animal products have played in a healthy traditional diet for many thousands of years. This one-sided perspective has lead to many extremist reactions against the human consumption of any and all animal products.

While this point of view is prevalent in many natural diet philosophies, it is most evident in the plant-based raw foods groups (there are animal-based raw foods groups as well) and the vegan groups. Ironically, it is within the vegan groups that we find the most extensive use of imitation animal products made from highly processed soy, fungi, and other ingredients.

The second common reason for choosing a natural diet and lifestyle is as a way to define one's personal identity. Human beings have a long history of identifying strongly with a wide variety of lifestyles. Religions, professions, and other cultural factors have long offered ways in which we can develop identities to which we can "belong" and with which we can label ourselves and others. Identifying with a particular diet group, even becoming a proud model for and example of what it represents, is a common path to distinction in today's world.

For many, the need to be part of a group with high ideals is very important; many diet groups offer unique combinations of philosophies and lifestyles. The foods that make up a particular diet are often used to feed the identity of an individual. At the same time, those foods prohibited by the diet are often the ones that end up actually defining the individual.

Even if diet groups with leanings toward moral, spiritual, or philosophical agendas are your thing, you still need to examine whether or not you are thriving while nourishing yourself with your chosen approach. It's easy to find support in subculture diet groups such as raw foods, vegan, macrobiotics, and others, but it is just as easy to lose this support if you question or challenge leadership or the basic dictates of the regime, or if you stray from the path. Intolerance of dissension, criticism, and even persecution are common within such groups. Knowing this in advance can be helpful for those exploring new paths to health with diet groups.

Another vitally important thing to know about diet groups is that when health issues arise, whether concerning oneself or others, it is essential to search for consistencies within the group before accepting stock answers from experienced group leaders. Nutritional deficiencies are common in natural diet groups and can manifest as hypothyroidism, loss of libido, loss of menstruation, premature aging, premature hair loss, arthritis, extreme weight loss or weight gain, and more.

It is not uncommon for nutritional deficiencies to be addressed (or dismissed) as a "cleansing experience," a "period of adjustment to the new diet" or as a reaction caused by "straying from the diet." It is even not uncommon for such predicaments to be criticized as being symptomatic of the individual adherent's ineptitude or lack of understanding. While some of these assertions can be true to some extent, if several cases of similar deficiencies show up among other followers in the group, it is important to consider making improvements and changes in your diet.

In fact, it makes the most sense to look for these problems *first,* before diving headfirst into something that could cause more problems than what you began with. Look first at the children, as they tend to be the first to be adversely affected by nutritional problems. Be cautious, stay grounded, and remember that while there can be many health benefits and much to learn from diet groups, your safest approach will be one where you seek out the rational and traditional aspects of the diet and avoid the extremes.

Reality Checks

Here are a few tips to help get you through the often confusing experiences of natural diet hopping. Start by asking yourself the following questions.

Does your diet consist of a wide variety of wholesome natural foods?

If you are interested in health, and not just weight loss, you need to consume a diet consisting of mostly natural whole foods and not prepackaged artificial products, which may in the short term help you lose weight but will do little to support your health.

Contrary to what many people think, not all fad diets are "health food" diets. Quite the contrary, most modern fad diets are comprised of fake foods loaded with preservatives and designed for the sole purpose of addressing the issue of overweight. Fad diets that are based on natural foods, on the other hand, should at least be made up of real foods— although this is not always the case either.

When a diet is said to be comprised of natural whole foods, it is important to understand that this does not mean natural "designer foods" that contain a natural ingredient or two but cannot be found anywhere in a traditional setting before fifty years ago. So far, modern food technology has not been able to improve on traditional natural foods, other than in the capacity to store foods through refrigeration and packaging. The addition of synthetic vitamins and nutrients to factory-farmed foods grown on depleted soils is not an improvement, nor are faster growing times or fatter animals derived from growth hormones, unnatural feed, and inhumane animal treatments.

For the most part, while some natural diets can lack important sources of nutrition commonly found in most traditional diets, natural foods–based diets are good places to begin one's journey to better health.

How much of your diet is comprised of "substitute foods"?

Having already established the importance of a diet based on natural foods, we will approach the remaining questions and comments from the basis of a natural food diet.

"Substitute foods" can be classified as foods that offer little quality nutrition but are eaten for fun, to satisfy hunger, to satisfy emotional states; junk foods or binge foods that are not on your particular diet (and if they are, then they may not necessarily be recognized as junk foods). For convenience, we can break down substitute foods into two categories.

- Commercial substitute foods: Packaged pastries, cakes, and cookies; ice cream; candy; fast food; soda; chips; some deli foods; flour products (breads, bagels, rolls); processed dairy products; etc. You may be thinking that this category does not apply to you, because you are on a "natural diet." Maybe so—but most people following natural diets of all types frequently indulge in large quantities of these food products.

- Natural substitute foods: Soy products made from soy protein isolates; soy milk; nondairy ice creams and cheese substitutes; margarine (all types); candy; coffee; nutrition bars (containing soy, refined oils, and synthetic vitamins); packaged foods (cookies, chips, breakfast cereals, etc.) made with soy, safflower, and canola oils. There are more, but these are the ones most commonly consumed in large quantities by natural food enthusiasts. These foods are typically found in natural food stores, and sometimes in specialized sections of grocery stores.

Keep in mind that this is simply a reality check and not some harebrained idea about making you either perfect or guilty of dietary sabotage. We all enjoy the freedom to explore and indulge in things that are not always beneficial to our health. While this rarely poses a problem with any healthy diet, a quantity of insalubrious foods, along with the common misunderstanding that some are healthy as compared to more traditional foods, can and often does contribute to problems.

Going back to the question, "How much of your diet is comprised of 'substitute foods'?" we can get more specific: *What percentage of your current diet* is made up of these foods: 10 percent, 30 percent, 50 percent, 75 percent, 100 percent? What can be said about these percentages?

If you answered "10 percent," congratulations! Your diet is probably quite balanced and satisfying on many levels. It is perfectly normal to consume things that do not fit your ideal diet; everyone does it.

If you answered "30 percent" or "50 percent," either you are confused about what is truly healthy for you or your diet is lacking important nutritional sources, and you may be unconsciously or consciously trying to compensate for a lack of higher-quality nutritional sources. This isn't going to work. Before long, you will begin to notice a decline in energy, and possibly other negative symptoms as well. Your diet needs some serious revision.

If you answered "75 percent" or "100 percent," you are fooling yourself: you are not eating a healthy diet. Not even close. It is time to start over.

Is your diet fulfilling the promises associated with it?

While you might think your diet is special as compared to others, when it comes to "diet promises," yours is exactly the same as all the other health diets. Healthy diets promise the following: youthful appearance, weight loss, increased energy and vitality, beautiful skin, optimal nutrition, minimal cravings, improved digestion, and more. These are reasonable promises that a truly healthy and balanced diet (along with moderate exercise and a positive attitude) should be able to fulfill, no? I think we can agree on that.

So what do you think? Has your diet fulfilled or is it fulfilling its promises?

If you have been on your diet for four to six months, there should be no reason why many of these criteria should not be starting to manifest in a positive light, unless you are seriously lacking exercise or very negative about life in general.

Granted, if you are suffering from chronic digestive disorders and have been for ten years or more, it may take a while before you are happy with your results. But even so, a healthy, balanced diet should result in some noticeable improvements within a relatively short time. The same goes for the other promises. If your diet is what it promises, you should be getting results.

Let's consider one of the above promises: increased energy and vitality. This one is a major appeal for many people choosing a new diet. How does yours fare in that department? Has your diet given you more energy and vitality on a regular basis? Hmm, think about that one carefully before answering. Got your answer? Good . . .

Now: remove coffee, tea, chocolate, and all other stimulants from your diet and answer the question again. Uh-huh. I know I may not have gotten *you* with that one, but I guarantee that I got at least 75 percent of those reading these words. These stimulants are a good barometer for gauging the "increased energy and vitality" factor of your diet.

The more you need of these stimulants, the less your diet is fulfilling its promise.

Again, I want to emphasize that these foods *used in moderation* do not define dietary characteristics—but when they comprise a large percentage of your natural diet, you are obviously dealing with false promises and will at some point have to face the reality check.

What keeps you inspired to stay on your diet?
Is it convenience? Have you figured out simple ways of incorporating the essentials into your lifestyle, or is your diet simply something you return to now and then for reassurance in some area of your life? Do you need your diet to help define who you are—a vegan, raw foodist, a macrobiotic, Atkins?

If so (even if only partly so), what does this definition do for you? Is it because you have made many friends through your dietary choice, and these friends make up most of your world? Is it because some admired celebrity proclaimed his or her allegiance to the diet? Is it the philosophical leanings, e.g., animal rights, a peaceful world, nonviolence, free love? How about weight control, energy, and the other reasons mentioned above?

Whatever your reasons, it is important to consider whether they still apply to you at this stage of your life, and how those reasons weigh in as priorities compared to the essentials of a healthy diet.

Essential Perspectives for Those on a Healthy Diet

1. Foods that have been consumed by traditional peoples for thousands of years and have contributed to robust health are not impure, bad, or "less spiritual" than other foods.
It is very common for some diet programs to outlaw certain traditional foods and preparation methods based on a particular agenda. Grains, beans, animal products, cooked foods, raw foods, and fats are some of the foods and preparation methods that can be taboo in some diets. Avoid judging real foods with simplistic terms such as "good and bad."

The question of what is *real food* is not a black or white issue. While you may choose to follow the dictates or ideals of a particular diet, always remember before making a judgment about any traditional food that there is the issue of *quality* to consider. People have thrived physically and spiritually for thousands of years on the very foods that may be taboo to your current diet.

Furthermore, there is no evidence that quality sources of these taboo foods, in and of themselves, when used in a balanced and healthy diet, have caused the problems your regime might accuse them of causing. Because many people judge food based on "good or bad" does not mean this judgment is correct.

For example: "Fat is bad." Not true. Fat is essential for metabolic functions, among other things. Some fats are very efficient at assisting in these functions, whereas others can inhibit these natural functions and are generally harmful to the human body. You always have a choice as to what you eat and do not eat, but be careful not to get caught up in the bad food/good food "diet agenda" to the point where you think you are better than someone else because of your newfound "diet identity."

2. Know your limitations and habits, understand balance, and remember that "more is not necessarily better."

This applies to any food. Falling for the "more is better" idea leads to extremes and contributes to eating disorders and a host of other problems.

What is familiar from the past will tend to be brought into the present. Be aware of how your old habits influence your new diet. For example, someone may have had a habit of eating a bag of potato chips for lunch with a soda. On his new diet, he eats a bag of "natural" potato chips with soy milk or a "natural" soda. This is not an improvement over the old diet.

Another example would be an individual whose past eating habits, consisting of large amounts of cold deli foods and iced beverages, have contributed to chronic constipation and digestive distress. On his new diet, he brings the same familiar pattern to the "natural" deli and does the same thing as before with better-quality foods. While the quality of the ingredients has changed, the eating pattern and habit has not, so the digestive distress continues unabated.

Other past influences one must be careful of bringing to a healthy diet include food fears, emotional eating (eating to compensate for emotional distress), fanaticism, and obsessive-compulsive eating. Some "natural diets" can actually contribute to these problems—so be careful.

3. Question your beliefs.

If you are not thriving on your diet and do not feel well, question *everything* about the diet and your practice of it until you find out where the problem lies.

It is okay to question the diet and the philosophy. In fact, it is *essential* that you do. Don't let yourself get to a place in your health where you will regret what you have done. Be prepared to make changes in your diet. Dietary changes are inevitable. Some of these changes may require that you explore and embrace ideas contrary to your present beliefs.

Remember the list of diet promises.

Most of all, give yourself permission to enjoy a wide variety of wholesome foods and celebrate life!

Acknowledgments

I would like to thank my good friend John David Mann for all of his work on the original manuscript and for his professional input every step of the way. Even though John was up to his ears in high-level professional work, writing, co-writing, and editing tomorrow's bestsellers with some of the hottest authors in publishing, he managed to take the time to tirelessly go through the material. John's practical suggestions and uncanny grasp of any material he works with are trademarks that helped to earn him the impeccable reputation in the field of publishing, as an author, interviewer, and editor that he deserves.

I also want to thank all of those wonderful good-hearted people from different parts of the world who have shared their home and hearth with me. The experiences and knowledge I have gained about food and natural living have been an educational experience that will forever be burned into my memory and I will continue to draw on those memories in times of reflection and contemplation. Even though many of these people will never see this book or even the written word in their lifetime, I will never forget and always cherish the generosity and love you showed this stranger from the West.

Notes

Chapter 37
The Origins of Agriculture

1. *A Dictionary of Quaternary Acronyms and Abbreviations,* www
.scirpus.ca/cgi-bin/dictqaa.cgi?option=b; May 5, 2004.
2. Bruce D. Smith, *The Emergence of Agriculture* (New York: W. H.
Freeman and Co., 1999), 165.
3. David Whitehouse, "World's 'Oldest' Rice Found," British
Broadcasting Corporation News (BBC), October 21, 2003.
4. David R. Harris, ed., *The Origins and Spread of Agriculture and
Pastoralism in Eurasia* (London: UCL Press 1999), 151.
5. Douglas T. Price and Anne Birgitte Gebauer, eds., *Last Hunters—
First Farmers: New Perspectives on the Prehistoric Transition to
Agriculture* (Santa Fe: School of American Research Press, 1995),
198.
6. Smith, *The Emergence of Agriculture,* 60.
7. Mary Settegast, *Plato Prehistorian* (Hudson, N.Y.: Lindisfarne Press,
1990), 3.
8. www.scientificamerican.com, June 22, 2004.
9. Smith, *The Emergence of Agriculture,* 60.
10. Jack Harlan, *The Living Fields: Our Agricultural Heritage.*
(Cambridge: University Press, 1998), 95.
11. Harris, *The Origins and Spread of Agriculture and Pastoralism in
Eurasia,* 154.
12. Ibid.

13. Smith, *The Emergence of Agriculture,* 47.
14. Harris, *The Origins and Spread of Agriculture and Pastoralism in Eurasia,* 194.
15. Harlan, *The Living Fields,* 34.
16. Price and Gebauer, *Last Hunters—First Farmers,* 126.

Chapter 39
Traditional Ancestral Diets

1. A familiar term used in place of *hunter-gatherer-scavengers,* the more correct term due to a recent scientific update.
2. Harlan, *The Living Fields,* 89, www.cup.org.
3. "Ancient Amazon Settlements Uncovered," *Seattle Times,* September 18, 2003.
4. "Amazonian Find Stuns Researchers," *Seattle Times,* September 20, 2003.
5. Harlan, *The Living Fields,* 179.
6. Graham Hancock, *Fingerprints of the Gods* (New York: Three Rivers Press, 1996).
7. www.westonaprice.org/nutrition_greats/price.html, May 24, 2004. Also see Weston A. Price, *Nutrition and Physical Degeneration* (La Mesa, Calif.: The Price-Pottinger Nutrition Foundation Inc., 2000).
8. *UPI Science News,* January 27, 2003.
9. Price, *Nutrition and Physical Degeneration.*
10. Viegas, Jennifer, "Study: Human DNA Neanderthal-Free," *Discovery News,* May 12, 2003, http://dc.discovery.com/news/briefs/20030512/neanderthal.html.
11. Reuters, March 27, 2000.
12. Marvin Harris, *Good to Eat: Riddles of Food and Culture* (Prospect Heights, Ill.: Waveland Press, 1998), 225.
13. Brian Hayden cited in "A New Overview of Domestication," *Last Hunters—First Farmers* by Price and Gebauer, 280.
14. Ibid.
15. Edgar Anderson, *Plants, Man and Life.*

16. "Mysteries of the Unexplained," *Readers Digest,* 36–38, 1982.

17. Michael A. Cremo, *Forbidden Archeology: The Hidden History of the Human Race* (Badger, Calif.: Torchlight Publishing), 1998.

Chapter 42
Dangerous Brains: The "Lo-Carb" Fad and Diet Extremism in the Twenty-First Century

1. *Associated Press,* April 29, 2004.

Selected Bibliography

Anderson, Edgar. *Plants, Man and Life*. Berkeley: University of California Press, 1967.

Brothwell, Don R. *Food in Antiquity (Expanded Edition)*. Baltimore: Johns Hopkins University Press, 1997.

Chan, Roman Pina. *The Olmec: Mother Culture of Mesoamerica*. New York: Rizzoli International Publications, 1989.

Clymer, Dr. R. Swinburne. *Your Health—Your Sanity in the Age of Treason*. Quakertown, Penn.: The Humanitarian Society, 1958.

Coe, Sophie D. *America's First Cuisines*. Austin: University of Texas Press, 1994.

Coe, Sophie D., and Michael D. Coe. *The True History of Chocolate*, reprint ed. London: Thames and Hudson, 2000.

Corliss, William R. *Ancient Man: A Handbook of Puzzling Artifacts*. Glen Arm, Md.: Sourcebook Project, 1994.

———. *Science Frontiers: Some Anamalies and Curiosities of Nature*. Glen Arm, Md.: Sourcebook Project, 1994.

Cousteau, Jacques. *The Ocean World*. New York: Abradale Press, 1979.

Creasy, Rosalind. *Cooking from the Garden*. San Francisco: Sierra Club Books, 1988.

Cremo, Michael A. *Forbidden Archeology: The Hidden History of the Human Race; The Full Unabridged Edition*. Badger, Calif.: Torchlight Publishing, 1998.

Deloria, Jr., Vine. *Evolution, Creationism, and Other Modern Myths*. Golden, Colo.: Fulcrum Publishing, 2002.

Deutsch, Ronald M. *Realities of Nutrition,* 2nd ed. Boulder: Bull Publishing Company, 1993.

Dunn, Christopher. *The Giza Power Plant: Technologies of Ancient Egypt.* Rochester, Vt.: Bear & Company, 1998.

Enig, Mary G., Ph.D. *Know Your Fats: The Complete Primer for Understanding the Nutrition of Fats, Oils and Cholesterol.* Silver Spring: Bethesda Press, 2000.

Fallon, Sally. *Nourishing Traditions: The Cookbook That Challenges Politically Correct Nutrition and the Diet Dictocrats,* 2nd ed. Winona Lake, Ind.: New Trends Publishing, 1999.

Feuerstein, George, Subhash Kak, and David Frawley. *In Search of the Cradle of Civilization.* Madras: Quest Books, 2001.

Gutteridge, Anne C., ed. *Barnes and Noble Thesaurus of Biology.* New York: Barnes & Noble Books, 1983.

Hancock, Graham, *Fingerprints of the Gods,* reissue ed. New York: Three Rivers Press, 1996.

———. *Underworld: The Mysterious Origins of Civilization.* New York: Three Rivers Press, 2003.

Hapgood, Charles Hutchins. *Earth's Shifting Crust.* New York: Pantheon Books, 1958.

Harlan, Jack Rodney. *The Living Fields: Our Agricultural Heritage.* Cambridge: University Press, 1998.

Harris, David R., *The Origins and Spread of Agriculture and Pastoralism in Eurasia.* London: UCL Press, 1999.

Harris, Marvin. *Cannibals and Kings: Origins of Cultures,* reissue ed. New York: Vintage, 1991.

———. *Good to Eat: Riddles of Food and Culture.* Prospect Heights, Ill.: Waveland Press, 1998.

Hauschka, Rudolf. *Nutrition: A Holistic Approach.* London: Rudolf Steiner Press, 1983, reprint 2002.

Huxley, Anthony Julian. *Plant and Planet.* New York: Viking Penguin, 1974.

Kiple, Kenneth F. *The Cambridge World History of Food.* Cambridge: University Press, 2000.

McGee, Harold, *On Food and Cooking: The Science and Lore of the Kitchen,* revised ed. New York: Scribner, 1984, 2004.

Milton, Richard. *Shattering the Myths of Darwinism.* Rochester, Vt.: Park Street Press, 2000.

Nicholson, Barbara Evelyn, Stephen G. Harrison, G. B. Masefield, and Michael Wallis. *The Oxford Book of Food Plants.* Oxford: Oxford University Press, 1969.

O'Brien, Christian, and Barbara Joy O'Brien. *The Shining Ones.* The Golden Age Project. www.goldenageproject.org.uk.

Price, T. Douglas, and Anne Birgitte Gebauer, eds. *Last Hunters—First Farmers: New Perspective on the Prehistoric Transition to Agriculture.* Santa Fe: School of American Research Press, 1995.

Price, Weston A. *Nutrition and Physical Degeneration.* La Mesa, Calif.: The Price-Pottinger Nutrition Foundation Inc., 2000.

Pye, Lloyd. *Everything You Know Is Wrong.* New York: The Disinformation Company, 2002.

Root, Waverly, *Food by Waverly Root: An Authoritative and Visual History and Dictionary of the Foods of the World.* New York: Simon & Schuster, 1980.

Rudgley, Richard. *Lost Civilizations of the Stone Age.* New York: Touchstone, 2000.

Russell, Dr. Walter. *The Secret of Light.* Waynesboro, Va.: University of Science and Philosophy, 1974.

Scott, Philippa. *Gourmet Game: Recipes and Anecdotes from Around the World.* New York: Simon & Schuster, 1989.

Smith, Bruce D. *The Emergence of Agriculture.* New York: W. H. Freeman and Co, 1999.

Trager, James. *The Food Book.* New York: Avon Books, 1970.

Tribe, Ian. *The Plant Kingdom.* New York: Bantam Books, 1971.

Tudge, Colin. *Neanderthals, Bandits and Farmers: How Agriculture Really Began.* New Haven: Yale University Press, 1999.

Visser, Margaret. *Much Depends on Dinner: The Extraordinary History and Mythology, Allure and Obsessions, Perils and Taboos, of an Ordinary Meal.* New York: Grove Press, 1986

About the Author

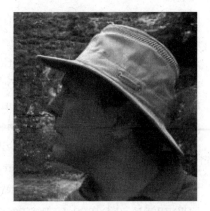

Steve Gagné describes himself as "an ordinary man investigating extraordinary information." He is an independent investigator/researcher as well as one of the most versatile and experienced teachers in whole-foods education.

Steve's long-standing fascination with theories of human origins and his passion for cultural dietary traditions have led him through exhaustive studies in multiple disciplines, both conventional and alternative—and have taken him all over the globe. Unconvinced by the accepted theory of human origins, Steve decided to investigate traditional cultures and the remains of ancient civilizations by experiencing them first-hand. Starting in 1995 and on through the present, he has embarked on a series of globe-circling expeditions to pursue his research, taking him to remote parts of the world to study traditional cultures, foods, and ancient archaeological mysteries.

These years of research and experience have made it increasingly clear to Steve that traditional peoples around the world are intimately linked by a consistent thread woven through their myths and legends, architecture, astronomy, and food traditions. This comprehensive understanding of art and culture, revealed through a wealth of evidence from lost civilizations, extends deep into prehistory—much further back than was originally thought possible.

Today Steve divides his time between continuing his investigations and speaking to audiences all over the world about his discoveries—about our extraordinary hidden heritage, commonsense whole-foods nutrition, and the fallacies of modern dietary and scientific trends.

Steve brings a lively, innovative intelligence to his work and, since 1972, has extended his teaching throughout America and Europe. His many years of research into traditional diets, along with his travel adventures to remote parts of the world to experience and explore ancient traditions, have justly earned him a reputation as one of the most progressive, popular, and informed holistic educators in the country. While well-known for his knowledge of many areas of holistic studies and alternative history, Steve is especially acknowledged as an expert and pioneer in food energetics—where ancient wisdom and dietary traditions merge with modern perspectives and breakthrough research in the field of nutritional science.

Steve lives in Colorado but is more apt to be found poking around making new discoveries in the cities, villages, countrysides, and jungles of the world. His website address is www.stevegagne.com.

Index